Ambulatory Gynecology

John V. Knaus
Marko J. Jachtorowycz
Allan A. Adajar · Teresa Tam
Editors

Ambulatory Gynecology

Springer

Editors
John V. Knaus
Gynecologic Oncology
Presence Saint Francis Hospital
Evanston, IL, USA

Department of Obstetrics and Gynecology
University of Illinois
Chicago, IL, USA

Allan A. Adajar
Medical Education
St. Francis Hospital
Evanston, IL, USA

Marko J. Jachtorowycz
Presence Saint Francis Hospital
Department of Medical Education
Evanston, IL, USA

Teresa Tam
Presence Saint Francis Hospital
Department of Obstetrics and Gynecology
Evanston, IL, USA

ISBN 978-1-4939-7639-3 ISBN 978-1-4939-7641-6 (eBook)
https://doi.org/10.1007/978-1-4939-7641-6

Library of Congress Control Number: 2018931427

Printed on acid-free paper

This Springer imprint is published by the registered company Springer Science+Business Media, LLC part of Springer Nature.
The registered company address is: 233 Spring Street, New York, NY 10013, U.S.A.

To those who have provided our past and present motivation to complete a text intended to improve women's healthcare.

Preface

In a little more than a decade, outpatient gynecologic practice has transitioned from a primarily screening environment to a specialty nearly unto itself. Genetic counseling, minor surgical procedures, advanced diagnosis (ultrasound, urodynamic, office hysteroscopy, endometrial ablations, etc.), cancer preventative strategies, and the like now complement the annual breast examination, pelvic examination, and Pap smear. Entire practices are devoted to care of the ambulatory gynecologic patient. Indeed, the scope of this text, which stemmed from *Office Gynecology* published in 1993, demonstrates the evolution and importance of this type of patient care practice.

It has taken more than 5 years to finish this volume, a testament to the ever-changing management of the ambulatory gynecologic patient. Most chapters were rewritten several times as edition deadlines approached and significant new changes in patient care standards were published. The format variability of each chapter is intentional with each authored by a practicing physician(s). The editors challenged each author to produce a chapter integrating their practice patterns with current guidelines.

Chapter authors were chosen for their demonstrated expertise. The variety of chapter titles should provide the practitioner with a ready resource for the most common to the most difficult ambulatory gynecologic patient care problem.

Evanston, IL, USA

John V. Knaus
Marko J. Jachtorowycz
Allan A. Adajar
Teresa Tam

Acknowledgements

The editors wish to acknowledge with sincere thanks the significant contribution of Ms. Farheen Z. Syeda for her assistance with the myriad of tasks, including frequent communication with chapter authors, contributors and the publisher, to achieve completion of this project. The editors also wish to thank Mr. Michael Griffin of Springer publishers for his continued encouragement and suggestions throughout the process of this texts creation.

Contents

Contributors

Doreen M. Agnese The Ohio State University, Surgical Oncology and Human Genetics, Columbus, OH, USA

Gloria A. Bachmann Rutgers Robert Wood Johnson Medical School, Department of OB/GYN and Reproductive Sciences, New Brunswick, NJ, USA

Michele Bucciero Saint Anthony Hospital, Chicago, IL, USA

Joseph D. Calandra Presence Saint Francis Hospital, Department of Radiology, Evanston, IL, USA

Shambhavi Chandraiah Quillen College of Medicine, Department of Psychiatry and Behavioral Sciences, East Tennessee State University, Johnson City, TN, USA

Migdalia Cortina St. Francis Hospital, Department of Obstetrics and Gynecology, Evanston, IL, USA

Carolyn B. Coulam Reproductive Medicine Institute, Evanston, IL, USA

Janelle Foroutan Rutgers Robert Wood Johnson Medical School, Saint Peter's University Hospital, Department of OB/GYN, New Brunswick, NJ, USA

Valerie P. Grignol Ohio State University, Department of Surgery, Columbus, OH, USA

James A. Hall Memorial Hospital, Women's Health Center, Logansport, IN, USA

Cassing Hammond Department of Obstetrics and Gynecology, Northwestern Memorial Hospital, Northwestern University Feinberg School of Medicine, Chicago, IL, USA

Megan Harrington Stanford Hospital, Stanford, CA, USA

Marko J. Jachtorowycz Presence Saint Francis Hospital, Department of Medical Education, Evanston, IL, USA

Janice L. Johnson University of Illinois at Chicago, College of Medicine, Presence St. Francis Hospital, Department of Obstetrics and Gynecology, Skokie, IL, USA

Sara Kostant Hackensack University Medical Center, Department of Obstetrics and Gynecology, Hackensack, NJ, USA

John V. Knaus Department of Obstetrics and Gynecology, University of Illinois at Chicago, Chicago, IL, USA

Gynecologic Oncology, Presence Saint Francis Hospital, Evanston, IL, USA

Elliot M. Levine Advocate Illinois Masonic Medical Center, Department of Obstetrics and Gynecology, Chicago, IL, USA

Obstetrics and Gynecology, Rush University Medical Center, Chicago, IL, USA

Barbara Levy The American College of Obstetricians and Gynecologists, Washington, DC, USA

Edward S. Linn Cook County Health and Hospitals System, Northwestern University Feinberg School of Medicine, Department of OB/GYN, Chicago, IL, USA

Melissa J. Miller Advocate Sherman Hospital, Elgin, IL, USA

Sheila Mody Department of Obstetrics and Gynecology, Northwestern Memorial Hospital, Northwestern University Feinberg School of Medicine, Chicago, IL, USA

Michael D. Moen Rosalind Franklin University Chicago Medical School, Advocate Lutheran General Hospital,

Department of Obstetrics and Gynecology, Park Ridge, IL, USA

Katherine A. O'Hanlan Laparoscopic Institute for Gynecology and Oncology, Department of Gynecologic Oncology, Portola Valley, CA, USA

Soraya Ong Presence Saint Francis Hospital, Department of Radiology, Evanston, IL, USA

Jennifer Ozan Women's Hospital-Cone Health, Department of Obstetrics and Gynecology, Greensboro, NC, USA

Magdalena Parda-Chlebowicz St. Francis Hospital, Evanston, IL, USA

Nancy Phillips Rutgers Robert Wood Johnson Medical School, Saint Peter's University Hospital, Department of OB/GYN, New Brunswick, NJ, USA

John S. Rinehart Division of Reproductive Endocrinology and Infertility, Department of Obstetrics and Gynecology, NorthShore University HealthSystem, Evanston, IL, USA

Pritzker School of Medicine, University of Chicago, Department of Obstetrics and Gynecology, Section of Reproductive Endocrinology and Infertility, Evanston, IL, USA

Steven Rockoff Presence Saint Francis Hospital, Department of Radiology, Evanston, IL, USA

Sharon Beth Rosenberg Saint Francis Hospital Evanston, Department of Internal Medicine, Evanston, IL, USA

Sondra L. Summers University of Illinois Hospital at Chicago, Department of Obstetrics and Gynecology, Chicago, IL, USA

Teresa Tam Presence Saint Francis Hospital, Department of Obstetrics and Gynecology, Evanston, IL, USA

Maria B. Thomas Kaiser Permanente Signal Hill Medical Offices, Department of Obstetrics and Gynecology, Signal Hill, CA, USA

Kevin Ward Presence Saint Francis Hospital, Department of Obstetrics and Gynecology, Evanston, IL, USA

Lara Weyl Saint Francis Hospital Evanston, Department of OB/GYN, Evanston, IL, USA

Chapter 1
Breast Cancer Screening

Steven Rockoff and Joseph D. Calandra

Introduction

Breast cancer is the most commonly diagnosed cancer and the second leading cause of cancer death among women in the United States. Approximately one out of every eight American women will be diagnosed with breast cancer in their lifetime [1]. Since the turn of the century, an abundance of guidelines for breast cancer screening has been put forth by numerous medical organizations, each with its own variations. These include the government organization known as USPSTF (US Preventive Services Task Force), as well as non-governmental professional medical societies such as (in alphabetical order) American Cancer Society (ACS), American College of Radiology (ACR), the American Congress of Obstetricians and Gynecologists (ACOG), and the National Comprehensive Cancer Network (NCCN).

With an emphasis on screening and diagnostic imaging, this chapter describes the methods of breast cancer screening and summarizes the recommendations of these prominent

S. Rockoff, MD (✉) · J. D. Calandra, MD, FACR
Presence Saint Francis Hospital, Department of Radiology, Evanston, IL, USA

J. V. Knaus et al. (eds.), *Ambulatory Gynecology*, https://doi.org/10.1007/978-1-4939-7641-6_1

organizations in order to provide a practical and concise clinical approach for the early detection of breast cancer.

Screening Evaluation

Overview

Breast cancer screening has been consistently demonstrated to decrease morbidity and mortality [2]. Figure 1.1 illustrates the number of breast cancer cases and deaths in the United States in 2015. Between 1989 and 2012, breast cancer death rates declined by 36%, and an estimated 249,000 breast cancer deaths were avoided, due to advances in detection and treatment [3]. The goal of a screening exam, whether radiographic or clinical, is to detect and diagnose breast cancer before it produces symptoms or spreads throughout the body.

Traditionally, the pillars of screening were imaging, clinical breast exam, and breast self-examination. Over time, evidence has steered screening recommendations to heavily emphasize the role of imaging and de-emphasize or even discourage the practice of physical examination by some.

Age	In situ cases	Invasive cases	Deaths
<40	1,650	10,500	1,010
40-49	12,310	35,850	3,690
50-59	16,970	54,060	7,600
60-69	15,850	59,990	9,090
70-79	9,650	42,480	8,040
80+	3,860	28,960	10,860
All ages	**60,290**	**231,840**	**40,290**

Fig. 1.1 Estimated new female breast cancer cases and deaths by age, US 2015*. *Rounded to the nearest 10 (American Cancer Society, Inc., Surveillance Research 2015)

The breast cancer screening recommendations regarding the frequency and modality of such screening vary based on the patient population. The method of screening should be tailored to an individual patient's risk factors, taking into account items such as age, family history, and many other factors that will be described below. There are accelerated screening regimens for women who have certain high-risk factors.

Breast Self-examination

Breast self-examination (BSE) was traditionally advocated as a method of self-screening. Over the years, evidence has demonstrated that self-examination does not reduce breast cancer-related mortality and is associated with an increased rate of benign biopsies [4]. Beginning in 2009, the USPSTF specifically recommended against clinicians teaching the practice of breast self-examination (awarding that service a "D" grade), concluding with a moderate or high certainty that BSE did not have a net benefit for patients. This recommendation went unchanged in the USPSTF's 2016 update [5] and is now perhaps the least controversial recommendation regarding breast cancer screening.

The new mantra being advocated, in place of the traditional practice of BSE, is the concept of "breast self-awareness," which is being promoted by essentially all organizations, including the ACOG, ACS, and NCCN [6]. Rather than a methodically and routinely performed self-exam, this recommendation emphasizes the importance of patients being aware of the way their breasts normally appear and feel. The patient is encouraged to be aware of any change that may occur in their own body and to discuss these changes with their physician. A breast finding brought to a clinician's attention by the patient may be appropriately followed up with either reassurance, clinical breast exam, and/or imaging.

Clinical Breast Exam

The practice of a physician-performed clinical breast exam (CBE) remains a widely adopted practice. While CBE can detect some breast cancers that are not found by screening mammography, the sensitivity is dependent on the technique and experience of the examiner. As with the self-exam, the intent is to evaluate for the presence of new or abnormal breast findings, which can be detected by palpation (such as a new mass) or inspection (such as dimpling, erythema, etc.). Since 2002, the USPSTF has adopted the position that there is insufficient evidence to recommend the practice of routine CBE, going unchanged in the USPSTF's 2016 update (grade "I"). The ACS similarly was not able to recommend the clinical breast exam as providing a clear net benefit for average-risk women, as stated in its revised recommendations in late 2015 [7]. The ACOG continues to advocate the use of CBE beginning at the age of 19 [8].

Figure 1.2 provides an overview of societal recommendations regarding the practices of the clinical breast exam and breast self-awareness.

Summary of Societies' Non-Imaging Screening Recommendations in Asymptomatic Women of Average Risk				
USPSTF	ACR	NCCN	ACOG	ACS
Breast self-awareness		Breast self-awareness	Breast self-awareness	Breast self-awareness
Insufficient evidence regarding Clinical Breast Exam (CBE)	No recommendations	25 - 40 years: CBE every 1-3 years ≥40 years: CBE annually	> 19 years: CBE annually	Recommend against CBE

FIG. 1.2 Summary of societies' non-imaging screening recommendations in asymptomatic women of average risk

Mammography Overview

Mammography is the primary modality of breast cancer screening for most women 40 years of age or older, and its use as a screening tool has been consistently proven to lower mortality among women [2]. Its primary benefit is in its ability to detect small breast cancers before the onset of symptoms. The sensitivity of screening mammography to detect breast cancers has historically ranged from approximately 70% to 90%; one recent large study found a sensitivity of 83.8% [9]. Traditional film mammography has almost been completely replaced by digital mammography in the United States, allowing comparisons between a patient's exams over time to be made more easily. This helps avoid unnecessary additional imaging or intervention, as a potentially worrisome finding seen on an exam can usually be confidently determined to be benign if it has been demonstrated as stable over several years.

Risk Assessment

Risk factors affect a woman's chances of developing breast cancer in her lifetime. Potentially controllable factors which portend to an increased risk include being overweight or obese, use of hormone therapy, physical inactivity, and use of alcohol. Noncontrollable risk factors include not only the two most important overall risk factors of female gender and older age but also a myriad of other features such as a personal or family history of breast cancer, certain inherited genetic mutations, ethnicity, personal history of certain benign or precancerous breast conditions, and dense breast tissue, among others [10]. Additionally, hormonal states of relatively increased estrogen such as early menarche, late menopause, and nulligravid status have all been linked to an increased risk of developing breast cancer [11]. Conversely, the risk of breast cancer is decreased in women who have breastfed for at least 1 year, have exercised regularly, and have a healthy body weight.

Several modeling tools which estimate a woman's risk of developing breast cancer are available to clinicians. The calculated risk produced for any one patient will likely vary depending on which model is used, as they each use different aspects of a patient's history. The "Breast Cancer Risk Assessment Tool," based on the Gail model, is one of the more widely used applications in practice, developed by the National Cancer Institute (http://www.cancer.gov/bcrisktool) [12]. With this tool, by answering numerous questions regarding a patient's history, her 5-year and lifetime risk of developing breast cancer can be estimated. Note that the Gail model is not validated or appropriate for a patient who already has a history of breast cancer, DCIS, or LCIS, as well as those with a *BRCA1* or *BRCA2* gene mutation.

The ACS divides the population into three broad categories based on the risk of developing breast cancer in a lifetime: average risk (<15%), moderate risk (15–20%), and high risk (>20%) [7, 13]. For the purposes of making coherent recommendations, these risk categories will be used below, with the understanding that even each of these groups is quite heterogeneous and there is no "one size fits all" recommendation.

Asymptomatic Women of Average Risk

Most women can be considered to have an average risk of developing breast cancer, which is generally considered a less than 15% lifetime risk. In the absence of risk factors which would place a patient in the moderate- or high-risk categories (as described in upcoming sections), the majority of asymptomatic women may follow the standard guidelines for screening. Unfortunately, the recommendations and statements from the various cancer, women's health, and imaging professional societies have noticeable differences which have resulted in confusion for the patient and their doctor. These

Summary of Societies' Recommendations for Screening Mammography in Asymptomatic Women of Average Risk

	USPSTF	ACR	NCCN	ACOG	ACS
< 40 years	Screening not appropriate	Screening not appropriate	Screening not appropriate	Screening not appropriate	Screening not appropriate
40-49 years	Small net benefit (moderate certainty); decision to screen should be an individual one (Grade C)				40-44 years: Choice to begin annual screening
50-74 years	Biennial screening (Grade B)	Annual Screening	Annual Screening	Annual Screening	45-54 years: Annual Screening
> 75 years	Insufficient evidence for a recommendation (Grade I)				> 55 years: Biennial screening with the option for annual

FIG. 1.3 Summary of societies' recommendations for screening mammography in asymptomatic women of average risk

various guidelines have changed over time and will undoubtedly be subject to more changes as new evidence is synthesized. Guidelines for mammography screening in women of average risk are summarized in Fig. 1.3, representing the most up-to-date information as of early 2016.

As Fig. 1.3 demonstrates, the most significant guideline discrepancies involve the screening recommendations for women in the 40–49 age group. Traditionally, annual mammography screening in the 40–49 age group was a near-universal recommendation, which, as of this writing, is a position still advocated by the ACR, NCCN, and ACOG groups, as well as the authors [8, 14, 15]. Since the update of the USPSTF recommendation statement in 2009, the recommendations in this age group have been subject to considerable controversy among physicians and various professional organizations. The USPSTF 2009 guidelines recommended against routine screening in average-risk women between the ages of 40 and 49. The USPSTF update in 2016 partially softened this stance, clarifying that there is a clear positive net benefit of screening mammography in this 40–49 age group, although it is small when compared to the net benefit that women of age 50–74 receive. USPSTF language stated that "the decision to start screening mammography in women prior to age 50 years should be an individual one. Women who place a higher value on the potential benefit than the potential harms may choose to begin biennial screening between the ages of 40 and 49 years (C recommendation)" [5].

The primary justification for this more conservative recommendation in the 40–49 age group is related to the evidence regarding the harms of mammography, particularly overdiagnosis and overtreatment. These concepts can be summarized as the detection and treatment of breast cancers through screening mammography that otherwise would never have become clinically apparent or contribute to early mortality. The USPSTF points to evidence that the rates of overdiagnosis/overtreatment have risen, resulting in increased harms to women, while other organizations such as the ACR and ACS propose that these apparently increased overdiagnosis rates are artificially inflated by the inclusion of DCIS. It should be noted that one proposed harm of mammography screening, which is the increased anxiety that may result from a false-positive mammogram, has been shown to be real in the short term but with no detrimental effect on intention to undergo future breast cancer screening or anxiety in the long term [16].

New studies composed of populations which have been exposed to more modern standards of care in surgery and adjuvant treatment continue to provide evidence that detection of cancer at the earliest tumor stages can still improve overall survival rates [17]. At the very least, even if a patient is not given the outright recommendation by her physician to begin screening at age 40, the authors advocate that women should be made aware that beginning annual mammography screening at the age of 40 saves the most lives—it is estimated that almost 65,000 additional lives would be saved in the United States for screening starting at 40 years (compared to 50 years) under current compliance rates [18].

Beyond the numerous scientific criticisms of the USPSTF guidelines, another effect of those particular recommendations has been a generalized anxiety among the medical community regarding patients' ability to afford screening mammograms from the ages of 40 to 49. As the USPSTF designated a "C" grade to their recommendation for that age group, private insurance providers and Medicare are not currently obligated to provide coverage for mammography in women of those age. The Affordable Care Act mandates that only preventive services with a grade of "A" or "B" must be covered by insurers [19]. Whether this particular concern will have a long-term effect on screening rates remains to be seen.

Magnetic resonance imaging (MRI) does not currently have a role as a routine screening tool for women of average risk. The ACS recommends against MRI screening for women with a calculated lifetime breast cancer risk of less than 15% [7]. A higher rate of false positives when compared to mammography is one reason that MRI has not entered the clinical algorithm for screening in average-risk women.

Asymptomatic Women of Moderate Risk

A woman can be said to have a moderate (or "intermediate") risk of developing breast cancer if she has a 15–20% lifetime

Asymptomatic Women of Moderate Risk (15-20% Lifetime Risk)

- A personal history of breast cancer
- A personal history of DCIS or LCIS
- A personal history of ADH or ALH (atypical ductal & lobular hyperplasia)
- Extremely dense breasts
- Lifetime risk of 15-20% as calculated by a risk model

FIG. 1.4 Asymptomatic women of moderate risk (15–20% lifetime risk)

risk of developing breast cancer or has one of the risk factors described in Fig. 1.4. For this subset of moderate-risk women, the evidence regarding screening recommendations is less developed, with no general concordance as to whether supplementary or alternate screening methods provide a clear net benefit. In particular, the ACS states that there is insufficient evidence to make a recommendation regarding the use of screening MRI in this population [7]. At the very least, for women with these risk factors, supplementary MRI can be considered, but may not be appropriate for all women.

Asymptomatic Women of High Risk

A woman can be said to have a "higher than average risk" if she has a 20% or greater lifetime risk of developing breast cancer (as calculated by one of numerous statistical models such as the Gail model) or has any of the risk factors described in Fig. 1.5.

Most societies advocate using a combination of mammography and MRI as screening tools for these high-risk women. For women of high risk (20–25% or greater), the ACS recommends screening MRI [20], specifically combined mammo-

Asymptomatic Women of High Risk (>20% Lifetime Risk)

- A personal BRCA1 or BRCA2 gene mutation
- A first degree relative with a BRCA1 or BRCA2 gene mutation, with the patient's own genetic status unknown
- A personal history of a genetic syndrome associated with an increased breast cancer risk (i.e. Li-Fraumeni, Cowden, & Bannayan-Riley-Ruvalcba syndromes), or a first degree relative with one of these syndromes
- A personal history of radiation to the chest wall between the ages of 10 and 30 years (i.e. prior treated Hodgkin's lymphoma)
- Lifetime risk of >20% as calculated by a risk model

Fig. 1.5 Asymptomatic women of high risk (>20% lifetime risk)

grams and MRI beginning at 30 years old and continuing while in good health [13].

MRI has been shown to be a more sensitive modality than mammography and particularly more sensitive for detecting breast cancers in certain high-risk women, such as those with the BRCA1 or BRCA2 mutation [21]. MRI has some practical disadvantages compared to mammography, as it is more costly, time-consuming, and sometimes less tolerable. Current standards of practice necessitate the administration of IV contrast, which is associated with its own risks and contraindications.

If MRI is utilized in a high-risk patient, it should be in addition to mammography, as MRI can still miss some cancers that mammography would otherwise detect. The method of combining the two modalities may vary; one commonly advocated schedule is to alternate MRI and mammography exams every 6 months.

An overview of the screening imaging recommendations for the average-, moderate-, and high-risk categories of women, as well as diagnostic imaging recommendations, is outlined in Fig. 1.6.

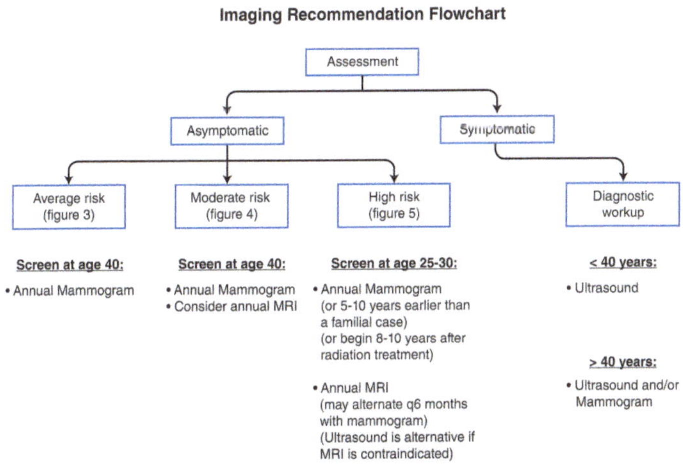

FIG. 1.6 Imaging recommendation flowchart

BI-RADS Breast Density Categories

- Breast composition is almost entirely fatty
- Breasts have scattered fibroglandular elements
- Breast tissue is heterogeneously dense
- Breasts are extremely dense

FIG. 1.7 BI-RADS breast density categories

Women with Dense Breasts

Increased breast density is associated with an increased chance of developing breast cancer [22]. The BI-RADS system of mammography reporting should be used to categorize a patient's breast density into one of four categories, as listed in Fig. 1.7.

Most studies show that approximately half of all women have a breast composition that places them in the third or fourth categories listed above, which are generally considered the "dense breast" categories [23]. Unfortunately, not only is dense breast tissue independently linked to increased risk, but the sensitivity of mammography to detect breast cancer worsens with increasing breast density, from approximately 78% to as low as 48% in women with extremely dense breasts [24]. The transition from traditional film mammography to modern digital mammography has slightly alleviated the masking effect of dense breast tissue to hide breast cancers [25]. However, the increased risk conferred by dense breasts remains very real and has been subject to great attention in both the medical community and media.

Numerous studies have been performed in an attempt to develop adequate and cost-effective supplementary screening methods in women with dense breasts [26]. However, there has yet to have been widespread evidence-based adoption of any one particular method for supplementary screening in these women. Indeed, most professional societies do not currently recommend supplementary screening for women with dense breasts but who are of otherwise average risk.

The combination of mammography and traditional ultrasound in this population has a higher sensitivity than the combination of mammography and physical exam (97% vs. 74%) [24]. However, the addition of screening ultrasound produces a greater number of false positives [27]. Implementing widespread use of screening ultrasound may also be impractical, as it is a time-consuming and an operator-dependent modality. Similarly, implementing widespread supplementary MRI for all women with dense breasts has its own drawbacks, such as cost. There has not yet been a randomized controlled study evaluating the use of supplemental MRI in women with dense breasts but who are of otherwise average risk. Newer modalities such as digital breast tomosynthesis and automated whole-breast ultrasound are showing promise as supplementary screening methods for women with dense breasts, but the evidence for these techniques is still under investigation [28]. As of yet, there are no evidence-based guidelines for recommending these new technologies, but this may change in the near future.

As of early 2016, almost half of US states have enacted the so-called “breast density” laws, which require that a patient be informed if it is determined that she has dense breasts on a mammography exam. The patient can then be informed that she can consider or pursue additional imaging. The practical implications of these laws are uncertain. This is an area that continues to evolve, both clinically and legislatively.

Diagnostic Evaluation

Overview

A diagnostic exam is performed to determine whether a new breast symptom represents breast cancer, or to further evaluate whether a finding detected on a screening exam represents breast cancer. After undergoing physical exam by the clinician, initial imaging evaluation is almost always performed with ultrasound or mammography. Ultrasound is usually the appropriate modality in women younger than 40 years old, as these younger women tend to have dense breast tissue, which greatly lowers the sensitivity of diagnostic mammography. In women of age 40 or older, diagnostic mammography or ultrasound may be pursued in either one or both breasts. After the first diagnostic imaging exam is performed, the method and frequency of follow-up will depend on the results as reported by the BI-RADS system, which is described later in this chapter.

Signs and Symptoms

Breast cancer typically produces no symptoms when small. However, there are many potential breast symptoms which may lead a patient to pursue diagnostic imaging. The most common symptom of breast cancer is a palpable mass, which is typically but not always painless. Other breast symptoms which may prompt a patient to seek medical evaluation include nipple changes (such as discharge or retraction), axillary changes (such as swelling), or skin changes (such as thickening or erythema). Of note, mastodynia (breast pain) is a common symptom that is rarely a sign of breast cancer, especially if it is an isolated symptom and/or self-resolving. Focal breast pain, however, may require diagnostic evaluation.

BI-RADS Assessment Categories

- **BI-RADS 0:** Incomplete, Additional Imaging Evaluation is needed
- **BI-RADS 1:** Negative
- **BI-RADS 2:** Benign
  - Essentially 0% probability that an identified finding is malignant
- **BI-RADS 3:** Probably Benign
  - Less than 2% probability that an identified finding is malignant
- **BI-RADS 4:** Suspicious
  - 4A: Low suspicion for malignancy (2-10%)
  - 4B: Moderate suspicion for malignancy (10-50%)
  - 4C: High suspicion for malignancy (50-95%)
- **BI-RADS 5:** Highly Suggestive of Malignancy
  - Greater than 95% probability that an identified finding is malignant
- **BI-RADS 6:** Known Biopsy-Proven Malignancy

FIG. 1.8 BI-RADS assessment categories

After the Imaging Exam: BI-RADS and Follow-Up

Regardless of the patient's risk factors and the type of imaging exam performed, a patient's screening exam should be evaluated by a radiologist using the Breast Imaging Reporting and Data System (BI-RADS), which is a standardized reporting system developed by the American College of Radiology [29].

BI-RADS has many components; for practical purposes, the most important features are the use of standardized lexicon and the provision of a BI-RADS assessment category at the end of the report. This assessment should always include a recommendation regarding follow-up, whether imaging or intervention. Assessment categories are described in Fig. 1.8.

It may be useful to emphasize to the patient that mammography alone can usually not determine whether a newly identified finding is benign or malignant. With the rare exception of certain masses which have a highly suspicious and unequivocal mammographic appearance that warrant a BI-RADS 5 designation, the determination of benignity vs. malignancy can only be definitively ascertained by biopsying the finding or, in some cases, demonstrating a stable imaging appearance of the finding over a long period of time (at least 2 years).

Approximately 10% of women who undergo a screening mammography exam will be recommended to return for additional imaging, such as ultrasound or additional mammographic views [30]. The majority of these recalled women will be found to have normal or benign findings on the subsequent follow-up exam, but 1–2% of screened women will undergo a needle biopsy as a result of a suspicious finding on their initial exam and/or follow-up images, and approximately 0.5% of screened women will be ultimately diagnosed with breast cancer as a result of the screening exam [31].

If a screening mammogram exam is designated as BI-RADS 0, or BI-RADS 3 or higher, then the patient will be recommended to pursue either additional imaging or biopsy, depending on the specific findings. If subsequent diagnostic imaging demonstrates a more clearly benign and reassuring appearance, then the need for additional follow-up imaging may cease, and the patient may resume annual screening mammograms. If suspicious findings persist or are found to be more worrisome on follow-up imaging, biopsy is generally recommended. The results of biopsy should always be correlated with the clinical picture; there are low but real rates of discordance between the tissue diagnosis provided by the pathologist and the clinical or imaging presentation [32]. Unfortunately, breast cancers may either be initially missed during biopsy or be upgraded during subsequent excision [33].

Conclusion

Breast cancer screening with mammography in women of average risk has been consistently demonstrated to save lives [2, 3]. While there is no universally agreed upon set of guidelines, annual screening mammography should be strongly considered at the age of 40, as beginning screening at that age saves the most lives [18]. Women with dense breasts should be informed of such status and be made aware that additional screening options can be considered, such as ultrasound or MRI. Women with particular high-risk factors are recommended to undergo screening with both mammography and MRI.

Regardless of risk status, women should be aware of changes in their breasts and report such changes to their physician. When additional diagnostic imaging evaluation is recommended or pursued, women should be counseled as to what to expect and how to interpret their imaging reports. The collection of new evidence continues to influence screening guidelines, which are sure to undergo further changes in the future, particularly in regard to women with dense breasts.

References

1. Howlader N, Noone AM, Krapcho M, et al., editors. SEER cancer statistics review, 1975–2009 (Vintage 2009 Populations). Bethesda: National Cancer Institute; 2012.
2. Nelson HD, Tyne K, Naik A, et al. Screening for breast cancer: an update for the U.S. preventive services task force. Ann Intern Med. 2009;151(10):727–37. W237–42.
3. American Cancer Society. Cancer facts & figures 2016. Atlanta: American Cancer Society; 2016.
4. Thomas DB, Gao DL, Ray RM, et al. Randomized trial of breast self-examination in Shanghai: final results. J Natl Cancer Inst. 2002;94(19):1445–57.

5. Siu AL, on behalf of the U.S. Preventive Services Task Force. Screening for breast cancer: U.S. Preventive Services Task Force recommendation statement. Ann Intern Med. 2016;164:279–96.
6. American College of Obstetricians and Gynecologists. Frequently asked questions: mammography and other screening tests for breast problems; 2016. https://www.acog.org/-/media/For-Patients/faq178.pdf . Retrieved Feb 2016.
7. Oeffinger KC, Fontham ET, Etzioni R, et al. Breast cancer screening for women at average risk: 2015 guideline update from the American Cancer Society. JAMA. 2015;314(15):1599–614.
8. American College of Obstetricians and Gynecologists. ACOG statement on revised American Cancer Society recommendations on breast cancer screening; 2015. http://www.acog.org/About-ACOG/News-Room/Statements/2015/ACOG-Statement-on-Recommendations-on-Breast-Cancer-Screening. Retrieved Feb 2016.
9. Ichikawa LE, Barlow WE, Anderson ML, et al. Time trends in radiologists' interpretive performance at screening mammography from the community-based breast cancer surveillance consortium, 1996–2004. Radiology. 2010;256(1):74–82.
10. American Cancer Society. Breast cancer facts & figures 2015–2016. Atlanta: American Cancer Society; 2015. Retrieved Feb 2016.
11. Singletary SE. Rating the risk factors for breast cancer. Ann Surg. 2003;237(4):474–82.
12. National Cancer Institute. Breast cancer risk assessment tool; 2011. http://www.cancer.gov/bcrisktool/. Retrieved Feb 2016.
13. American Cancer Society. American Cancer Society recommendations for early breast cancer detection in women without breast symptoms; 2015. http://www.cancer.org/cancer/breastcancer/moreinformation/breastcancerearlydetection/breast-cancer-early-detection-acs-recs. Retrieved Feb 2016.
14. Mainiero MB, Lourenco A, Mahoney MC, et al. American College of Radiology appropriateness criteria for breast cancer screening; 2012. https://acsearch.acr.org/docs/70910/Narrative. Retrieved Feb 2016.
15. National Comprehensive Cancer Network. Breast cancer screening and diagnosis, Version 1.2015; 2015. http://www.nccn.org/professionals/physician_gls/pdf/breast-screening.pdf. Retrieved Feb 2016.

16. Tosteson AN, Fryback DG, Hammond CS, et al. Consequences of false-positive screening mammograms. JAMA Intern Med. 2014;174(6):954–61.
17. Saadatmand S, Bretveld R, Siesling S, Tilanus-Linthorst MM. Influence of tumour stage at breast cancer detection on survival in modern times: population based study in 173,797 patients. BMJ. 2015;351:h4901.
18. Hendrick RE, Helvie MA. United States Preventive Services Task Force screening mammography recommendations: science ignored. AJR Am J Roentgenol. 2011;196(2):W112–6.
19. The Henry J. Kaiser Family Foundation. Preventive services covered by Private Health Plans under the Affordable Care Act; 2015. http://kff.org/health-reform/fact-sheet/preventive-services-covered-by-private-health-plans/. Retrieved Feb 2016.
20. Saslow D, Boetes C, Burke W, et al. American Cancer Society guidelines for breast screening with MRI as an adjunct to mammography. CA Cancer J Clin. 2007;57(2):75–89.
21. Warner E, Plewes DB, Hill KA, et al. Surveillance of BRCA1 and BRCA2 mutation carriers with magnetic resonance imaging, ultrasound, mammography, and clinical breast examination. JAMA. 2004;292(11):1317–25.
22. Harvey JA, Bovbjerg VE. Quantitative assessment of mammographic breast density: relationship with breast cancer risk. Radiology. 2004;230(1):29–41.
23. Kerlikowske K, Zhu W, Hubbard RA, et al. Outcomes of screening mammography by frequency, breast density, and postmenopausal hormone therapy. JAMA Intern Med. 2013;173(9):807–16.
24. Kolb TM, Lichy J, Newhouse JH. Comparison of the performance of screening mammography, physical examination, and breast US and evaluation of factors that influence them: an analysis of 27,825 patient evaluations. Radiology. 2002;225:165–75.
25. Pisano ED, Gatsonis C, Hendrick E, et al. Diagnostic performance of digital versus film mammography for breast-cancer screening. N Engl J Med. 2005;353:1773–83.
26. Sprague BL, Stout NK, Schechter C, et al. Benefits, harms, and cost-effectiveness of supplemental ultrasonography screening for women with dense breasts. Ann Intern Med. 2015;162(3):157–66.
27. Berg WA, Zhang Z, Lehrer D, et al. Detection of breast cancer with addition of annual screening ultrasound or a single screening MRI to mammography in women with elevated breast cancer risk. JAMA. 2012;307(13):1394–404.

28. Brem RF, Tabár L, Duffy SW, et al. Assessing improvement in detection of breast cancer with three-dimensional automated breast US in women with dense breast tissue: the SomoInsight study. Radiology. 2015;274(3):663–73.
29. D'Orsi CJ, Sickles EA, Mendelson EB, Morris EA, et al. ACR BI-RADS atlas, breast imaging reporting and data system. Reston: American College of Radiology; 2013.
30. Schell MJ, Yankaskas BC, Ballard-Barbash R, et al. Evidence-based target recall rates for screening mammography. Radiology. 2007;243(3):681–9.
31. Rosenberg RD, Yankaskas BC, Abraham LA, et al. Performance benchmarks for screening mammography. Radiology. 2006;241(1):55–66.
32. Liberman L, Drotman M, Morris EA, et al. Imaging-histologic discordance at percutaneous breast biopsy. Cancer. 2000;89(12):2538–46.
33. Foster MC, Helvie MA, Gregory NE, et al. Lobular carcinoma in situ or atypical lobular hyperplasia at core-needle biopsy: is excisional biopsy necessary? Radiology. 2004;231(3):813–9.

Chapter 2
Breast Disorders: Age-Based Management

James A. Hall

Primary care providers have the responsibility of investigating breast complaints and encouraging screening protocols. Although most women with breast complaints fear they have cancer, benign etiologies far outnumber malignant ones. Every breast complaint requires a thorough evaluation until a definitive diagnosis is established. Breast cancer is the most frequent malignancy diagnosed in US women with 192,370 estimated cases in 2009. Breast cancer results in approximately 40,000 deaths per year, which is second only to lung cancer. There are more breast cancer deaths each year than ovarian, uterine, fallopian tube, cervical, and vulva combined.

[1] An accurate history of the patient's complaint, family history, and age is essential. Although the presence or absence of risk factors is important, each complaint should be evaluated on its own merits without undue bias from risk factors.

Risk Factors

The two most important risk factors for breast cancer are female gender and advancing age. The lifetime risk of breast cancer for American women through age 85 is one in eight.

J. A. Hall (✉)
Memorial Hospital, Women's Health Center, Logansport, IN, USA
e-mail: jim.kylehall@comcast.net

J. V. Knaus et al. (eds.), *Ambulatory Gynecology*,
https://doi.org/10.1007/978-1-4939-7641-6_2

Only 1% of breast cancers occur in men. Breast cancer is rare before age 30 and increases with age until declining at 80. Other factors associated with an increased risk include early menarche, late menopause, nulliparity, first birth after age 35, positive family history, and radiation exposure especially in younger women. Five to ten percent of women with breast cancer have an associated autosomal dominant suppressor gene mutation BRCA. The risk of BRCA mutation is highest in younger women with cancer especially less than age 30, bilateral disease, or family history of breast or ovarian cancer. The lifetime risk for women with a known BRCA mutation is between 40% and 85%. Women with a personal history of breast cancer have a 1% per year risk of a new primary cancer and a lifetime risk of approximately 20%. Oral contraceptive use has not conclusively been shown to increase breast cancer risk.

Postmenopausal hormone replacement therapy (HRT) and breast cancer risk have been the heavily debated subjects. The Women's Health Initiative (WHI) study demonstrated an increased risk with estrogen/progesterone HRT(PremPro) after 4-year use and no increased risk with estrogen replacement therapy (ERT) alone. Any increased risk from HRT is gone after discontinuation for 5 or more years. Review of the WHI reveals the 1.26 increased relative risk of HRT and breast cancer results in only 8 more cancers per 10,000 women per year than nonusers, and this small difference was not statistically significant [2]. The average age of women entering the WHI was 63, and therefore the risk in younger women was not addressed. The only HRT used was equine estrogen and medroxyprogesterone (PremPro), and thus the risk with other estrogens or progesterones is not known. Another concern of the WHI is that 84% of breast cancer cases were found in the first 5 years of the study. Given the average growth rate takes a breast cancer tumor 8 years to reach a detectable 1 cm, it is probable that a high percentage of cancers were present but undetectable before the study began and would not be a result of HRT use. It is safe to conclude that if any HRT risk to breast cancer exists, it is small and does not manifest itself until several years of use. ERT has not been shown to increase risk. Benefits of HRT need to be considered when discussing breast cancer risk.

Proliferative breast lesions without atypia confirm a small increased risk of breast cancer and include tissue-proven fibroadenoma, ductal hyperplasia, papilloma, sclerosing adenosis, and radial scar. Proliferative breast lesions with atypia have a greater risk and include atypical ductal hyperplasia, atypical lobular hyperplasia, and lobular carcinoma in situ.

Screening

Screening with mammography has improved the chances of survival through early diagnosis when tumors are more likely to be smaller, low grade, and treatable with a less aggressive approach. Breast cancer death rates for US women have decreased 37% between 1991 and 2005 [3] largely due to screening mammography. Screening programs result in >50% of cancers that are stage O or I at diagnosis, >30% are <1 mm or in situ, and <25% are node positive. The mammographic window [4, 5] (Fig. 2.1) illustrates the importance of screening as tumors can be discovered before they would become clinically evident and have metastatic potential. The mammographic window is the time sequence when a breast cancer may be discovered only by mammogram imaging. Tumors are generally pre-mammographic until they reach at least 1 mm and are usually not clinically palpable until at least 1 cm. Screening mammography should begin at age 40 and continue annually [6]. Diagnostic mammography for a specific problem may be obtained at any time and at any age. Dense

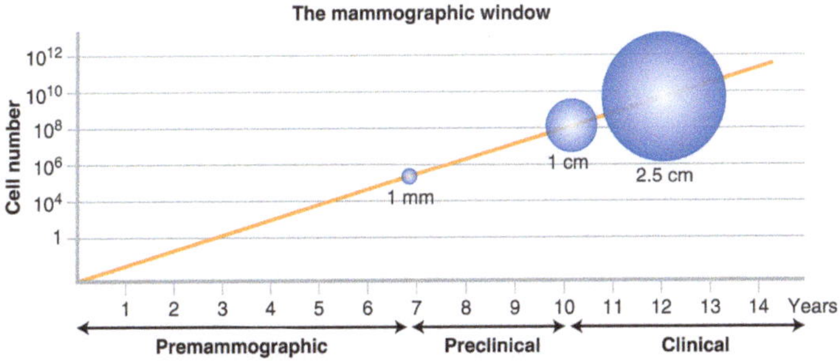

FIG. 2.1 Mammographic window

breasts are found in many women before age 40 and may make mammography less sensitive. Abnormal areas requiring biopsy are best sampled by image-guided core-needle technique. It is mandatory that the pathology result is in concordance with the mammogram appearance. Because the core-needle biopsy takes a representative sample, some pathology findings require an open excisional biopsy to more completely sample the area (Fig. 2.2). Breast ultrasound is an adjunct to mammography and is used to detect cystic from solid or complex cystic masses. Simple cysts confirmed by sonar do not need to be removed or aspirated.

Complex or solid masses require tissue sampling to exclude malignancy. Ultrasound may also be used to complement screening mammography for women with radiographic dense breasts. Breast MRI is not recommended for screening women with average breast cancer risk. MRI is considered as an adjunct to mammography for women at high risk especially BRCA mutations.

Breast MRI is also considered for suspected implant rupture and radiographic dense breast. MRI may also be part of the evaluation and staging in patients with known cancer.

Multifocal or contralateral disease may be found in at least 10% of patients and discovery allows individual specific treatment. BRCA testing is recommended for women with high risk

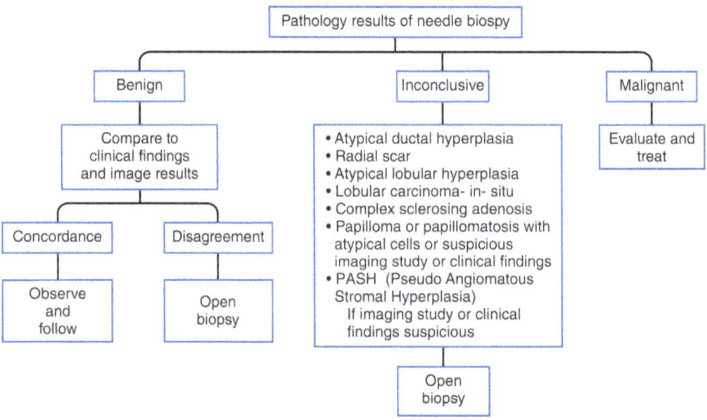

FIG. 2.2 Pathology results of needle biopsy

due to family history of breast or ovarian cancer. The complete BRCA gene profile is best obtained on a family member who has been affected by cancer. Remaining family members would not need testing in the absence of a BRCA gene mutation.

Medical Malpractice

Delayed or missed breast cancer diagnosis remains a frequent source of malpractice litigation. While most suits have little merit, it is still an expensive, time-consuming, and anxiety-provoking task to defend. Following screening guidelines, evaluating each complaint to a conclusive diagnosis and making an appropriate referral and accurate charting are essential steps for malpractice defense. It is important to chart all recommendations especially if the patient fails to comply. Conclusions based on phone messages from the patient regarding physical findings should never overshadow the importance of a clinical exam. Vague or confusing terms and diagrams in the chart are often difficult to defend and explain years later. Vague clinical findings such as thickening or tender areas should not be labeled a "mass" or "lump." Diagrams and drawings should be avoided unless there are positive findings such as a dominant mass. An outside reviewer will suggest that drawings and diagrams describe positive findings even if the physician later denies there was anything but vague findings. It is better to avoid diagrams and drawings unless there is a thorough evaluation of the complaint. Refrain from being overly descriptive.

Locations of abnormalities are best noted using references to the hours of a clock and distance from the areola edge. Make sure it is clearly stated which breast is involved.

Diagnostic Triad

The diagnostic triad (Fig. 2.3) serves as a visual of the concordance needed with the basic breast complaint evaluation including the clinical exam, imaging studies, and needle aspiration or biopsy. Each area's finding should agree with the others or the diagnosis remains in doubt.

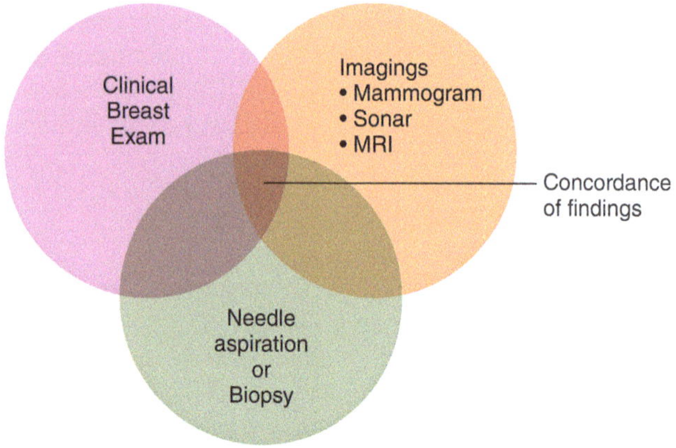

FIG. 2.3 Diagnostic triad

Abnormal Mammogram

A thorough clinical exam with history is a necessary part of the evaluation. The presence or absence of findings such as nipple discharge, palpable mass, skin changes, nipple retraction, or axillary adenopathy is an essential information. Steps to follow and diagnostic options are presented in Fig. 2.4.

Fine Needle Aspiration

Needle aspiration of a dominant mass (Fig. 2.5) with a 22-gauge needle and 10-cc. syringe can be done in the office without anesthesia and before obtaining imaging tests. Discovery of a simple cyst gives the patient immediate feedback that she does not have cancer.

Cytology of tissue aspirate can be obtained from a solid mass and correlates well with tissue biopsy if an adequate number of ductal cells are recovered.

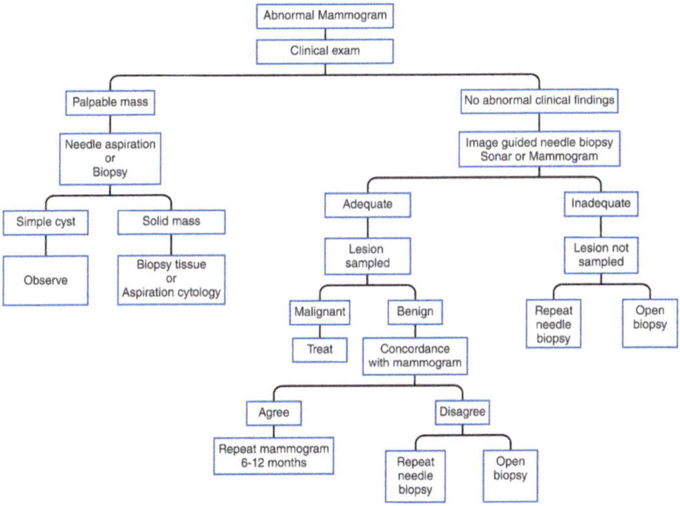

FIG. 2.4 Abnormal mammogram – clinical exam

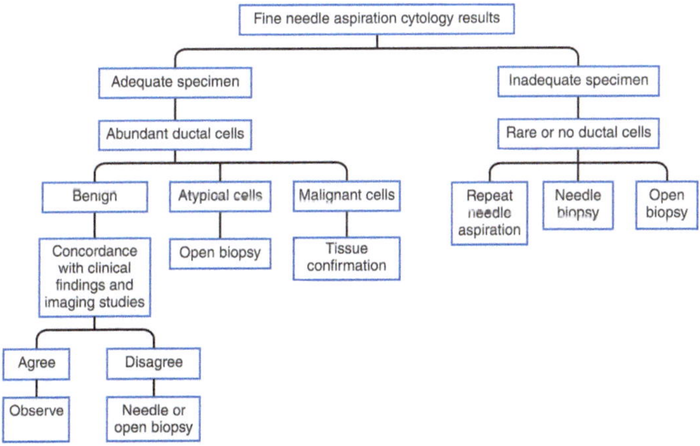

FIG. 2.5 Fine needle aspiration cytology results

Needle Biopsy Pathology Reports

Tissue diagnosis (Fig. 2.2) results must be in concordance with the clinical and imaging findings. Some pathology findings require open biopsy to further sample the abnormality. A sampling error may occur as the neoplasm may have heterogeneous histology with atypical cells immediately adjacent to malignancy. Approximately 15% of open biopsies following needle biopsy indicating only atypical changes will reveal malignancy.

Nipple Discharge

It is important to differentiate between pathologic nipple discharge and physiologic galactorrhea (Fig. 2.6). Each duct opening on the nipple drains a unique isolated area of the breast, which also geographically corresponds to the duct's location on the nipple. Observing the location of the duct opening allows mapping of the abnormal area producing the nipple discharge. Cytology of nipple discharge gives unreliable results and is not recommended.

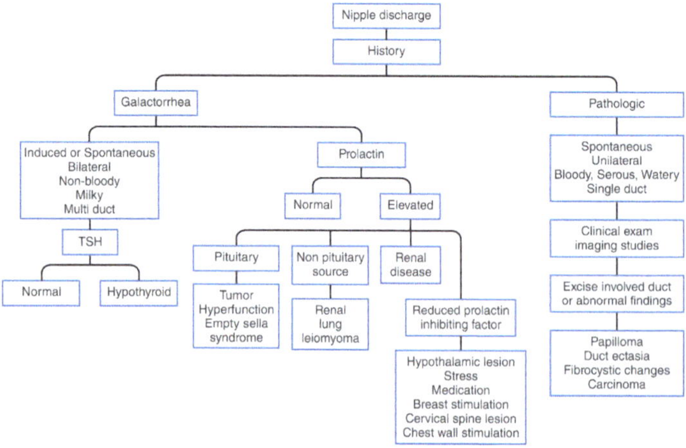

FIG. 2.6 Nipple discharge – history

Breast Mass

The evaluation of a dominant mass (Fig. 2.7) should proceed until there is a definite diagnosis. The diagnostic triad requires agreement between findings of the clinical exam, imaging studies, and needle aspiration or biopsy.

Mastalgia

Malignancy rarely presents with pain or tenderness. However, this cannot be used to exclude clinical findings or give reassurance without a thorough evaluation (Fig. 2.8). There is no evidence that caffeine is responsible for breast cysts, pain, or tenderness.

Non-puerperal Mastitis

Non-puerperal breast infection (Fig. 2.9) is rare. Lack of rapid improvement requires consideration of inflammatory carcinoma. Antibiotics with serial needle aspirations, if there is an

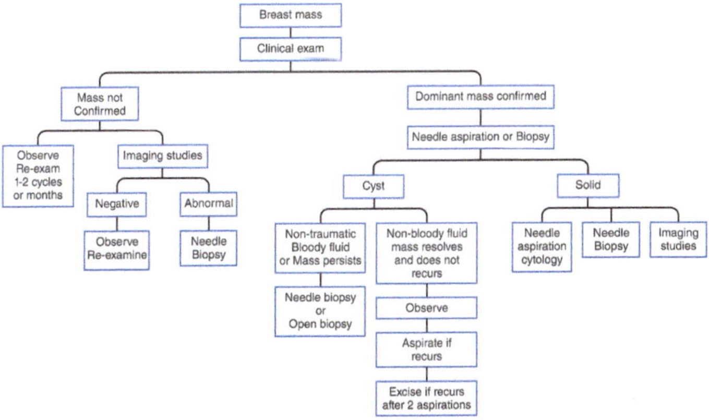

FIG. 2.7 Breast mass – clinical exam

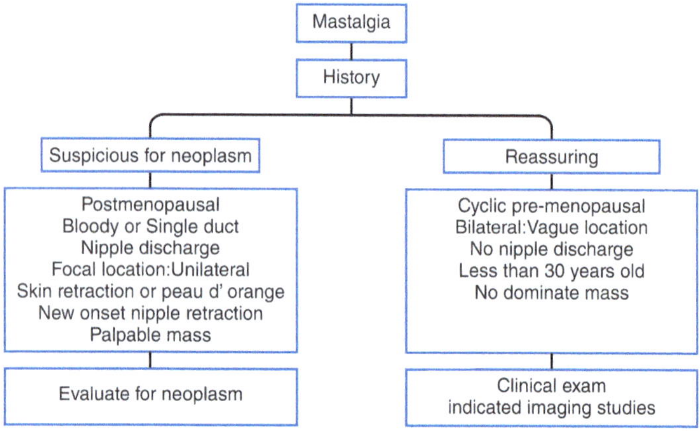

FIG. 2.8 Mastalgia – history

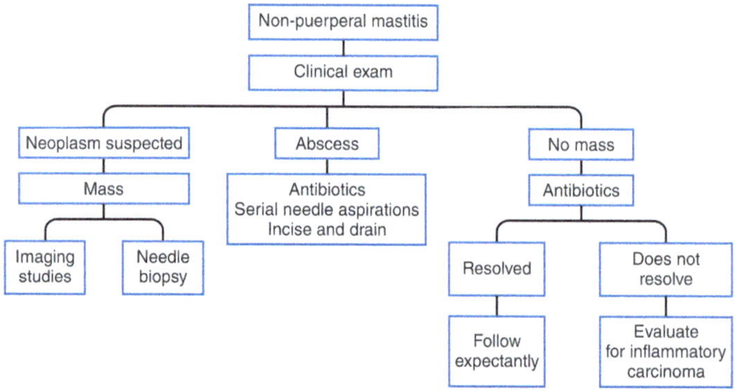

FIG. 2.9 Non-puerperal mastitis – clinical exam

abscess, usually prevent the need for an open drainage procedure with resulting poor cosmetic result. Inflammatory carcinoma can be confirmed with needle biopsy.

Punch biopsy of the skin may also reveal malignant cells in the dermal lymphatic channels.

References

1. Pearlman M, Griffin J. Benign breast disease. Obstet Gynecol. 2010;116:747–58.
2. Editorial. Women's health initiative results: breast cancer risk in perspective. Breast J. 2003;9:449–51.
3. Jemel A, Siegel R, Ward E, et al. Cancer statistics 2009. CA J Clin. 2009;59:225–49.
4. Werthheimer M, Constanza M, Dodson T, et al. Increasing the effort toward breast cancer detection. J Am Med Assoc. 1986;255:1311.
5. Hall J, Knaus J. An atlas of breast cancer. New York: Parthenon; 2003.
6. Screening FS. Mammography controversies: resolved, partly resolved, and unresolved. Breast J. 2005;11(Suppl. I):3–6.

Chapter 3
Contraception: Overview

Michele Bucciero and Magdalena Parda-Chlebowicz

Introduction

Women have used some type of birth control method for thousands of years. Despite this, nearly one half of all pregnancies in the United States still remain unplanned [1]. Adolescent pregnancy rate in the United States is the highest among developed countries, with a rate in 2010 of 57 per 1,000 girls aged 15–19. Three quarters of adolescent pregnancies are unintended [2]. There is no "best" method of birth control, and the choice depends on multiple factors including: women's overall health, age, frequency of sexual activity, number of sexual partners, desire for future fertility, family history of certain diseases, possible side effects, and women's comfort level with using the method, whether it helps protect against HIV and other STDs and whether the chosen method offers additional health benefits besides birth control. A clear understanding of the available contraceptive methods permits a clinician to counsel women about methods that are most consistent with their health status, lifestyles, and comfort and therefore most likely to be successful.

M. Bucciero, MD, MBA-HCM (✉)
Saint Anthony Hospital, Chicago, IL, USA
e-mail: mbucciero@sahchicago.org

M. Parda-Chlebowicz, MD
St. Francis Hospital, Evanston, IL, USA

J. V. Knaus et al. (eds.), *Ambulatory Gynecology*,
https://doi.org/10.1007/978-1-4939-7641-6_3

Office Evaluation

ROUTINE DISCUSSION OF CONTRACEPTION
All reproductive age women including adolescents.
Ideal time during annual preventative health visits.
⇓
HISTORY AND PHYSICAL
Gynecologic history including menstrual cycle, sexual activity, and history of STIs.
⇓
EXPLAIN IMPORTANCE OF CONTRACEPTION & DISPEL MYTHS
Enforce safety of planned pregnancy
⇓
HELP YOUR PATIENT IN CHOOSING APPROPRIATE METHOD
Using data gathered in the H&P portion of evaluation, considering age, weight, medical problems, sexual behaviors/risks, smoking status, and socioeconomic status
⇓
OFFER CONTRACEPTION
Obtain pregnancy test.
Encourage condom use to protect against STIs.
⇓
DISCUSS POTENTIAL SIDE EFFECTS
⇓
USE 'QUICK START'
⇓
PROVIDE EDUCATION MATERIALS

Birth Control Methods (www.womenshealth.gov – Birth Control Methods, ACOG Patient Education Booklet, ACOG-Long-Acting Reversible Contraception, and www.emedicinehealth.com)[3]

1. **Continuous Abstinence**
2. **Behavioral Methods**
   (a) **Coitus Interruptus**
   (b) **Natural Family Planning**
3. **Barrier Methods**
   (a) **Contraceptive Sponge**
   (b) **Diaphragm, Cervical Cap, and Cervical Shield**
   (c) **Female and Male Condom**
   (d) **Spermicide**

4. **Hormonal Methods**
   (a) **Oral contraceptives**
      - **Combined pill ("The Pill")**
      - **Progestin-only pill ("Mini-pill")**
   (b) **The Patch**
   (c) **Injectables**
   (d) **Vaginal Ring**
5. **Implantable Devices**
   (a) **Intrauterine Devices (IUD)**
   (b) **Implantable Rods**
6. **Permanent Birth Control Methods**
   (a) **Male Sterilization**
   (b) **Female Sterilization**
      (i) **Postpartum**
      (ii) **Laparoscopic**
      (iii) **Hysteroscopic**
7. **Emergency Contraception**
8. **Special Populations**

Continuous Abstinence

This involves completely refraining from sexual intercourse (vaginal, anal, or oral) at any time, and it is the only way to completely prevent pregnancy and protect against sexually transmitted diseases, including HIV (www.womenshealth.gov).

Behavioral Methods

Coitus Interruptus

This involves the withdrawal of the entire penis from the vagina before male ejaculation occurs in the hopes of preventing sperm from reaching the egg and thus fertilization.

Effectiveness of this method largely depends on the man's ability to withdraw prior to ejaculation with failure rate estimated to be ~4% in the first year with "perfect use." With typical use, the failure rate approaches 19% during the first year of use. Advantages of this method include ability to be used at any time with no involvement of medications/devices and no cost. Disadvantages include abovementioned high risk of unintended pregnancy and no protection against STIs (www.emedicinehealth.com).

Natural Family Planning

Natural family planning remains one of the most widely used methods of fertility regulation for women whose religious or cultural beliefs do not allow medications or devices for contraception.

A woman who has a regular menstrual cycle has approximately 9 or more days each month, about 5 days before and 3 days after ovulation, when she is able to achieve highest pregnancy rate. Rhythm method involves not having sexual intercourse or using a barrier method on these fertile days.

It also involves educating the patient about her menstrual cycle to help her predict the fertile days. The current method thought by the Couple to Couple League and many other teaching organizations is the symptothermal method that involves checking cervical mucus for consistency as well as recording basal waking body temperature. A clear, slippery, stretchy discharge indicates period of highest fertility. Basal body temperature with rise by 0.4–0.8 °F from baseline basal body temperature before ovulation of 97–97.5 °F indicates first day of ovulation. Quoted effectiveness of this method varies with the Couple to Couple League (the primary agency endorsing the method) reporting a failure rate of 1%, the FDA reporting the failure rate of 20%, and with ACOG reporting the failure rate of 25% (these figures did not differentiate for type of periodic abstinence) (Table 3.1).

Table 3.1 Barrier methods

Barrier method	Mechanism of action	Length of use	Effectiveness (within first year of typical use)	Benefits	Risks	Side effects
Contra-ceptive sponge	A soft, disk-shaped device made out of polyurethane foam and contains the nonoxynol-9 spermicide which is released in small amounts for 24 h A wetted sponge with loop side down is placed in the vagina to cover the cervix before having intercourse	Remains effective for more than one act of intercourse for up to 24 h and it must be left in for at least 6 h after to prevent pregnancy Must be taken out within 30 h from insertion	12–24 out of 100: 12 out of 100 women who have never given birth will become pregnant It is less effective in women who have given birth: 24 out of 100 will become pregnant	• Over the counter • No effect of woman's natural hormones • May be used while breast feeding beginning 6 weeks after childbirth	• Toxic shock syndrome -rare (should not be used during: menstrual period, if given birth less than 6 weeks prior, or with prior history of TSS • No protection from STDs and with frequent use increased risk of acquiring HIV from infected partner (see below[a])	• Vaginal irritation • Allergic reaction to polyurethane, spermicides, or sulfites (all found in the sponge)

(continued)

TABLE 3.1 (continued)

Barrier method	Mechanism of action	Length of use	Effectiveness (within first year of typical use)	Benefits	Risks	Side effects
Diaphragm, cervical cap, and cervical shield	• Diaphragm: a shallow dome-shaped latex or silicone cup that comes in different sizes and requires fitting before use • Cervical cap: thimble-shaped silicone cup that comes in different sizes and requires fitting before use • Cervical shield: a silicone cup that has a one-way valve that creates suction and helps it fit against the cervix. It comes in one size and does not require fitting before use All three are used in adjunct with spermicide. Recent pregnancy and child-birth; large weight gain or weight loss, may require a refitting	All three must be left in place for 6–8 h after intercourse to prevent pregnancy Diaphragm can be inserted up to 2 h before intercourse and should be taken out within 24 h Cap and the shield should be taken out within 48 h	• Diaphragm with spermicide: 12 out of 100 women will become pregnant Cervical cap with spermicide: 17–23 out of 100 women will become pregnant –13 out of 100 women who have never given birth will become pregnant –23 out of 100 women who have given birth will become pregnant	• No effect of woman's natural hormones • May be used while breastfeeding beginning 6 weeks after child birth	• Increased risk of toxic shock syndrome if left in for more than the recommended length • Increased risk of urinary tract infection • No protection from STDs and with frequent use can increase the risk of acquiring HIV from infected partner (see below[a])	• Allergic reaction • Vaginal irritation

Condoms female and male	• Female condom: thin, flexible, synthetic rubber pouch that lines the vagina and is held in place by a closed inner ring at the cervix and an outer ring at the opening of the vagina • Male condom: thin sheath made out of latex, polyurethane, or "natural/lamb skin" that is placed over an erect penis to keep sperm away More effective in preventing pregnancy when used in conjunction with spermicide All protect from STIs except for the natural membrane type	Female condom: can be inserted into the vagina for up to 8 h before intercourse; Need to use new condom with each sex act Latex condoms should only be used with water-based or silicone lubricants to avoid weakening and tearing the condom	Without spermicide: • Male condom: 18 out of 100 women will become pregnant • Female condom: 21 out of 100 women will become pregnant With spermicide: Male condom: As affective as using the combination BCP	• Not expensive • Over the counter • No effect of women natural hormones • May be used while breastfeeding • Can be carried in pocket or purse • Latex and polyurethane male condoms provide the best available protection against STIs	• None	• Allergic reaction to latex or polyurethane

(continued)

TABLE 3.1 (continued)

Barrier method	Mechanism of action	Length of use	Effectiveness (within first year of typical use)	Benefits	Risks	Side effects
Spermicide	A chemical barrier in a form of a foam, cream, jelly, suppository, or film that is placed in the vagina, close to the cervix, before each attempt of intercourse By inactivating the sperm, it prevents it from passing through cervical canal into the uterus and fallopian tubes and thus fertilizing the egg	May be used with all available barrier methods except the sponge, which already contains a spermicide Needs to be placed in the vagina 5–90 min before intercourse. Need to leave it in at least 6–8 h after intercourse	28 out of 100 women will become pregnant	• Easy to use • Not expensive • Over the counter • No effect of women natural hormones • May be used while breastfeeding	• When used alone, do not protect against STIs including HIV • Frequent use may cause changes in the lining of the vagina and rectum that can increase the risk of acquiring HIV from an infected partner (see below[a])	Allergic reaction Vaginitis UTI

ACOG Educational Pamphlet AB020—Birth Control
www.womenshealth.gov
www.emedicinehealth.com
www.fda.gov/birthcontrol

[a]Important information about spermicides and protection against STDs

Nonoxyno-9 (N-9) is found in all spermicides sold in the United States

N-9 has not been shown to protect against HIV or other STDs. Also, frequent use of N-9 may cause changes in vaginal lining and rectum that increases the risk of getting HIV from an infected partner. N-9 is not recommended for protection against STDs and HIV infection. You should use a spermicide for birth control by itself or with another barrier only if you are at low risk of HIV infection

You are at high risk of HIV infection if you have any of the following:

- Have had more than one sexual partner since your last HIV test or a sexual partner who has had more than one partner since the partner's last HIV test
- Have been diagnosed with an STD in the past year
- Have a history of prostitution of injected drug use
- Have had a past or present partner who is HIV positive
- Had a blood transfusion from 1979 to 1985
- Have a history of invasive cervical cancer
- Live in an area where there is a high rate of HIV infection

Hormonal Methods

QUICK START TO INITIATE CONTRACEPTION AT INITIAL VISIT

FIRST DAY OF LMP <5DAYS?

⇓ ⇓

YES → ⇓ → **INITIATE CONTRACEPTION**

NO → ⇓ → **DO URINE PREGNANCY TEST IF NEGATIVE:** ⇓

1. **Initiate contraception**
2. **Back up method for a week**
3. **Discuss Emergency contraception if patient had unprotected intercourse in the past 5 days.**

Oral Contraceptive Pills/Birth Control Pills

Oral contraceptives are widely used and are generally safe and effective contraceptive method for many women. They have been marketed in the United States since 1962, and over the past 40 years, there have been changes made in the type and dose of estrogen and progesterone formulations to improve safety profile and reduce side effects (www.emedicinehealth.com).

The choice of pill formulation is influenced by many clinical considerations. By choosing the appropriate available pill formulation, the physician can minimize any associated negative side effects and also maximize the noncontraceptive benefits for their patients. The World Health Organization has developed a risk stratification system to aid physicians in advising their patients about the safety of oral contraceptive pills.

Mechanism of Action

Combination oral contraceptive pills consist of estrogen and progestin components and prevent ovulation by inhibiting gonadotropin secretion at both pituitary and hypothalamic levels. The progestin component in the pill primarily suppresses luteinizing hormone (LH) secretion and thus prevents ovulation. The estrogen component of the pill suppresses follicle-stimulating hormone (FSH) secretion and thus prevents the formation of a dominant follicle. The estrogen component in the pill serves two other purposes as well. It stabilizes the endometrium and thus reduces unwanted spotting, and it potentiates the action of the progestin component allowing for reduction of the progestin dose in the pill [4].

Types of Oral Contraceptives

Over 30 different combinations are available in the United States. Majority of these pills have 21 hormonally active pills followed by 7 placebo pills.

Monophasic pills: have constant dose of both estrogen and progestin in each of the hormonally active pills.

Phasic pills: can alter either or both hormonal components to try to mimic the natural menstrual cycle.

91-day pill: FDA-approved regimen of 12-week duration with 84 days of hormone active and 7 days of hormone-free pills with menstruation occurring during the hormone-free week, every 3 months.

Absolute Contraindications to the Use of Oral Contraception

1. Thrombophlebitis, thromboembolic disorders (including a close family, parent, or sibling, suggestive of an inherited susceptibility for venous thrombosis), cerebral vascular disease, coronary occlusion, or a past history of these conditions or conditions predisposing to these problems.
2. Markedly impaired liver function. Steroid hormones are contraindicated in patients with hepatitis until liver function tests return normal.
3. Known or suspected breast cancer.
4. Undiagnosed abnormal vaginal bleeding.
5. Known or suspected pregnancy.
6. Smokers over the age of 35.

7. Severe hypercholesterolemia or hypertriglyceridemia.
8. Elevated blood pressure.

Relative Contraindications to the Use of Oral Contraception Requiring Clinical Judgment and Informed Consent

1. Migraine headaches
2. Hypertension
3. Uterine leiomyoma
4. Gestational diabetes
5. Diabetes mellitus
6. Elective surgery
7. Seizure disorder
8. Obstructive jaundice in pregnancy
9. Sickle cell disease or sickle C disease
10. Gallbladder disease
11. Mitral valve prolapse
12. Systemic lupus erythematosus
13. Hyperlipidemia
14. Smoking
15. Hepatic disease

Side Effects

1. Headaches
2. Breast tenderness
3. Nausea
4. Irregular bleeding
5. Missed menstrual cycles
6. Weight gain (progestin-only pills)
7. Anxiety or depression (progestin-only pills)
8. Excessive body hear growth (progestin-only pills)
9. Acne (progestin-only pills)

Pill Taking

Effective contraception is present during the first cycle of pill use, provided the pills are started no later than the fifth day of the cycle and no pills are missed (Figs. 3.1 and 3.2).

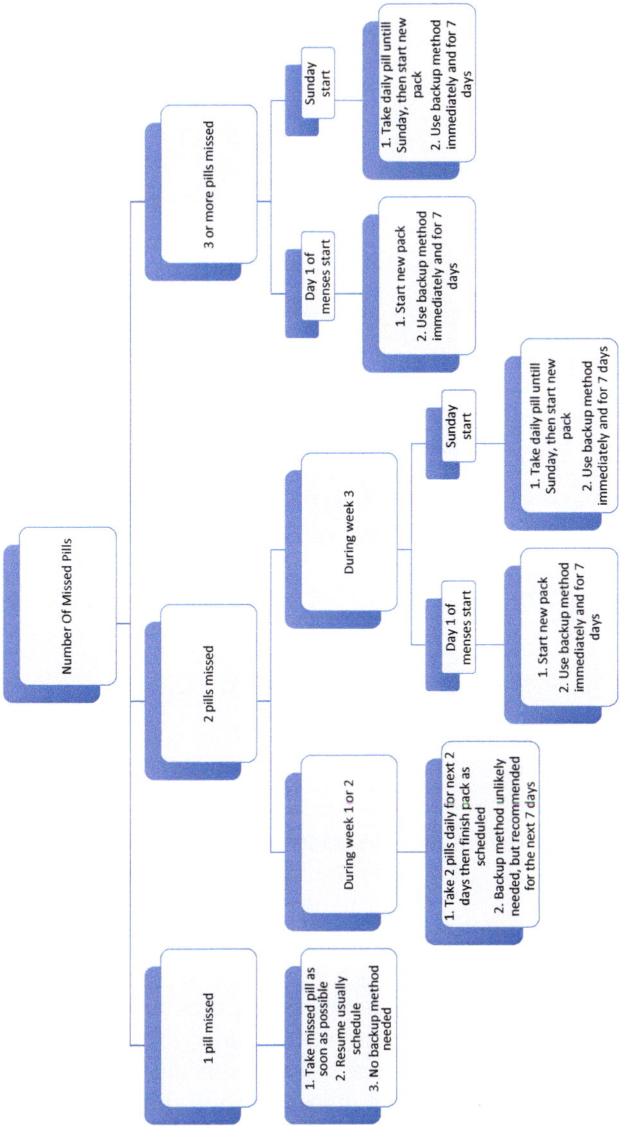

FIG. 3.1 Algorithm: missed combined oral hormonal contraceptive

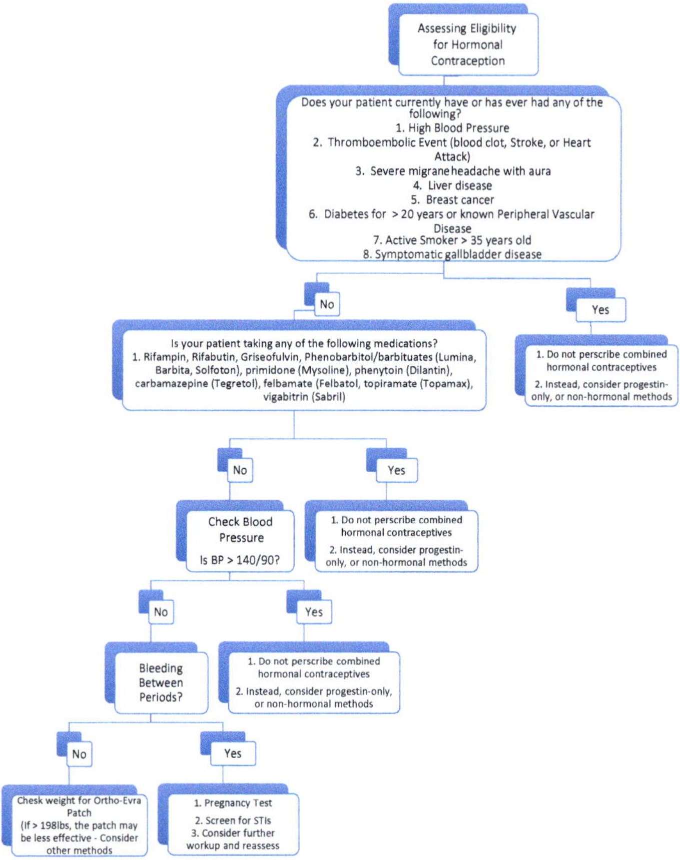

FIG. 3.2 Algorithm: assessing eligibility for hormonal contraception

Types of Oral Contraceptives

(a) Combined pill

Contain both the hormones estrogen and progesterone and are taken daily to prevent the ovary from releasing the egg. It also caused the changes in the lining of the uterus and the cervical mucus to keep the sperm from joining the egg.

(b) Progestin-only pill
Only contain the hormone progesterone. It is taken daily to thicken cervical mucus and thus preventing the sperm from joining the egg. Less often, it stops the ovaries from releasing the egg. It must be taken at the same time each day, and if taken more than 3 h late, a backup method must be used to prevent pregnancy.

The Patch (Ortho Evra or Xulane)

A skin patch that is worn on the lower abdomen, buttocks, outer arm, or upper body and releases the hormones progestin and estrogen into the bloodstream. It works in similar fashion to oral contraceptives by stopping the ovaries from releasing eggs and thickening the cervical mucus. A patch is placed once a week for 3 weeks with the fourth week being the hormone-free period when menses occur.

Vaginal Ring (NuvaRing)

A thin flexible ring that releases the hormones progestin and estrogen. It works by preventing the ovaries from releasing the egg and by thickening the cervical mucus and thus keeping the sperm from joining the egg.

Injectables (Depo-Provera)

A birth control method that involves intramuscular injection of the hormone progestin in the buttock or arm every 3 months. It works by preventing the ovary from releasing an egg and changing the cervical mucus to stop the sperm from joining with the egg. It should not be used for more than 2 years in a row because it can cause a temporary loss of bone density. Bone regrowth occurs after stopping it, but the risk of fracture and osteoporosis increases the longer it is used.

Implantable Devices

1. Implantable Rod (Nexplanon)
   A matchstick-size, flexible rod that is put under the skin of the upper arm. It releases the hormone progestin and works by inhibition of ovulation, thickening of cervical mucous, and alteration of endometrial thickness. It remains effective for up to 3 years.
2. Intrauterine Devices (IUDs)
   Worldwide, IUDs are the most common reversible contraceptive method utilized with estimated use by 90 million women. Intrauterine contraception became popular in the United States in the 1960s and 1970s and, at its height of popularity, was used by 11% of women. Its use has significantly decreased soon after reports of septic abortion and pelvic infections led to class action lawsuit against IUD manufacturers. By 1988, all but one IUD type had been removed from the US market. The National Survey of Family Growth, in 1995, reported that less than 1% of women who use contraception use an IUD.
   Currently, five types of IUDs are FDA approved and available for use in the US market, the copper IUD and four hormonal IUDs. All are small "T"-shaped devices that are placed in the uterus to prevent pregnancy. Multiple mechanisms of action for these intrauterine devices have been proposed and include inhibition of sperm migration and viability, change in transport speed of the ovum, and damage to or destruction of the ovum. In addition, the levonorgestrel-releasing IUDs prevent pregnancy by suppressing the endometrium and changing the amount and viscosity of the cervical mucus. All of these effects occur before implantation occurs. Return of fertility is rapid after IUD removal.
   The copper T380A IUD (Paragard) is made out of polyethylene wrapped with copper wire around the stem and arms. The Paragard IUD is FDA-approved for ten consecutive years, with a 10-year cumulative pregnancy rate comparable to that of sterilization. It can also be utilized for

postcoital contraception with failure rate of less than 1% with placement within 5 days after unprotected intercourse.

LNg-releasing IUD (Mirena) is made out of polydimethylsiloxane sleeve and contains 52 mg of levonorgestrel on its stem of which approximately 20 ug is released daily. It has been approved for continuous use for up to five consecutive years.

LNg-releasing IUD (Skyla) consists of a polyethylene frame with a steroid reservoir containing 13.5 mg levonorgestrel which releases 14 mcg/day and prevents pregnancy for up to three years.

LNg-releasing IUD (Liletta) contains 52 mg LNg at initial placement and with an initial LNg release rate of 18.6 mcg/day, and the FDA approved its use for four years.

LNg-releasing IUD (Kyleena) contains 19.5 mg LNg. Release rate of levonorgestrel is 17.5 mcg/day after 24 days and declines to 7.4 mcg/day after 5 years. Kyleena is FDA approved for five years

For device comparison, please refer to Table 3.2.

Candidate selection:

1. Women who desire the most effective contraception
2. Women who are not considering pregnancy in the next 1–2 years but desire a reversible method
3. Desire or need to avoid estrogen (LNg IUDs) or hormone-free contraception (copper IUD)
4. Women at low risk for STDs to minimize risk of PID

Permanent Birth Control Methods

Female sterilization can be performed by several different techniques but mostly involve interruption of the fallopian tubes to prevent sperm from coming into contact with an oocyte. These techniques are intended to be permanent with a documented failure rate of < 1%. It is the second-most common form of contraception in the United States and the most common form of contraception worldwide.

TABLE 3.2 Long-acting reversible contraceptives (LARC)

Contraceptive method	Duration of action	Administration	Mechanism of action	Efficacy	Side effects
Depot medroxy-progesterone acetate (Depo-Provera)	12–14 weeks	150 mg IM or 104 mg SQ every 3 months	Inhibits the secretion of gonadotropins, preventing ovarian follicle maturation and ovulation and causing endometrial thinning. It thickens cervical mucus and slows tubal mobility	99.7%	1. Decreased BMD 2. Change in menstrual bleeding pattern 3. Weight gain
Etonogestrel implant (Nexplanon)	3 years	68 mg implant placed in SQ tissue of the arm	Suppresses ovulation by inhibition of LH surges Thickens the cervical mucus Thins the endometrium	99%	1. Changes in bleeding patterns 2. Weight gain

Levonorgestrel intrauterine system (Kyleena)	5 years	19.5 mg IUD placed in uterine cavity	Inhibition of sperm migration and viability Change in transport speed of the ovum Damage to or destruction of the ovum Suppressing the endometrium Changing the amount and viscosity of the cervical mucus	99%	1. Changes in bleeding patterns 2. Weight gain 3. Pelvic pain (dysmenorrhea or dyspareunia)
Levonorgestrel intrauterine system (Skyla)	3 years	13.5 mg IUD placed in uterine cavity	Inhibition of sperm migration and viability Change in transport speed of the ovum Damage to or destruction of the ovum Suppressing the endometrium Changing the amount and viscosity of the cervical mucus	99%	1. Changes in bleeding patterns 2. Weight gain 3. Pelvic pain (dysmenorrhea or dyspareunia)

(continued)

Table 3.2 (continued)

Contraceptive method	Duration of action	Administration	Mechanism of action	Efficacy	Side effects
Levonorgestrel intrauterine system (Liletta)	4 years	52 mg IUD placed in uterine cavity	Inhibition of sperm migration and viability Change in transport speed of the ovum Damage to or destruction of the ovum Suppressing the endometrium Changing the amount and viscosity of the cervical mucus	99%	1. Changes in bleeding patterns 2. Weight gain 3. Pelvic pain (dysmenorrhea or dyspareunia)
Copper intrauterine device (Paragard)	10 years	Hormone-free IUD placed in uterine cavity	Inhibition of sperm migration and viability Change in transport speed of the ovum Damage to or destruction of the ovum	99%	1. Changes in bleeding patterns 2. Pelvic pain (dysmenorrhea or dyspareunia)

Federal funding in the United States prohibits sterilization in women under the age of 21 and requires a consent to be reviewed, signed, and dated between 30 and 180 days prior to the procedure. Waivers do exist in some states and these restrictions generally do not apply to patients with private insurance.

Male sterilization: Vasectomy has been shown to be the safest and most cost-effective method of permanent sterilization. It has similar efficacy rates to female sterilization and is significantly underutilized. While 25% of women rely on female sterilization, only about 8% rely on male sterilization.

Female sterilization: Procedures vary by timing, surgical route, and tubal occlusion method.

Postpartum sterilization: Typically performed at the time of cesarean delivery or within 24–48 h after vaginal delivery. If it is performed after a vaginal delivery, an infraumbilical minilaparotomy is usually performed as the uterine fundus is near the umbilicus. The method usually involves excision of a segment of the fallopian tube.

Interval sterilization: Typically performed outside the postpartum period and may be accomplished via hysteroscopic or laparoscopic routes.

Laparoscopy is currently the most common surgical approach and typically involves placement of clips or rings on the tubes or electrosurgery. Hysteroscopy involves placement of a device into the fallopian tube lumen that stimulates tissue growth until tubal occlusion is confirmed.

Postabortion sterilization: Typically performed via laparoscopy immediately following uterine evacuation. Hysteroscopy cannot be performed until 6 weeks following an induced or spontaneous abortion.

Patients need to weigh the risks versus benefits when considering type of tubal ligation as well as timing. Laparoscopy is associated with an increased risk of perioperative complications but hysteroscopy requires the confirmatory study in 3 months postoperatively and also runs the risk of need for reoperation.

Safety concerns do exist for hysteroscopic sterilization in the long term especially with pelvic pain and menstrual abnormalities. Any patient requesting sterilization with a nickel allergy or chronic pelvic pain, should proceed with laparoscopic sterilization if possible. Evidence is also increasing that some ovarian cancers are actually primary fallopian tube malignancies. Complete salpingectomy is becoming more common in an attempt to reduce the risk of ovarian, tubal, and peritoneal cancers [5].

Emergency Contraception

Emergency contraception, also known as postcoital contraception, is widely used to prevent unintended pregnancy after an unprotected or inadequately protected act of sexual intercourse. It is sometimes confused with medical abortion which is the term used to terminate an existing pregnancy. Emergency contraception can only prevent a pregnancy and is completely ineffective after implantation.

The most commonly used regimen is the progestin-only pill (Plan B) that can be purchased over the counter and is available without any age restriction. The pill contains 1.5 mg of levonorgestrel and can be used for up to 72 h after unprotected intercourse. This has largely replaced the two-dose regimen of 0.75 mg and is equally as effective.

A second emergency contraceptive contains 30 mg of ulipristal acetate and requires a prescription. It can be used up to 120 h after unprotected intercourse.

The copper IUD may also be used as emergency contraception and is effective if it is placed within 5 days of sexual intercourse but is not currently FDA approved for this indication.

Mechanism of Action

The mechanism of action varies depending on the days of the menstrual cycle the method is used. Both levonorgestrel and ulipristal inhibit or delay ovulation. It is unlikely that they prevent implantation of a fertilized egg. The copper IUD has been shown to affect sperm viability and function and therefore prevents fertilization.

Adverse Effects

Significant adverse effects are rare and consist mostly of nausea, headache, and irregular bleeding. No deaths or serious complications have occurred.

Barriers to Use

Providing access to emergency contraception has never been shown to encourage sexual behavior or increase the risk of unintended pregnancy. Access to this method still remains a challenge in some areas despite it being approved for over-the-counter use. Another significant barrier is education for both providers and patients. Many women are unaware that this option exists and is easily available to them. Surveys of practitioners have repeatedly demonstrated a failure to educate patients about their options with less than half of eligible women receiving emergency contraception when appropriate [6].

Special Populations

Adolescents

In the United States, 80% of pregnancies in patients age 15–19 years are unintended. It has been shown that only about one-third of sexually active students use an effective method of contraception. Sexually active teens are more likely to seek contraception if they see pregnancy as a negative outcome, have long-term goals regarding their careers or education, have a higher maturity level, have friends or family who advocate contraceptive use, or have had a pregnancy or pregnancy scare in the past.

Barriers to contraceptive use include cost, concerns about confidentiality, and lack of education regarding pregnancy and contraceptive options.

All contraceptive options should be discussed with these patients, especially with regard to what they prefer and are able to use correctly. Barrier methods should also be discussed to prevent transmission of sexually transmitted diseases [7].

Obesity

No contraceptive method is restricted in use for obese patients. However, there is concern about decreased effectiveness of the contraceptive pill, patch, and ring, and this possibility should be addressed with patients during counseling. IUDs and etonogestrel implants should be considered first in these patients due to their high efficacy [8].

Medical Issues

1. The CDC published *The United States Medical Eligibility Criteria for Contraceptive Use* in 2016 which provides contraceptive recommendations for patients with various medical conditions. When possible, LARCs are the preferred contraceptive for medically complex women due to their efficacy and ability to avoid surgery [9]. Similar recommendations were made by the World Health Organization in 2015 [10].
2. The Society for Family Planning (SFP) published guidelines for contraception in women with cancer in 2012.
   - In general, women with active cancer, treated cancer within the last 6 months, or with a history of chest wall radiation should avoid all estrogen-progestin contraceptives due to increased risk of venous thromboembolism and breast cancer.
   - Women with a history of breast cancer should use the copper IUD unless they are taking tamoxifen. These patients should consider use of a levonorgestrel-releasing

IUD to reduce the risk of endometrial changes without increasing the risk of recurrence [11].
3. Women with anemia should consider using a levonorgestrel-releasing IUD to minimize blood loss with menses.
4. Women with osteopenia or osteoporosis should avoid injectable progestin-only contraception and should be considered for estrogen-containing contraception unless contraindicated due to its positive effect on bone density.
5. Immunosuppression – IUDs are not contraindicated in these patients.
6. Risk for breast cancer or recurrence – Emergency contraception is not contraindicated in these patients.

References

1. Finer LB, Zolna MR. Unintended pregnancy in the United States: incidence and disparities, 2006. Contraception. 2011;84(5):478–85.
2. Counseling Adolescents About Contraception. ACOG Committee Opinion No. 710. The American College of Obstetrics and Gynecologists. Obstet Gynecol. 2017;130:e74.
3. Long-acting reversible contraception: implants and intrauterine devices. Practice Bulletin No. 186. American Collage of Obstetricians and Gynecologists. Obstet Gynecol. 2017;130:e251.
4. Speroff L, et al. Clinical Gynecologic Endocrinology and Infertility. 7th ed; 2005. Chapters 22, 23, 24, 25 and 26.
5. Braaten KP, Dutton C. Overview of female sterilization. UpToDate; 2016.
6. Emergency Contraception. ACOG Practice Bulletin. Number 152; 2015.
7. Chacko M. Contraception: overview of issues specific to adolescents. UpToDate; 2016.
8. Edelman A, Kaneshiro B. Contraception counseling for obese women. UpToDate; 2016.
9. Centers for Disease Control. U.S. Medical Eligibility Criteria for Contraceptive Use 2016.
10. World Health Organization. Medical Eligibility Criteria for Contraceptive Use. 5th Edition, 2015. Geneva, Switzerland.
11. Patel A, Schwarz EB, Society of Family Planning. Cancer and contraception. Release date May 2012. SFP Guideline #20121. Contraception. 2012;86:191.

Chapter 4
Abnormal Uterine Bleeding

Teresa Tam

There are many different causes of abnormal uterine bleeding (AUB), and it accounts for majority of gynecological consults with most office visits among peri- and postmenopausal women. Although there is variation within cycles, a normal menstrual cycle typically lasts between 21 and 35 days, lasting an average of 5 days [1]. Traditionally, abnormal uterine bleeding has been described as menorrhagia, metrorrhagia, and menometrorrhagia. These terms are inaccurate because abnormal bleeding patterns are very dependent on a patient's perception of her bleeding.

The widespread confusion on terminologies used to describe uterine bleeding abnormalities led to a formation of an international panel of obstetricians and gynecologists, clinicians, and scientists. The participants consulted and provided recommendations on terminologies and definitions of AUB [2]. In 2011, the International Federation of Gynecology and Obstetrics (FIGO) formulated a new classification system to provide a universally accepted nomenclature to describe AUB. This system is called "PALM-COEIN" and was endorsed by the American College of Obstetricians and Gynecologists (ACOG).

T. Tam (✉)
Presence Saint Francis Hospital, Department of Obstetrics and Gynecology, Evanston, IL, USA
e-mail: drtam@allforwomenhealthcare.com

J. V. Knaus et al. (eds.), *Ambulatory Gynecology*,
https://doi.org/10.1007/978-1-4939-7641-6_4

Table 4.1 PALM-COEIN classification system for abnormal uterine bleeding in reproductive-aged women

PALM: structural causes
Polyp (AUB-P)
Adenomyosis (AUB-A)
Leiomyoma (AUB-L)
Submucosal myoma (AUB-L_{SM})
Other myoma (AUB-L_O)
Malignancy and hyperplasia (AUB-M)
COEIN: nonstructural causes
Coagulopathy (AUB-C)
Ovulatory dysfunction (AUB-O)
Endometrial (AUB-E)
Iatrogenic (AUB-I)
Not yet classified (AUB-N)

Data from Munro et al. [3]

Causes of abnormal uterine bleeding were categorized to be either due to structural or systemic causes. The acronym "PALM" signifies structural causes. Structural causes include P for polyps, A for adenomyosis, L for leiomyoma, and M for malignancy and hyperplasia. "COEIN" indicates nonstructural or systemic causes. "COEIN" include C for coagulopathy, O for ovulatory disorders, E for endometrial causes, I for iatrogenic, and N for not yet classified [3] (Table 4.1).

Discontinuation of the phrase "dysfunctional uterine bleeding" is further recommended. The PALM-COEIN system indicates the etiology of AUB with a letter qualifier to signify the cause of bleeding, for example, abnormal uterine bleeding (AUB) due to polyps (P) could be qualified as AUB-P, while AUB-O means abnormal uterine bleeding due to ovulatory dysfunction.

In addition to providing the etiology of AUB, the PALM-COEIN classification also provides description of the bleeding pattern. The new system classifies the bleeding abnormality as either heavy menstrual bleeding instead of the term menorrhagia or intermenstrual bleeding versus the term metrorrhagia. The FIGO classification leads to an enhanced and standardized methodology for effective diagnosis and appropriate management of AUB.

Pathophysiology

Normal menstrual cycles could last between 21 days and 35 days with a normal duration of 5 days and the first 3 days associated with most blood loss [4]. A normal ovulatory cycle depends on an intact hypothalamus producing gonadotropin-releasing hormone, which then stimulates the anterior pituitary gland to produce follicle-stimulating hormone (FSH) and luteinizing hormone (LH). Estrogen and progesterone production by the ovary depends on the feedback regulation of the gonadotropic hormones. Proliferation of the uterine endometrium and shedding is in response to ovarian production of estrogen and progesterone.

Ovulatory dysfunction typically occurs in adolescents and perimenopausal women causing AUB-O. Physiologic anovulation during puberty due to the immature hypothalamic-pituitary-ovarian axis causes AUB. In the perimenopausal women, anovulation occurs because of abnormal follicular development resulting from reduction of ovarian reserve.

Evaluation for Diagnosis

A thorough history and physical examination is essential to evaluate and treat a patient with AUB. Another important question is to determine whether the bleeding episode is acute or chronic. Anovulation or immaturity/dysfunction of the hypothalamic-pituitary-ovarian axis is the most common cause of AUB in adolescents. Other causes include infection, pregnancy, hormonal contraception, and coagulopathies. It is important to rule out pregnancy in patients who have child-bearing capabilities. For patients with risk factors such as obesity and comorbidities associated with endometrial hyperplasia and malignancy, an endometrial biopsy is warranted. Medical conditions such as thyroid disease and prolactinoma require testing in patients with associated medical conditions or symptoms. Laboratory testing needs to be adapted according to the possible cause of AUB in conjunction with a

TABLE 4.2 Laboratory testing for the evaluation of patients with acute abnormal uterine bleeding

Laboratory evaluation	Specific laboratory tests
Initial laboratory testing	Complete blood count
	Blood type and cross match
	Pregnancy test
Initial laboratory evaluation for disorders of hemostasis	Partial thromboplastin time
	Prothrombin time
	Activated partial thromboplastin time
	Fibrinogen
Initial testing for von Willebrand disease[a]	von Willebrand factor antigen[b]
	von Willebrand factor ristocetin cofactor assay[b]
	Factor VIII[b]
Other laboratory tests to consider	Thyroid-stimulating hormone
	Serum iron, total iron binding capacity, and ferritin
	Liver function tests
	Chlamydia trachomatis

Data from James et al. [5], National Heart, Lung, and Blood Institute [6], *and* American College of Obstetricians and Gynecologists [1]

[a]Adult women who receive positive results for risk of bleeding disorders or who have abnormal initial laboratory test results for disorders of hemostasis should undergo testing for von Willebrand disease. Adolescents with heavy menses since menarche who present with acute abnormal uterine bleeding also should undergo testing for von Willebrand disease

[b]Consultation with a hematologist can aid in interpreting these test results. If any of these markers are abnormally low, a hematologist should be consulted

patient's age, acuity of symptoms, and findings on examination (Table 4.2).

Imaging studies such as transvaginal with or without transabdominal ultrasound (US) could diagnose uterine abnormalities such as leiomyomas and neoplasms. Vaginal and cervical pathologies causing postcoital bleeding may be diagnosed during a transvaginal ultrasound, but visualization is better during a speculum examination. Saline infusion sonohysterography (SIS) will provide evaluation of endometrial polyps, submucosal myoma, and other intrauterine pathologies. Hysteroscopy provides better accuracy because of complete visualization and the ability to perform directed biopsies [7] as in a "see and treat" approach.

Evaluation in Adolescents

AUB in adolescents is commonly caused by immaturity of the hypothalamic-pituitary-ovarian axis. Although normal adolescent physiology often explains anovulatory bleeding, other causes such as pregnancy, infection, and trauma have to be all ruled out. Inherited bleeding disorders such as von Willebrand disease need to be ascertained especially since as many as 50% of adolescents with heavy menstrual bleeding will be diagnosed with a coagulopathy [8].

Screening for coagulation disorders is important in this patient population if heavy menses occurs at menarche. Anovulatory bleeding is common in young adults. Family history of a bleeding disorder, heavy menses, nosebleeds, easy bruisability, and prolonged bleeding following small wounds, surgical, or dental procedures should all raise suspicion for von Willebrand disease [9].

Initial laboratory testing for women with a bleeding disorder includes complete blood count with platelets, activated partial thromboplastin time, and prothrombin time. Patients that have positive findings for possible inherited bleeding conditions should be further investigated for von Willebrand disorder. Specific testing for von Willebrand disease is best done in conjunction with a hematology consultation.

Evaluation in Women 19–39 Years

Pregnancy, leiomyomas, endometrial polyps, anovulation, and endometrial hyperplasia are all possible causes of AUB in young women. Management of AUB is tailored to the disorder causing abnormal bleeding. Initial laboratory testing is similar to AUB testing in adolescents and includes a pregnancy test and evaluation of coagulation profile if indicated. Although endometrial biopsy is reserved for women >45 years of age with AUB, endometrial biopsy is recommended even in younger women with risk factors for unopposed estrogen exposure such as obesity and polycystic ovarian syndrome.

Transvaginal and transabdominal US are common imaging modalities used to diagnose leiomyomas or endometrial polyps. Uterine pathologies could also be visualized with SIS or hysteroscopy with directed biopsies if warranted, depending on patient's risk factors.

Evaluation in Women >40 Years

Similar to the common reason for AUB seen in adolescents, anovulatory bleeding is also common in older women. AUB is evaluated with endometrial sampling in women >45 years old. Benign causes such as leiomyomas or endometrial atrophy are common causes. Endometrial hyperplasia or carcinoma is to be suspected in this population if postmenopausal bleeding is encountered.

Evaluation of intrauterine pathology could also be performed with imaging techniques with the primary imaging test being transvaginal ultrasonography. In cases where there is clinical suspicion for hyperplasia or carcinoma, endometrial biopsy is recommended.

Medical Management

Although conservative management with medical therapy is considered the first-line treatment for AUB, acuity of symptoms dictates treatment choice. Hormonal therapy either with combination hormonal contraceptive or progesterone-only medications is the preferred initial treatment option for treatment of chronic heavy bleeding. Estrogen maintains endometrial growth and stability, while the progestin component prevents ovulation and provides an atrophic endometrium.

For patients who are unable to tolerate or have contraindications to estrogen, progestogen-only formulations are recommended. Progesterone stabilizes the endometrium by inhibiting endometrial thickening. Oral medroxyprogesterone acetate (MPA), depot medroxyprogesterone acetate (DMPA), and levonorgestrel-releasing intrauterine system (LNG-IUS) have all been used for treatment of AUB/HMB.

Gonadotropin-releasing hormone (GnRH) agonists have also been used for treatment of heavy menstrual bleeding caused by leiomyomas. GnRH agonists create a hypogonadotropic state leading to endometrial atrophy. The medication decreases uterine volume for preoperative treatment of leiomyomas and increases the patient's blood count in preparation for surgery. Menopausal side effects such as hot flashes, bone loss, and vaginal atrophy limit their long-term use. Intramuscular leuprolide acetate injection is FDA approved and comes in two different doses: 3.75 mg monthly dose and 11.25 mg every 3 months. The second FDA-approved GnRH agonist is subcutaneous goserelin acetate. This medication produces amenorrhea and endometrial atrophy within 3–4 weeks of the drug's administration. Add-back therapy with norethindrone acetate (NETA) 5 mg minimizes GnRH agonists' adverse effects. Patients on anticoagulant therapy are good candidates for leuprolide acetate treatment to control heavy uterine bleeding [10].

The US Food and Drug Administration has approved intravenous (IV) conjugated equine estrogen for the treatment of acute heavy bleeding. Women who have acute excessive bleeding would require high-dose intravenous (IV) estrogen therapy of 25 mg IV every 4–6 h for 24 h.

Nonsteroidal anti-inflammatory drugs (NSAIDs) are well studied but underutilized nonhormonal therapies for AUB. Treatment with NSAID increases platelet aggregation resulting in vasoconstriction and decrease of menstrual bleeding. Both naproxen and mefenamic acid are NSAIDs that could be used in combination with medical therapy for the treatment of AUB/ HMB and associated dysmenorrhea.

Oral tranexamic acid is another medication to treat ovulatory cause of AUB. It is an antifibrinolytic medication that competitively blocks plasminogen-binding sites and inhibits fibrin degradation and clot breakdown. The most common dosage is 1300 mg orally three times a day during menses with 5 days of maximum use.

Medical Management in Adolescents

Hormonal contraceptive is a viable first-line treatment for AUB possibly skipping the placebo weeks. This allows recovery of heavy bleeding and facilitates rebuilding the patient's blood count. Iron therapy is also recommended if anemia is encountered. After resolution of anemia, cyclic or continuous hormonal contraceptives could be prescribed for menstrual regulation with added benefit of contraceptive effects.

Medical Management in Women 19–39 Years

Combined hormonal contraceptive and progestin-only therapy are common medical treatments for women who are hemodynamically stable. The Mirena levonorgestrel intrauterine device (LNG-IUD) and DMPA 150 mg injection are commonly used progesterone-only hormonal therapies for treatment of AUB/HMB.

Medical Management in Women >40 Years

Medical options mentioned earlier such as hormonal contraceptives, DMPA, LNG-IUD, GnRH agonists, and tranexamic acid are all available therapies for AUB.

Surgical Management

The surgical option is based on the patient's severity of bleeding and clinical stability. If the patient has contraindications to medical therapy, fails medications, or requests definitive

Table 4.3 Medical treatment regimens

Medical treatment regimens[a]				
Drug	**Source**	**Suggested dose**	**Dose schedule**	**Potential contraindications and precautions according to FDA labeling[b]**
Conjugated equine estrogen	DeVore et al. [11]	25 mg IV	Every 4–6 h for 24 h	Contraindications include, but are not limited to, breast cancer, active or past venous thrombosis or arterial thromboembolic disease and liver dysfunction or disease. The agent should be used with caution in patients with cardiovascular or thromboembolic risk factors
Combined oral contraceptives[c]	Munro et al. [12]	Monophasic combined oral contraceptive that contains 35 μg of ethinyl estradiol	Three times per day for 7 days	Contraindications include, but are not limited to, cigarette smoking (in women aged 35 years or older), hypertension, history of deep vein thrombosis or pulmonary embolism, known thromboembolic disorders, cerebrovascular disease, ischemic heart disease, migraine with aura, current or past breast cancer, severe liver disease, diabetes with vascular involvement, valvular heart disease with complications, and major surgery with prolonged immobilization

(continued)

TABLE 4.3 (continued)

Medical treatment regimens[a]

Drug	Source	Suggested dose	Dose schedule	Potential contraindications and precautions according to FDA labeling[b]
Medroxyprogesterone acetate[d]	Munro et al. [12]	20 mg orally	Three times per day for 7 days	Contraindications include, but are not limited to, active or past deep vein thrombosis or pulmonary embolism, active or recent arterial thromboembolic disease, current or past breast cancer, and impaired liver function or liver disease
Tranexamic acid	James et al. [5]	1.3 g orally[e] or 10 mg/kg IV (maximum 600 mg/dose)	Three times per day for 5 days (every 8 h)	Contraindications include, but are not limited to, acquired impaired color vision and current thrombotic or thromboembolic disease. The agent should be used with caution in patients with a history of thrombosis (because of uncertain thrombotic risks), and concomitant administration of combined oral contraceptives needs to be carefully considered

FDA indicates US Food and Drug Administration, *IV* intravenously

[a]American College of Obstetricians and Gynecologists [13]

[b]The US Food and Drug Administration's labeling contains exhaustive lists of contraindications for each of these therapies. In treating women with acute abnormal uterine bleeding, physicians often must weigh the relative risks of treatment against the risk of continued bleeding in the context of the patient's medical history and risk factors. These decisions must be made on a case-by-case basis by the treating clinician

[c]Other combined oral contraceptive formulations, dosages, and schedules also may be effective

[d]Other progestins (such as norethindrone acetate), dosages, and schedules also may be effective.

[e]Other dosages and schedules also may be effective

treatment, there are several surgical alternatives. Dilation and curettage, endometrial ablation, and operative hysteroscopy with removal of submucosal leiomyomas are minimally invasive surgical options for the management of heavy uterine bleeding. For patients who have completed childbearing, endometrial ablation is a minimally invasive surgical option for AUB but requires a benign endometrial sampling prior to endometrial ablation. The other operative routes for pathology removal include vaginal surgery, laparoscopy or laparotomy. For patients who are no longer interested in fertility, a hysterectomy versus a myomectomy could be offered.

Conclusion

AUB is a usual complaint in women and commonly encountered in office gynecology. The PALM-COEIN classification assists medical providers in the diagnosis and management of AUB. The FIGO terminology provides guidance for clinicians on the etiology of AUB to enable prompt and accurate diagnosis for proper treatment management. Choosing the appropriate treatment plan ensures effective and timely treatment, facilitating a woman's return to normal activity and improving her quality of life.

References

1. American College of Obstetricians and Gynecologists. Diagnosis of abnormal uterine bleeding in reproductive-aged women. Practice bulletin no. 128. Obstet Gynecol. 2012;120:197–206.
2. Fraser IS, Critchley HO, Munro MG, Broder M. A process designed to lead to international agreement on terminologies and definitions used to describe abnormalities of menstrual bleeding. Writing Group for this Menstrual Agreement Process [published erratum appears in Fertil Steril 2007;88:538]. Fertil Steril. 2007;87:466–76.
3. Data fromMunro MG, Critchley HOD, Broder MS, Fraser IS. FIGO classification system (PALM-COEIN) for causes of

abnormal uterine bleeding in nongravid women of reproductive age. Int J Gyn Obstet. 2011;113:3–13.
4. American College of Obstetricians and Gynecologists. Menstruation in girls and adolescents: using the menstrual cycle as a vital sign. ACOG Committee opinion no. 349. Obstet Gynecol. 2006;108:1323–8.
5. James AH, Kouides PA, Abdul-Kadir R, Dietrich JE, Edlund M, Federici AB, et al. Evaluation and management of acute menorrhagia in women with and without underlying bleeding disorders: consensus from an international expert panel. Eur J Obstet Gynecol Reprod Biol. 2011;158:124–34.
6. National Heart, Lung, and Blood Institute. The diagnosis, evaluation, and management of von Willebrand disease, NIH Publication No. 08-5832. Bethesda: NHLBI; 2007. Available at http://www.nhlbi.nih.gov/guidelines/vwd/vwd.pdf. Retrieved 5 Dec 2012.
7. Clark TJ, Voit D, Gupta JK, Hyde C, Song F, Khan KS. Accuracy of hysteroscopy in the diagnosis of endometrial cancer and hyperplasia: a systematic quantitative review. JAMA. 2002;288:1610–21. (Meta-analysis).
8. Black A, Francoeur D, Rowe T, et al. Society of Obstetrics and Gynaecology of Canada. Canadian contraception consensus. J Obstet Gynaecol Can. 2004;26:347–87, 389–436.
9. National heart, Lung, and Blood Institute. The diagnosis, evaluation, and management of von Willebrand disease. NIH Pub. No. 08-5832; 2007. Available at: http://www.nhlbi.nih.gov/files/docs/guidelines/vwd.pdf. Retrieved 15 Feb 2016.
10. Bradley LD, Gueye N-A. The medical management of abnormal uterine bleeding in reproductive-aged women. Am J Obstet Gynecol. 2016;214:31–44.
11. DeVore GR, Owens O, Kase N. Use of intravenous Premarin in the treatment of dysfunctional uterine bleeding—a double-blind randomized control study. Obstet Gynecol. 1982;59:285–91.
12. Munro MG, Mainor N, Basu R, Brisinger M, Barreda L. Oral medroxyprogesterone acetate and combination oral contraceptives for acute uterine bleeding: a randomized controlled trial. Obstet Gynecol. 2006;108:924–9.
13. American College of Obstetricians and Gynecologists. ACOG committee opinion no. 557: Management of acute abnormal uterine bleeding in nonpregnant reproductive-aged women. Obstet Gynecol. 2013;121:891–6.

Chapter 5 Amenorrhea in the Adolescent

John S. Rinehart

Introduction

Amenorrhea in the adolescent presents a complicated diagnostic problem for a gynecologist since the etiologies are numerous, the frequency is low, and the treatments are varied. Organizing the approach into a simplified, easily remembered sequence can allow a gynecologist to adequately initiate the diagnostic pathway that leads to successful definition of the etiology and the correct treatment for amenorrhea. This brief chapter is designed to provide the gynecologist with a simple approach that will allow the physician to appropriately approach the adolescent patient with amenorrhea.

J. S. Rinehart (✉)
Division of Reproductive Endocrinology and Infertility, Department of Obstetrics and Gynecology, NorthShore University HealthSystem, Evanston, IL, USA

Pritzker School of Medicine, University of Chicago, Department of Obstetrics and Gynecology, Section of Reproductive Endocrinology and Infertility, Chicago, IL, USA
e-mail: jsrinehart@aol.com

J. V. Knaus et al. (eds.), *Ambulatory Gynecology*,
https://doi.org/10.1007/978-1-4939-7641-6_5

Definition

While many definitions for amenorrhea exist, the following from Speroff and Fritz (2005) is widely accepted:

1. No period by age 14 in the absence of growth or development of secondary sexual characteristics
2. No period by age 16 regardless of the presence of normal growth and development with the appearance of secondary sexual characteristics
3. In a woman who has been menstruating, the absence of periods for a length of time equivalent to a total of at least three of the previous intervals or 6 months of amenorrhea [1]

The etiologies of amenorrhea can be organized into problems with one or more of three areas:

1. Head	H
2. Ovaries	O
3. Outflow tract	OT

So give an HOOT to help remember how to begin the investigation of the adolescent with amenorrhea.

Outflow Tract

Problems with the outflow tract can broadly be divided in three categories:

1. Mullerian origin
   (a) Imperforate hymen
   (b) Transverse vaginal septum
   (c) Mullerian agenesis
2. Androgen insensitivity syndrome
3. Intrauterine adhesions (Asherman's syndrome)

Intrauterine Adhesions

Patients who present with secondary amenorrhea may have amenorrhea secondary to extensive or obstructive intrauterine adhesions. The patient will most frequently have a history which will suggest this diagnosis. The scarring is a result of injury to the basalis of the endometrium. Injury can result from surgery such as an abortion or dilation and curettage (D&C), from retained products of conception, or from an infection following some injury to the endometrium. Patients can have amenorrhea either from extensive adhesions throughout the uterus or from obstructive adhesion near the internal os of the cervix. Suspicion of the problem is the key element in defining the etiology.

Diagnostic procedures involve hysterosalpingography/saline infusion sonography or serial ultrasounds. Serial ultrasounds for a 1-month period help define that the patient is having menstrual cycles. During mense, the uterine cavity will be filled with blood and the cause becomes obvious. Treatment involves either dilation of the cervix with lysis of the obstructive lesions or surgical resection of the intrauterine adhesions. Ultrasound in the operating room can be helpful to guide the dilators so as to minimize the risk of perforation. Nonobstructive adhesions severe enough to cause complete absence of menses are rare and frequently not amenable to surgical correction. Milder presence of adhesions usually does not cause amenorrhea. The surgical resection of intrauterine adhesions has many different unresolved issues, namely: choice of cutting modality, the use of postoperative stents such as a Foley catheter, estrogen and/ or antibiotic use, and proper timing of the menstrual cycle to perform the procedure. None of these issues has been resolved with level I evidence [2].

Mullerian Anomalies

Mullerian anomalies occur because of abnormal formation or fusion and resorption of the Mullerian precursors. There can be complete absence of the upper portion of the vagina, the uterus, and the fallopian tube with Mullerian agenesis, or there can be partial to complete obstruction due to abnormal fusion and resorption of the Mullerian precursors resulting in conditions such as an imperforate hymen or a transverse vaginal septum. Other anomalies do not present as amenorrhea but may present in menstruating women as cyclic pain or vaginal/abdominal masses.

Patients with an imperforate hymen or a transverse vaginal septum will present with primary amenorrhea. Diagnosis can usually be inferred from a physical exam, but imaging such as ultrasound or MRI will confirm the presence and extent of the abnormality. Treatment is surgical, and the preoperative use of MRI or ultrasound will assist the surgeon in anticipating the correct approach based upon the patient's particular anomaly.

Mullerian agenesis (Mayer-Rokitansky-Kuster-Hauser {MRKH} syndrome) describes patient pathology that is characterized by absence of the uterus and upper 2/3 of the vagina. Other malformations are common including renal, skeletal, and occasionally hearing, cardiac, and digital anomalies. The incidence has been estimated to be 1 in 4500 females with the majority of cases being sporadic, but there have been described familial cases where the inheritance seems to be autosomal dominant [3]. The patients typically present with primary amenorrhea, are normally developed females with a shortened vagina, have normal ovarian function, and have an XX karyotype. Urinary tract malformations are common with MRKH syndrome occurring in as many as 40% of the patients [4]. Diagnosis utilizes MRI and ultrasonography to confirm the extent of the anomaly. The advantage of an MRI is that it can also identify renal and skeletal anomalies during the same examination. Other diagnostic efforts include screening for hearing deficits and cardiac abnormalities.

Treatment of MRKH involves psychological counseling. The treatment for a lack of vagina can be either nonsurgical or surgical with the current recommendations being an initial nonsurgical correction through the use of dilator therapy. Surgical creation of a neo-vagina can be accomplished through the use of skin grafts using the Abbe-McIndoe procedure. Fertility is possible since the patients have normal ovarian function through the use of gestation hosts to carry the fetus derived from embryos created with the patient's own oocytes.

Androgen Insensitivity Syndrome (Testicular Feminization Syndrome)

Androgen insensitivity syndrome (AIS) was described in 1953 by Morris as patients who present as female with normal breast development, scant to absent pubic hair, and normal external genitalia but a small vagina with the absence of a uterus or fallopian tubes [5]. AIS results from a genetic abnormality on the X chromosome inherited in many cases as an X-linked recessive resulting in either complete or partial inactivation of the androgen steroid receptor. Androgens exert their influence on the phenotype through the androgen receptor. The gene for the androgen receptor is located on the X chromosome. The variability in the phenotype has led to the classification of androgen insensitivity into three categories): complete, partial, and mild [6]. The gonads are normally functioning testis so both Mullerian-inhibiting hormone and testosterone are produced. External genitalia require proper testosterone functioning to develop male so an abnormal receptor leads to either no male development or partial development depending upon the severity of the genetic defect. The presence of MIH causes regression of the Mullerian structures resulting in the absence of upper 2/3 of the vagina, the uterus, and the fallopian tubes. Physical examination should alert the physician to the possibility of AIS when there is normal breast development and scant to no pubic hair. AIS is distinguished from MRKH through karyotyping with the AIS patient having an XY karyotype.

Diagnosis depends upon physical exam and laboratory findings which include a XY karyotype and elevated testosterone and LH levels. Gonadectomy is indicated after puberty due to the risk of malignancy. At some point, the patient may request the formation of a vagina. As with MRKH, formation of a vagina can be accomplished either through dilator therapy or surgery [7].

Ovary

Problems with ovarian function include the two extremes in the number of oocytes the ovary possesses. There can be no or too few or there can be too many oocytes. The most common problems presenting as amenorrhea in the adolescent of ovarian origins are:

1. Polycystic ovary syndrome (PCOS)
2. Gonadal dysgenesis
   (a) 50% – 45, X (Turner syndrome)
   (b) 25% – mosaics
   (c) 25% – XX
3. Premature ovarian failure

Adolescent polycystic ovary syndrome (PCOS) is an increasing problem as a result of the increasing frequency of overweight and obesity in the adolescent population. Data from the National Health and Nutrition Examination Survey has shown that the prevalence of overweight among women ages 2–19 years was 16.4% in 2003–2004 compared to 5% in the same group of women in the 1960s and 1970s [8].

The definition of PCOS has been problematic. The problem is magnified in the adolescent because the disease may still be evolving and the full clinical presentation may not yet have occurred. Presently, a commonly used definition of PCOS relies upon the Rotterdam criteria (2003) which have two parts [9]. The first part requires excluding diseases which mimic PCOS such as congenital adrenal hyperplasia. The second defines three criteria, two of which must be present for the diagnosis of PCOS. The three criteria are:

1. Oligo-anovulation
   (a) Fewer than nine menses per year

2. Clinical or biochemical hyperandrogenism
   (a) Acne
   (b) Hirsute
   (c) Elevated serum androgens
3. Ultrasound-documented polycystic ovaries
   (a) Greater than 12 antral follicles 2–9 mm in one or both ovaries in any pattern and/or an increased ovarian volume (>10 ml)

The Rotterdam criteria allow for four phenotypes, but where amenorrhea is the presenting symptom, only one of the other two criteria needs to be present to make the diagnosis. Serum gonadotropin levels and overweight/obesity are not used to make the diagnosis, but their presence adds support to the diagnosis. The definition does require a sophisticated ultrasound examination of the ovaries where attention needs to be directed to measuring all antral follicles and providing an antral follicle count.

Simply noting multiple ovarian cysts does not establish the ultrasound criteria for polycystic ovaries by ultrasound. The incidence of PCOS in adolescents is 11–26% and 50% are obese [10].

PCOS is a complex syndrome involving both a genetic and an environmental component with many possible presentations both physically and hormonally. The core problem for all PCOS patients is increased intraovarian androgens. However, the pathway to this increase is extremely complex and in many cases undefined. PCOS does not have a single easily definable cause. People with PCOS have a genetic makeup that puts them at risk. The genetic background is complex, involving many areas of the genetic code. Some of the problem areas include heredity (so there may be a family history of PCOS, obesity, or adult-onset diabetes) but often the genetic abnormalities arise anew during the genetic formation of the person with PCOS. However, having the genetic background does not mean that a person will automatically have PCOS. There needs to be certain environmental factors that trigger the problem. There is no agreement on what environmental factors exist or how important are known factors. One environmental factor which can trigger PCOS is overweight/obesity and the insulin resistance which often accompanies these conditions. PCOS is associated with certain metabolic disorders which are part of the metabolic syndrome. These include dyslipidemia and glucose intolerance. The prevalence of metabolic syndrome in adolescents has been estimated to be between 12% and 44% [11]. Primary amenorrhea as a presenting symptom in PCOS is uncommon since the usual history is one of secondary amenorrhea [12]. However, both presentations have similarities such as insulin resistance and increased intraovarian androgens. Obesity is present in 35–50% of adolescents with PCOS [13] and in some patients seems to be a risk factor for PCOS with the link being insulin resistance. The increased androgen production increases the incidence of hirsutism and acne. Included in the diagnosis is hormonal testing to eliminate other causes of the clinical picture of PCOS such as 17-0H progesterone for nonclassic adrenal hyperplasia and androgen profiles to eliminate the diagnosis of adrenal or ovarian tumors.

Adolescent patients have similar hormone profiles and physical findings as do adults with PCOS.

Ultrasound is required as part of the defining criteria for the diagnosis of PCOS. Assessment of the metabolic status of the patient requires a 2-h oral glucose tolerance test [14]. Fasting insulin levels are less reliable but may provide a baseline that can be used to follow the progress of the PCOS as the patient ages. Treatment for PCOS addresses the insulin resistance and the lack of menses. Weight loss and lifestyle changes such as exercise and carbohydrate restriction are the mainstays of non-pharmacological treatment. Insulin-sensitizing agents have been used but their continued use in the adolescent age patient is controversial. Menses can be normalized through the use of oral contraceptives which also reduces the risk of endometrial cancer. Hirsute patients will benefit with addition of antiandrogens of which spironolactone is the most frequently used. Hair removal techniques such as electrolysis or laser hair removal are needed to remove the hair which has already been masculinized. The identification and treatment of the adolescent with PCOS offer a chance to impact the lifetime health of these patients. Long-term health consequences of PCOS include obesity, adult-onset diabetes, cardiovascular disease, hypertension, endometrial hyperplasia/cancer, infertility, and depression. Short-term goals include regulation of menses, control of acne and hirsutism, and weight control.

Patients can present with amenorrhea as a result of too few oocytes or no oocytes. Patients with gonadal dysgenesis have no or a few oocytes with the most common and recognizable form being 45, X Turner syndrome. Less common forms with variable presentation include X chromosome mosaic karyotype or XX karyotype. Turner syndrome is the most common form of hypergonadotropic hypogonadism with an estimated incidence of 1 in 2500 female births. Women possess two X chromosomes, one of which is normally silenced during development so that the genetic complement is closer to that of a male. The X chromosome contains approximately 1000 genes, while the male has about 200. However, not all of the X chromosome is silenced, and about 15–25% of the genes, which are clustered near the tip of the short arm, continue to be active [15]. Many of these have homologues on the Y chromosome. Classically a patient with Turner syndrome lacks an entire chromosome, but some will have both X chromosomes, yet the tip of the short arm will be missing, and thus they will express the Turner phenotype.

Short statue is the most common physical finding in Turner syndrome, and this is caused by haploinsufficiency (reduced gene production) for the SHOX (a homeobox gene) [16]. Phenotypically, Turner syndrome results in short stature, gonadal dysgenesis, sexual infantilism, and multiple somatic abnormalities. Diagnosis relies upon karyotyping, but evaluation for skeletal abnormalities and cardiovascular problems is also required. Examination of all extremities for blood pressure disparities is recommended due to the risk of coarctation of the aorta. The prevalence of aortic coarctation and bicuspid aortic valve (BAV) is approximately 10% and 15%, respectively [17]. Using magnetic resonance angiography, Ho et al. [18] identified a number of vascular abnormalities such as an unusual angle of the aortic arch in 50%. The clinical significance of these is uncertain, but it seems that Turner patients treated with donor oocytes to achieve a pregnancy have a higher incidence of maternal death due to dissecting aortic aneurisms which may be as high as 2% [19]. Many patients with Turner syndrome will be diagnosed prior to their adolescent years due to short stature. Treatment with growth hormone under the care of a team experienced in the treatment of Turner patients can maximize the patient's adult height. For patients diagnosed over the age of 10, educational and psychosocial counseling are important. Screening should also include thyroid functions, renal imaging, skeletal imaging, hearing evaluation, and ovarian function testing [20]. Continuing care of these patients is complicated, and many patients will benefit from care provided through a multidisciplinary group specializing in the care of patients with Turner syndrome.

Premature Ovarian Failure

Premature ovarian failure (POF) is defined as the cessation of menses with elevated gonadotropins prior to the age of 40 years old. Most patients with POF remain menopausal for the duration of their lives. However, up to 50% of the patients may actually ovulate, menstruate, or even achieve a viable pregnancy [21]. A more accurate description for these patients would be ovarian insufficiency. It is not possible to accurately predict if a patient has POF or ovarian insufficiency. The incidence has been estimated to be <1% for women less than 40 years old, but an accurate estimate of the incidence for adolescents is not currently available. There are numerous etiologies for POF but for many no etiology can be discerned. Increasingly, genetic associations are becoming more common as potential etiologies for POF. Both X-linked and autosomal abnormalities have been implicated in the etiology of POF. The FMRI gene which is responsible for the fragile X syndrome has been associated with early ovarian failure [22]. Other potential etiologies include autoimmune causes and chemotherapy.

Autoimmune causes may be responsible for up to 30% of the cases of POF [23]. A small subset of patient with POF will have anti-adrenal antibodies. This information is important since some of them may develop adrenal insufficiency. An increasing number of adolescents treated for cancer are long-term survivors. Many of the chemotherapeutic protocols are gonadotoxic and can cause ovarian failure or ovarian insufficiency which may not manifest itself as POF until a number of years after the treatments.

The diagnosis of POF is frequently delayed especially in the clinical setting of secondary amenorrhea. Whenever there has been secondary amenorrhea of greater than 3 months, an FSH determination is warranted, and if elevated a repeat FSH will help in the diagnosis of POF. A very challenging aspect of the diagnosis of POF is the manner in which this information is relayed to the patient. The diagnosis of POF can have significant psychological consequences for both the patient and the parents so counseling is an important adjunct to diagnosis and treatment. Treatment consists of estrogen replacement therapy, but the timing and method are not well established [24]. The use of hormone replacement therapy in young patients with POF is not analogous to HRT in older menopausal women.

Head

Consideration of the head:

1. CNS tumors
2. Pituitary adenomas
3. Hypothalamic hypogonadism
    (a) Idiopathic constitutional delay
    (b) Eating disorders
    (c) Athlete triad

Lesions of the CNS can affect reproductive function in a number of ways including the physical location of the lesion, treatment for cancerous lesions, or hydrocephalus secondary to the lesion. The history will alert the physician to the possibility that amenorrhea is secondary to cancer treatment. Evaluation of the CNS can identify those patients with intracranial lesions that may affect reproductive function.

Tumors which have been associated with hypothalamic pituitary dysfunction include craniopharyngiomas, germ cell tumors, gliomas, hamartomas, and adenomas [25]. The majority of sellar and parasellar tumors in the pediatric patient population are craniopharyngiomas (80–90%) [26].

Craniopharyngiomas arise from remnants of Rathke's pouch. Presenting symptoms include endocrine abnormalities, headache, or visual disturbances. In general, craniopharyngiomas are slow-growing, benign tumors but do account for 6% of all expanding pediatric intracranial neoplasms [27]. Presenting signs and symptoms can include visual defects, growth retardation, headaches, and delayed puberty. The endocrine disturbances found most commonly include growth hormone deficiency (75%), gonadotropin deficiency (40%), and corticotrophin or thyrotropin deficiency (25%) [28]. Diagnosis relies upon MRI imaging and treatment is surgical resection.

Pituitary adenomas are uncommon in the adolescent population, and when they do occur, the most common forms release prolactin [17]. Recent advances in the molecular biology of adenomas have initiated the possibility of defining the functional characteristics of the adenoma using molecular biology so that prognosis and treatment can be tailored for a particular patient's adenoma. Patients with prolactinomas commonly present with growth failure, headaches, visual disturbances, and either primary amenorrhea or galactorrhea and secondary amenorrhea depending upon the size of the tumor. Diagnosis is achieved using serum prolactin levels (fasting, resting), TSH, and MRI imaging. Even mild elevations of prolactin warrant pituitary imaging since larger tumors can cause a mild elevation of prolactin due to the "stalk effect" where there is a loss of tonic inhibition. Treatment is medical if indicated and consists of dopamine agonists. Bromocriptine and cabergoline are two possible choices for treatment, but cabergoline has the advantage of weekly administration which is usually better tolerated in the adolescent population. Treatment should result in normalization of prolactin levels and arrest of tumor growth. If medical treatment is unsuccessful, then transsphenoidal surgery is an option. Remission for transsphenoidal surgery is approximately 50%. For patients presenting with amenorrhea, treatment is necessary for proper reproductive functioning including estrogen for secondary sexual characteristics development and bone growth. There is no consensus about how long to treat but for some patients, the treatment can be stopped, and if reproductive functioning is maintained, no further treatment is necessary. Continued monitoring of prolactin levels is necessary since many will enlarge producing increasing level of prolactin necessitating restarting medical management. Surgery is rarely indicated [29]. Long-term follow-up is required but exact protocols are not defined.

Hypothalamic Hypogonadism (HH)

While there are numerous etiologies for HH, common etiologies can be categorized into:

1. Idiopathic constitutional delay of puberty
2. Kallmann syndrome
3. Secondary HH
   (a) Anorexia nervosa
   (b) Bulimia
   (c) Exercise triad

Delayed Puberty

Delayed puberty occurs when there is amenorrhea in the absence of secondary sexual characteristics in an adolescent who is 14 years of age or older. The onset of puberty is an ordered sequence of developmental stages initiated by nocturnal increases in the pulsatile release of GnRH combined with increased adrenal functioning. Many pediatric endocrinologists consider that the average age for the onset of puberty is between 8 and 13 years of age [30]. The normal sequence of developmental events is an increase in height velocity followed by breast development, but the breast development is noted first clinically. This is followed by the development of pubic hair and finally menses. The sequence of development for idiopathic constitutional delay of puberty is the normal sequences for puberty occurring within the proper age range. For many of these patients, no definite etiology will be found, and they are categorized as constitutional delayed puberty. In a study by Sedlmeyer and Palmert [31] which included 74 females, 22 (30%) were diagnosed with constitutional delayed (CD) puberty. Constitutional delay of puberty is a variation of normal; however, the patients usually will be short for their age. Their growth velocity and height are consistent with their bone age, but the final height is usually less than predicted. Frequently there will be a family history of delayed puberty. When the bone age reaches 11–13 years of age, the patient will demonstrate early signs of sexual maturation. Since development matches their genetic potential, there is usually no indication for treatment for the patients with CD puberty [32].

Kallmann Syndrome

Kallmann syndrome, a genetic disorder, is a combination of hypogonadotropic hypogonadism and anosmia [33]. The frequency for females is estimated to be 1 in 50,000 women. The etiology involves a failure of the proper neuronal migration of the GnRH-secreting and olfactory neurons. The mode of inheritance can be X-linked, autosomal recessive, or autosomal dominant.

Patients with this syndrome present with primary amenorrhea and/or delayed sexual maturation. They have normal adrenal androgens so pubic and axillary hair develops normally. Anosmia may need to be solicited since the patient is often unaware that they have anosmia. While they may have eunuchoid proportions, they have normal structure and growth in childhood. There may be midline defects, and frequently an MRI can detect aplasia or hypoplasia of the olfactory bulb and/or sulci.

Kallmann syndrome is associated with a number of somatic abnormalities including unilateral renal agenesis, imperfect facial fusion defects, epilepsy, and cerebellar ataxia [34]. Initiation of puberty is accomplished by the administration of estrogen and supported by estrogen replacement therapy. After breast development, oral contraceptives can be used for hormonal replacement.

Secondary Hypothalamic Hypogonadism

Eating disorders can result in hypothalamic hypogonadism. The DSM-IV categorizes eating disorders in three broad categories: anorexia nervosa, bulimia, and atypical eating disorders. Frequently, these disorders begin in the adolescent and thus provide an opportunity to intervene early in the progression of the disease. Eating disorders frequently have both medical and psychiatric comorbidities. Eating disorders are common in adolescents with the estimated frequency about 13% [35]. The highest incidence for eating disorders is between 10 and 19 years of age [36]. The etiology of eating disorders is poorly understood.

Anorexia nervosa is characterized by amenorrhea, weight loss, and psychiatric disturbances. The definition found in DSM-IV requires four criteria [37]:

1. Refusal to maintain weight within a normal range for height and age (more than 15% below ideal body weight)
2. Intense fear of gaining weight or getting fat
3. Severe body image disturbance or denial of the seriousness of the current low body weight
4. Absence of menstrual cycles for greater than three cycles.

Anorexia nervosa has a peak incidence in adolescent females ages 15–19 and has been increasing since 1935 [38]. Patients with anorexia have clinical features of cold intolerance, dry skin, constipation, hair loss, hypotension, and bradycardia. Hormonal features included low gonadotropin levels, low estrogen and androgen levels, and elevated cortisol.

Bulimia nervosa (the diagnosis for Bulimia nervosa (DSM-IV) [21]):

1. Recurrent episodes of binge eating with a sense of lack of control.
2. Recurrent inappropriate compensatory behavior to prevent weight gain such as self-induced vomiting, laxatives, diuretics, or excessive exercise.
3. The binge eating and compensatory behavior to occur at least twice per week for 3 months.
4. Self-evaluation unduly influenced by body shape and weight.
5. These disturbances must not occur exclusively during episodes of anorexia nervosa.

The weight for these patients may fluctuate but usually not to dangerously low levels. Bulimia is often associated with impulsive behavior: alcohol or drug use, promiscuity, and stealing or shoplifting. Clinical features for bulimia include parotid gland enlargement due to vomiting, erosion of the enamel on the teeth due to vomiting, and Russell's sign which is skin lesions on the fingers from induced vomiting.

Hormonally these patients have low gonadotropins but normal estrogen levels.

Treatments for eating disorders are more successful in the adolescent than in the adult. There are, however, no long-term studies to assess the lifetime success of treatment for eating disorders [39]. Anorexia is a chronic disease with a relapsing course and a high mortality rate. Common comorbidities include depression, substance abuse, anxiety disorders, and personality disorders. Overall, when diagnosed in an adolescent, the 10–15-year recovery rate is about 70% [40]. The treatment for bulimia is usually more favorable than for anorexia nervosa.

Female Athlete Triad

The American College of Sports Medicine had defined the female athlete triad as:

1. Eating disorder
2. Amenorrhea
3. Osteoporosis

The problem is found in athletes who compete in sports that emphasize a lean body build or subjective scoring performance. The common underlying problem is a reduction in the body's total energy stores which leads to amenorrhea [41]. Amenorrhea found in these women seems to be due to a disruption of the hypothalamic-gonadal axis, but the actual cause is unknown. There appears to be a number of factors involved in the etiology of amenorrhea including nutritional deprivation, stress, and excessive exercise [42]. Amenorrhea may result in osteopenia since the majority of bone mass is acquired during the early adolescent years. Many female athletes will have one or two of the components but very few have all three. Screening for the athlete triad includes a history of the athletic activity, intensity level, and time commitment. Bone density measurements by DEXA scans will establish the presence of osteoporosis. Treatment relies heavily on prevention which includes diet modification and altering the patient's exercise levels. A weight gain to bring the patient to 90% of her ideal body weight will result in the resumption of menses [43]. Osteoporosis may require estrogen replacement therapy, but bisphosphonates should not be used in this young population.

References

1. Speroff L, Fritz MA. Clinical gynecologic endocrinology and infertility. 7th ed. Philadelphia: Lippincott, Williams, & Wilkins; 2005. p. 402. Ch.10.
2. Berman JM. Intrauterine adhesions. Semin Reprod Med. 2008;26:349–55.

3. Marcel K, Camborieux L, Programe de Recherches sur Jes Aplasies Mulleriannnes (PRAM), Guerrier D. Mayer Rokitansky-Kuster-Hauser (MRKH) syndrome. Orphanet J Rare Dis. 2007;2:12–21.
4. Strubbe EH, Willemsen WN, Lemmens JA, Thijn JA, Rolland R. Mayer-Rokitansky-Kuster-Hauser syndrome: distinction between two forms based on excretory urographic, sonographic, and laparoscopic findings. Am J Roentgenol. 1993;160:331–4.
5. Morris JM. The syndrome of feminization in male pseudohermaphrodites. Am J Obstet Gynecol. 1953;65:1192.
6. Galani A, Kitsiou-Tzeli S, Sofokleous C, Kanavakis E, Kalpini-Mavrou A. Androgen insensitivity syndrome: clinical features and molecular defects. Hormones. 2008;7:217–29.
7. Oakes MB, Eyvazzadeh AD, Quint E. Complete androgen insensitivity syndrome- a review. J Pediatr Adolesc Gynecol. 2008;21:305–10.
8. Rossi B, Sukalich S, Droz J, Griffin A, Cook S, Blumkin A, Guzick D, Hoeger KM. Prevalence of metabolic syndrome and related characteristics in obese adolescents with and without polycystic ovary syndrome. J Clin Endocrine Metab. 2008;93:4780–6.
9. The Rotterdam ESHRE/ASRM- Sponsored PCOS consensus workshop group. Revised 2003 consensus on diagnostic criteria and long-term health risks related to polycystic ovary syndrome (PCOS). Hum Reprod. 2004;19:41.
10. Driscoll DA. Polycystic ovary syndrome in adolescence. Ann N Y Acad Sci. 2003;997:49–55.
11. Cool S, Auinger P, Li C, Ford ES. Metabolic syndrome rates in United States adolescents, from the National Health and Nutrition Examination Survey 1999–2002. J Pediatr. 2008;152:165–70.
12. Rachmiel M, Kives S, Atenafu E, Hamilton J. Primary amenorrhea as a manifestation of polycystic ovarian syndrome in adolescents: a unique subgroup? Arch Pediatr Adolesc Med. 2008;162:521–5.
13. Buggs C, Rosenfield RL. Polycystic ovary syndrome in adolescence. Endocrinol Metab Clin N Am. 2005;34:677–705.
14. Pfeifer SM, Kives S. Polycystic ovary syndrome in the adolescent. Obstet Gynecol Clin. 2009;36:129–52.
15. Davenprot ML. Approach to the patient with Turner syndrome. J Clin Endocrinol Metab. 2010;95:1487–95.
16. Vlement-Jones M, Schiller S, Roa E, Blaschke RJ, Zuniga A, Zeller R, Robson SC, Binder G, Glass I, Strachan T, Lindsay S, Rappold GA. The short stature homeobox gene SHOX is

involved in skeletal abnormalities in Turner syndrome. Hum Mol Genet. 2000;9:695–702.
17. Gotzsche C, Krag-Olsen B. Prevalence of cardiovascular malformations and association with karyotypes in Turner's syndrome. Arch Dis Child. 1994;71:433–6.
18. Ho VB, Bakalov VK, Cooley M, Hood MN, Burklow TR, Bondy CA. Major vascular anomalies in Turner syndrome: prevalence and magnetic resonance angiographic features. Circulation. 2004;110:1694–700.
19. The Practice Committee of the American Society for Reproductive Medicine. Increased maternal cardiovascular mortality associated with pregnancy in women with Turner syndrome. Fertil Steril. 2008;90(suppl 3):5185–6.
20. Bondy CA. The Turner syndrome consensus study group care of girls and women with Turner syndrome: a guideline of the Turner syndrome study group. J Clin Endocrinol Metab. 2007;92:10–25.
21. Nelson LM, Covington SN, Rebar RW. An update: spontaneous premature ovarian failure is not an early menopause. Fertil Steril. 2005;83:1327–32.
22. Murray A, Webb J, Grimley S, Conway G, Jacobs P. Studies of FRAXA and FRAXE in women with premature ovarian failure. J Med Genet. 1998;35:637–40.
23. Conway GS, Kaltsas G, Patel A, Davies MC, Jacobs HS. Characterization of idiopathic premature ovarian failure. Fertil Steril. 1996;65:337–41.
24. Rebar RW. Premature ovarian "failure" in the adolescent. Ann N Y Acad Sci. 2008;1135:138–45.
25. Brauner R, Adan L, Souberbielle JC. Hypothalamic- pituitary function and growth in children with intracranial lesions. Childs Nerv Syst. 1999;15:662–9.
26. Jagannathan J, Dumont AS, Jane JA. Diagnosis and management of pediatric sellar lesions. In: Laws ER, Sheehan JP, editors. Pituitary surgery- a modern approach. Front Harm Res. Basel, Karger. 2006;34:83–104.
27. Hayward R. The present and future management of childhood craniopharyngiomas. Childs Nerv Syst. 1999;15:764–76.
28. Keil MF, Stratakis CA. Pituitary tumors in childhood: an update in their diagnosis, treatment and molecular genetics. Expert Rev Neurother. 2008;8:563–74.
29. Fideleff HL, Boquete HR, Suarez MG, Azaretzky M. Prolactinoma in children and adolescents. Harm Res. 2009;72:197–205.

30. Carel J, Leger J. Precocious puberty. N Engl J Med. 2008;358:2366–77.
31. Sedlmeyer IL, Palmert MR. Delayed puberty: analysis of a large case series from an academic center. J Clin Endocrinol Metab. 2002;87:1613–20.
32. Viswanathan V, Eugster EA. Etiology and treatment of hypogonadism in adolescents. Endocrionol Metab Clin N Am. 2009;38:719–38.
33. Hoffman B, Bradshaw KO. Delayed puberty and amenorrhea. Semin Reprod Med. 2003;21:353362.
34. Winters SJ. Expanding the differential diagnosis of male hypogonadism. N Engl J Med. 1992;326:193–5.
35. Neumark-Sztainer D, Hannan PJ. Weight-related behaviors among adolescent girls and boys from a national survey. Arch Pediatr Adolesc Med. 2000;154:569–77.
36. Currin L, Schmidt U, Treasure J, Jick H. Time trends in eating disorder incidence. Br J Psychiatry. 2005;186:123–35.
37. WHO. International statistical classification of diseases and related health problems (ICD-10). Geneva: World Health Organization; 1992.
38. Hoek HW, van Hoeken D. Review of the prevalence and incidence of eating disorders. Int J Eat Disord. 2003;34:383–96.
39. Treasure J, Claudina AM, Zucker N. Eating disorders. Lancet. 2010;375:583–93.
40. Miller CA, Golden NH. Introduction of eating disorders: clinical presentation, epidemiology, and prognosis. Nutr Clin Pract. 2010;25:110–5.
41. Edwards JE, Lindeman AK, Nujesjtm AE. Energy balance in highly trained female endurance athletes. Med Sci Sports Exerc. 1993;25:1398–404.
42. Brunet M. Female athlete triad. Clin Sports Med. 2005;24:623–36.
43. Golden HN, Jacobson MS, Schebendach J. Resumption of menses in anorexia nervosa. Arch Pediatr Adolesc Med. 1997;151:16–21.

Chapter 6
Chronic Pelvic Pain

Sondra L. Summers

Chronic pelvic pain is defined as pain below the umbilicus, which lasts for at 6 months, is debilitating enough to affect the patient's ability to function, and causes her to seek medical care. The evaluation and management of chronic pelvic pain in women can be a challenge for many clinicians. Women seeking care for chronic pelvic pain (CPP) can account for as much as 25% of gynecologic office visits, and it has been estimated that this debilitating condition can affect as many as one out of seven women in the United States [1]. As with many chronic pain conditions, such as migraine or back pain, the complex psychosocial components involved make evaluation and treatment for these women and their physicians a challenge.

For women presenting with CPP, there are many characteristics which are similar to other chronic pain conditions; however, there can be unique characteristics that the clinician should be aware of in order to provide optimal therapy. It is well known that patients presenting with CPP have a higher incidence of childhood sexual abuse than the general population [2]. It has been postulated that these women suffer from a type of post-traumatic stress disorder and remodeling of

---

S. L. Summers (✉)
University of Illinois Hospital at Chicago, Department of Obstetrics and Gynecology, Chicago, IL, USA
e-mail: sondras@uic.edu

J. V. Knaus et al. (eds.), *Ambulatory Gynecology*,
https://doi.org/10.1007/978-1-4939-7641-6_6

their neurological response to pain, especially if the subsequent painful stimulus involves the anatomical region of the pelvis [2]. It is understandable that women suffering with CPP also have a higher incidence of anxiety and depression than the general population which affects not only their ability to respond to treatments but must be considered in the holistic approach to care for these women [2, 3].

The Evaluation of a Patient with Chronic Pelvic Pain

The Office Evaluation

The Importance of Collecting a Thorough History

The evaluation of CPP involves the typical components of a history and physical including a visual analogue scale (VAS) for the objective assessment of pain. When completing a history in these patients, it is imperative to include thorough documentation of previous therapies and evaluations, imaging, and surgical procedures. Validated questionnaires such as the McGill Pain Questionnaire can be useful for a thorough documentation of pertinent history.

A complete history of the pain should also include the description of the pain such as location, description, exacerbating and alleviating activities, and radiation pattern [4].

The patient's description of exacerbating and alleviating events is an important piece of the clinical puzzle. Symptoms worsened by events in the menstrual cycle or "cyclic" pain can be an indication that the pain is due to the presence of endometriosis. The clinical significance of cyclic versus noncyclic pain is discussed in more detail below. If the patient endorses that movement elicits pain, this history may suggest either musculoskeletal origin or adhesive disease is a causative or contributing factor. Another common exacerbating event for women with pelvic pain is intercourse, a complaint known as "dyspareunia"; the cause of this type of pain can be due to musculoskeletal tenderness or pelvic organ pathology.

A careful physical examination, as described below, can often differentiate between the two origins of tenderness.

For many patients with chronic pelvic pain, they will complain of symptoms involving multiple organ systems including the pelvic organs as well as the gastrointestinal and urinary tract [5, 6]. It has been postulated that CPP, for some women, can be a type of regional pain syndrome with an association with painful or frequent urination, urinary urgency or incontinence, irritable bowel syndrome, or chronic constipation [5–7]. It is imperative that the history for these patients includes a review of systems approach which incorporates gastrointestinal and urinary functioning and associated pain in order to fully evaluate women presenting with CPP [1].

As mentioned previously, many women presenting with CPP have a history of sexual abuse as a child so, although it can be traumatic to enquire about this history, many are relieved to share this history and to learn that it may be associated with their present condition [8]. A history of psychological conditions and treatments is also important; many patients with PTSD self-medicate with alcohol or recreational drugs so a thorough social history is important to gather. Spend a few minutes finding out about how the CPP affects their quality of life and ability to function at home and work. The Female Sexual Functioning Inventory questionnaire can be used to determine if this quality of life metric is affected [6].

Other medical conditions associated with CPP in women include psychosocial factors such as depression and anxiety [2, 8]. The occurrence of CPP in adult women has been associated with childhood sexual trauma and abuse which many experts believe leads to a type of post-traumatic syndrome changing the neurological response to painful stimuli (Fig. 6.1).

When the History Suggests Cyclic Pattern of Pain

Women complaining of pain that is exacerbated by events in the menstrual cycle demonstrate a cyclic pattern. For instance, pain that occurs in mid-cycle for a limited time, i.e., for 1 or

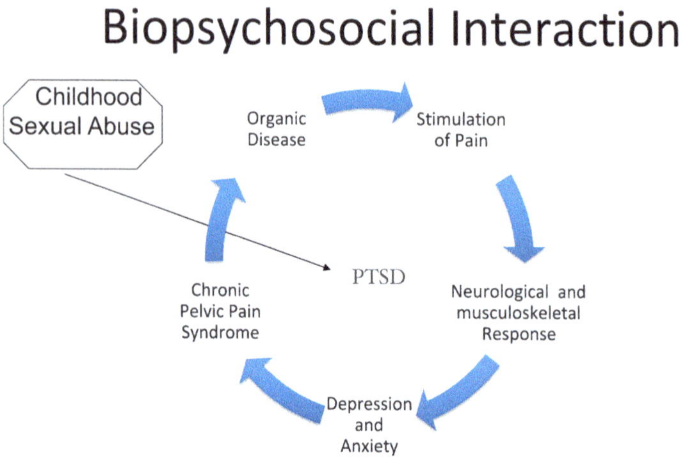

FIG. 6.1 Biopsychosocial interaction

2 days, can be pain that is associated with ovulation, also known as "mittelschmerz" [9]. This condition can be treated with anti-inflammatory pain medications or hormonal suppression of ovulation, such as with oral contraceptives.

Cyclic pain that occurs with the menses is known as "dysmenorrhea" and many times is caused by the presence of endometriosis. Endometriosis is defined as the presence of endometrial glands outside the uterine cavity and is thought to originate from a process known as retrograde menstruation although many experts believe that the implants may exist as embryonic rests in some patients [10]. The ectopic endometrial tissue may have histologic characteristics of uterine endometrium but reacts differently to hormonal stimulus which produces inflammatory cytokines and induces growth of vascular and neurological tissue, all of which are most likely responsible for the pain women experience [11].

The diagnosis of endometriosis is made histologically, when implants are visualized and biopsied at the time of surgery, such as laparoscopy [1]; however, a careful history and examination can provide clues to the diagnosis. Women suffering from endometriosis many times have a familial history of endometriosis and will have first- and second-degree relatives with diagnoses of infertility, dysmenorrhea, and early surgical intervention [12]. The ectopic endometriosis implants can be found growing on the colon, causing GI complaints such as diarrhea, cramping, and pain with defecation and intercourse, especially if the implants are in the rectovaginal fossa [1, 13].

A variant of endometriosis occurs when the endometrial glands are found in the myometrium of the uterus. This condition is known as "adenomyosis" and causes painful heavy bleeding during menses. The pathophysiology of these implants is not well understood although there are genetic, immunological, and anatomic factors; women with previous uterine surgery and presence of leiomyomas are at risk for adenomyosis as well [14]. The ultrasound findings for both endometriosis and adenomyosis can be normal although implants of adenomyosis can be seen as cystic spaces on ultrasound; MRI findings can be diagnostic with a diminished transition zone [14].

When the History Suggests Noncyclic Pattern of Pain

When evaluating a woman presenting with recurring pain that is not typically exacerbated with menstrual cycle, it can be helpful to consider the site or origin of her symptoms. Table 6.1 lists the conditions of the female pelvic organs that can cause chronic pain conditions. The following is a descriptive list of pelvic organs that can be involved with a CPP syndrome:

I. *Vulva*: A condition known as "vulvodynia" is defined as pain and tenderness localized to the structures of the vulva. The cause of the symptoms is multifactorial and can include neurological, hormonal, or dermatological changes such as caused by skin conditions or atrophy [16].

II. *Vagina*: Synthetic mesh that is placed transvaginally for urinary incontinence, also known as "tension-free vaginal tape" or TVT, can lead to postoperative pain, sometimes from erosion and fibrosis caused by the mesh [15].

Table 6.1 Anatomic sites for chronic pelvic pain

Anatomic site of pain	Recurrent cyclic pain	Chronic noncyclic pain
I. Vulva		Dermatoses such as lichen sclerosus Neuropathy (pudendal nerve) Atrophy Vulvodynia
II. Vagina	Endometrial implants	Granulation tissue Mesh erosion Chronic vaginitis Pelvic floor myofascial pain
III. Cervix		Cervical polyp Cervical cancer Granulation tissue
IV. Uterus	Adenomyosis Leiomyoma	Chronic endometritis Adenomyosis Leiomyoma
V. Adnexa	Endometriosis Intermittent torsion Post-ablation syndrome Post-Essure placement	Endometrioma or endometriosis Ovarian neoplasm Hydrosalpinx Adhesive disease Ovarian remnant Tubo-ovarian abscess
VI. Abdominal wall	Endometriosis	Scar restriction Neuroma Hernia Myofascial pain disorder
VII. Pelvic floor	Myofascial pain disorder	Myofascial pain disorder Neuropathy (pudendal nerve)

(continued)

Table 6.1 (continued)

Anatomic site of pain	Recurrent cyclic pain	Chronic noncyclic pain
VIII. Vascular structures	Pelvic congestion syndrome	Pelvic congestion syndrome
IX. Lower urinary tract		Interstitial cystitis Chronic infection Nephrolithiasis Hydroureter Neoplasia Foreign body
X. Gastrointestinal	Irritable bowel syndrome Endometriosis	Irritable bowel syndrome Diverticulitis Colitis Constipation

Many retrospective reports have noted that the occurrence of pain is higher in women post-TVT placement if they had a presurgical diagnosis of CPP [15].

III. *Cervix*: Structural causes of pain from the cervix can include polyps and erosive changes after surgical procedures such as conization of the cervix for dysplasia.

IV. *Uterus*: Leiomyomas do not generally cause CPP unless they undergo degeneration and torsion or are impacted into the pelvic brim. Adenomyosis is a painful condition which is worsened by menses but also causes tenderness in the uterus so that the pain may be more noncyclic in nature.

V. *Adnexa* (*ovary*): Endometriosis in the ovary, known as endometrioma, is a unique type of ovarian cyst which may cause chronic pain. Other types of ovarian cysts or neoplasms can produce a more prolonged pain pattern with intermittent torsion or if the ovary is encased in adhesive disease. Another ovarian source of CPP is the ovarian remnant syndrome, which occurs after surgery on the ovary, typically for endometriosis, with a small portion of functioning ovarian tissue left behind [17].

VI. *Adnexa (fallopian tubes)*: When the fallopian tubes are swollen or twisted, as can happen after surgery, infection, or tubal ligation, this may cause chronic pain. A syndrome known as "post-ablation syndrome" occurs in a woman who undergoes endometrial ablation after a tubal occlusion for sterilization; theoretically, this can cause menstruation to be trapped in the fallopian tube causing swelling and pain [18]. Sterilization with coils placed into the uterine cornua (Essure) has also been shown in a minority of women to cause post-procedural pain, especially if the coils become misplaced outside of the fallopian tube [19].

VII. *Abdominal wall*: The presence of hernias, scar restriction, or endometriosis implants or neuroma should be considered in women presenting with CPP.

VIII. *Pelvic floor*: The pelvic floor consists of musculoskeletal and neurological structures which can become inflamed and cause a chronic type of pain [20]. The systematic evaluation of this anatomy will be described in detail below.

IX. *Vascular structures*: Pelvic congestion syndrome is defined as enlarged or tortuous venous structures in the pelvis. Inflammation and swelling may increase during menstruation so that symptoms may be noncyclic in nature but worsened by menses [21].

X. *Lower urinary tract (LUT)*: Chronic LUT infections can cause painful voiding and suprapubic pain. Interstitial cystitis is a condition of the bladder which causes urinary frequency, urgency, and painful voiding [6]. A cystoscopy can be of assistance in order to make this diagnosis and can also rule out more worrisome pathology such as neoplasia. Nephrolithiasis in the ureter or foreign body in the LUT can be a cause of CPP.

XI. *Gastrointestinal*: Irritable bowel syndrome and chronic constipation have a known association with CPP [5]. These symptoms can be associated with a history of pain worsening with bloating which improves with bowel movements.

The Physical Exam

When a clinician is evaluating a woman presenting with chronic pelvic pain, it is important to recognize that this can be a traumatic and anxiety-provoking exam for the patients. It is important to note that patients will respond to a painful examination with guarding which may thus render a full exam of pelvic organs difficult to interpret. We prefer a systematic, gentle approach only as tolerated by the patient and in a manner which elicits maximum pain reserved for the end of the exam.

The exam typically starts with the patient seated on the exam table. The back is carefully inspected for vertebral or sacroiliac joint tenderness. The examination of the abdomen begins with visual inspection; note abdominal scars and any superficial masses or skin retraction. It can be helpful to ask the patient to find the tender points so the examiner will know prior to the exam. The patient is then asked to engage her abdominal wall muscles by lifting her head or legs off of the exam table. This maneuver, known as Carnett's test, will allow the examiner to evaluate the anterior abdominal wall for causes of pain such as trigger points in the rectus muscles, abdominal wall endometriomas, neuromas, or entrapped nerves near incisions [22]. The Valsalva effect will also elicit a bulge if there is a hernia present. If there is significant tenderness with this portion of the exam, allow the patient to relax prior to any deep palpation.

Deep palpation should begin at the point furthest away from the site of pain. Ask the patient to point out the site of maximum pain with one finger, if possible. The patient can press down to demonstrate the amount of pressure required to elicit the pain which can provide helpful information for the examiner without increasing anxiety. The examiner can palpate to look for an abdominal or pelvic mass, constipated stool in the colon, and bladder distention as he or she is isolating the location of the tenderness and checks for guarding as clinically indicated.

Inspection of the female genitourinary exam is performed in the dorsal lithotomy position with the physician seated. The external genitalia, specifically the vulva and the perineum, should be inspected for any visible lesion or skin breakdown. If the pain is localized, the patient may be asked to point out the site of symptoms. Any suspicious skin lesion should be biopsied or referred for consultation to rule out malignancy. A Q-tip test is used to faintly stroke the vulva and hymenal opening in order to note any dysesthesia which can be found with many chronic pain syndromes of the vulva, vulvodynia, or vestibulodynia.

Once the vulva is evaluated, the examiner can begin the evaluation of the perineal muscles and pelvic floor. Tell the patient that you are going to push on some muscles in her vagina to check for tenderness. Demonstrate the amount of pressure you will use by firmly pushing on her thigh muscles. Ask her to rate her tenderness on a scale of 0–10 where 0 is no pain and 10 is the worst pain imaginable. Use a single digit to firmly palpate the muscles of the posterior, lateral, and anterior pelvic walls looking for trigger points or myofascial tenderness [23, 24]. Sweep anteriorly to evaluate the urethra, anterior vaginal, and abdominal wall for similar findings. The digital exam concludes with isolation of the posterior cul-de-sac and cervix: cervical motion tenderness can be a sign of pelvic inflammatory disease, and nodularity of the cul-de-sac may be a sign of rectovaginal endometriosis.

A bimanual exam should be performed as tolerated to complete the pelvic exam in order to complete a comprehensive evaluation for masses and tenderness. If the patient cannot tolerate this examination, imaging with ultrasound can be performed to screen for structural causes. Place two fingers of the dominant hand beneath the cervix to allow palpation of the anteverted uterus and to assess its size. The vaginal cavity can also be palpated for the presence of foreign body such as an extruded mesh. By sweeping these digits anterolaterally, one can evaluate for tenderness or mass in the adnexal region.

After the bimanual exam is completed, the clinician can determine whether the clinical presentation requires *and* patient can tolerate a speculum examination. The use of a bivalve speculum allows the visualization of vagina and cervix for evaluation of possible infections, mesh erosion, or lesions as described above. However, there are many CPP patients who cannot tolerate a speculum examination and in whom this evaluation will offer no helpful information.

Office Testing

Evaluation of women during the office visit can include (1) urinalysis and culture, (2) vaginal and cervical specimens for infectious etiologies, and (3) cervical cytology that should be sent routinely if the patient is not up to date on her cervical cancer screening or evaluate any cervical lesions. Laboratory testing should be reserved for specific diagnoses; there are no blood biomarkers that have been shown to be accurate for the diagnosis of endometriosis [25].

Imaging

Pelvic ultrasound can be used to identify structural causes of pelvic pain such as uterine fibroids or adnexal masses. Pelvic endometriosis, with the exception of endometrioma, rectosigmoid implants, or deeply infiltrating endometriosis in the rectovaginal tissue, is not usually seen with imaging such as magnetic resonance imaging or transvaginal ultrasound [25–27].

CT scan of the pelvic structures is not as specific or sensitive for structural disorders of the pelvis but can be used to diagnose other causes of pain such as diverticulosis, hernia, and abdominal wall mass such as endometrioma [26].

Pelvic MRI scan can be helpful in identifying adnexal masses (endometrioma, hydrosalpinx), uterine mass such as adenomyosis or fibroid, or, less frequently, retroperitoneal neoplasms not imaged with ultrasound [27].

Surgical Evaluation

Laparoscopy can be an important tool in the evaluation of women with CPP, especially if medical treatment has not improved symptoms [1]. While most experts agree that laparoscopic visualization and directed biopsy are considered the gold standard methods to diagnose endometriosis, the specificity and sensitivity for etiology of CPP have not been well established [27, 28]. Women with CPP who undergo laparoscopy have findings consistent with endometriosis 33% of the time with adhesive disease found in 24% and 44% with no findings to explain the patient's CPP. Conversely, up to 40% women undergoing laparoscopy for sterilization are found to have endometriosis with no symptoms of pain at all [1, 27, 28].

Treatment of Chronic Pelvic Pain of Gynecologic Origin

Medical Therapy

For many women with CPP, a holistic, multidisciplinary approach including therapy for all components of their pain can offer the best results [30, 31]. An important line of therapy for women with CPP is hormonal control of cyclic exacerbation of pain or menses such as combined or continuous combination oral contraceptive agents; other agents include progesterone-only medications (such as Depo-Provera, norethindrone, levonorgestrel-coated IUD) or gonadotropin-releasing hormone (GnRH) agonists [32]. Analgesics such as nonsteroidal anti-inflammatory agents can be effective pain relievers. Opioids and narcotics should be used with caution and are best utilized for self-limited painful episodes and not for chronic use because this can lead to dependence and addiction [32, 33].

Regardless of the cause, CPP can be viewed as other chronic pain ailments which require attention to the central nervous systems' neuroregulation of pain with the use of neuromodulators such as Lyrica, amitriptyline, or gabapentin [34, 35].

Surgical Treatments

Laparoscopic Approach

The use of laparoscopic procedures for the evaluation and treatment of chronic pelvic pain has been the subject of much discussion and investigation. Investigators have found in some series that there was no significant difference in relief from dysmenorrhea between women undergoing laparoscopic excisional surgery versus diagnostic laparoscopy; however, some surgical outcome studies show that excisional removal of endometriosis is beneficial to ablation or treating with postoperative medical therapy without surgical excision [28, 29].

The beneficial effect of laparoscopic adhesiolysis for CPP is controversial; although there is some evidence to suggest that significant relief of pain occurs with lysis of severe adhesive disease involving bowel [28, 36, 37], other studies have failed to show that the presence of adhesive disease is associated with CPP or that adhesiolysis provides significant relief [36, 37]. Other laparoscopic procedures specific for CPP such as laparoscopic uterosacral nerve ablation (LUNA) have not been shown to provide effective relief [38]. Other specialized laparoscopic procedures such as presacral neurectomy have been shown to be effective for midline pain which can be helpful for a select few women with CPP [39]. Many experts feel that the laparoscopic procedures involving adhesiolysis, LUNA and PSN, and incidental appendectomy should not be routinely performed for CPP as they have not been shown definitively to help with CPP and require an expert level of surgical expertise with a potential for significant morbidity.

Hysterectomy

The removal of the uterus, or hysterectomy, can be considered when patients have a surgical cause of their CPP such as uterine leiomyoma or adenomyosis, if medical therapy has failed and the patient has completed her childbearing. Hysterectomy alone appears to offer relief from pelvic pain for the majority of women studied and for a prolonged time period [32, 33, 42].

However, if there is endometriosis, especially implants outside of the pelvic organs, there may be recurrence unless there is removal of ovaries at the time of hysterectomy or postoperative treatment with ovulation suppression medications such as gonadotropin-releasing hormones [40, 41]. Many observers have noted that, while there is commonly pelvic organ pathology such as leiomyoma (60%) and adenomyosis (40%) [43], there is a significant percentage of women who continue to have pain after hysterectomy with rates reported to be 21–40% [43, 44].

If the preoperative evaluation finds that there is a component of myofascial disorder (MFD) as a contributor to the pelvic pain, the CPP may continue postoperatively. It is important to identify the women with MFD and counsel them preoperatively that they may require continued medical treatment and/or physical therapy after surgery.

As stated previously, uterine leiomyomas do not generally cause CPP unless they undergo degeneration and torsion or are impacted into the pelvic brim. Degeneration of the solid leiomyoma, a process characterized by pain, tenderness of the fibroid, fever, and leukocytosis, is usually a self-limited process but which may require treatment with nonsteroidal anti-inflammatory agents and, at times, antibiotics. In the event that a uterine fibroid requires surgical excision for pain relief, a discussion with the patient can determine whether myomectomy or hysterectomy is warranted given her desire for future childbearing or other concerns.

Adnexal Surgery

Adnexal causes of CPP include endometriomas, benign and malignant neoplasms, and inflammatory conditions. Many or most of these causes require surgical intervention to remove the pathology. The ovarian remnant syndrome can be challenging to diagnose, and surgical removal of this ovarian remnant tissue can be difficult due to adhesive disease and inability to identify the ovarian tissue. Ovarian suppression with hormonal agents may sometimes offer symptomatic relief of this syndrome. The distention of the fallopian tube or hydrosalpinx or its involvement in adhesive complex is an example of a benign, chronic cause of pelvic pain which has no treatment other than surgery but which can easily be followed expectantly without removal.

Foreign Body Removal

The finding of a foreign body as a possible etiology for pain, whether it is mesh placed transvaginally for incontinence or for prolapse, micro-inserts in fallopian tubes for sterilization, or even a misplaced intrauterine device, should be addressed with possible removal of the material necessary in order to provide relief from pain.

Interventional Radiology

Interventional radiology (IR) procedures such as uterine artery embolization, by helping to reduce the size of uterine fibroids, can help with pain in a certain subset of women [45]. IR therapy can also provide embolization of pelvic varicosities found in pelvic congestion syndrome and provide relief for this condition.

Psychological Treatments

It has been well established that there is an association between a history of abuse, depression, anxiety, and pelvic pain [2, 3, 8]. Due to this psychological component of CPP, it is imperative that these needs are addressed in any treatment protocol. The patient should be receiving therapy from a mental health-care provider concurrent with medical and/or surgical intervention.

Physical Therapy and Other Nonmedical Therapies

For patients with myofascial trigger points, a program of physical therapy incorporating biofeedback and trigger point release has been shown to be helpful with alleviation of pain.

An NIH-funded trial of urologic symptoms of urinary urgency associated with CPP in men found that physical therapy was better than manual therapy for these symptoms [47].

There are some nontraditional treatments which have been shown also to be effective in relieving pelvic pain. Acupuncture, herbal and dietary therapies, biofeedback, physical therapy, and relaxation techniques have been used with some success [46]. The use of medical marijuana for chronic pain syndromes, such as CPP, has not been well studied, but many experts feel that there is promise with this treatment modality and preferred to the use of opiates for chronic pain [48].

There have been published reports that multispecialty clinics with providers specializing in chronic pain conditions has resulted in improvement in care for patients with other chronic pain syndromes [31]. Although this has not yet been proven to be beneficial for women with CPP, many organizations are recommending that women with CPP be referred to a pain specialized team for management of their challenging and multifocal disease with a multispecialty CPP clinic with physical and psychological therapists, gynecologists, urologists, and physical medicine specialists that can provide a patient with multiple resources for treatment [49].

References

1. Howard F. The role of laparoscopy in chronic pelvic pain: promise and pitfalls. Obstet Gynecol Surv. 1993;48:357–87.
2. Harrop-Griffiths J, Katon W, Walker E, Holm L, Russo J, Hickok L. The association between chronic pelvic pain, psychiatric diagnoses, and childhood sexual abuse. Obstet Gynecol. 1988;71:589–94.
3. Metzer-Brody S, et al. Psychiatric comorbidity in women with chronic pelvic pain. CNS Spectr. 2011;16:29–35.
4. Howard F. Pelvic pain. Diagn Manag. 2000;2–22.
5. Cheung, et al. Irritable bowel syndrome and chronic pelvic pain: a population-based study. J Clin Gastroenterol. 2010;44:696–701.
6. Bassaly L, et al. Myofascial pain and pelvic floor dysfunction in patients with interstitial cystitis. Int Urogynecol J. 2011;22:413–8.

7. Nickel JC, Tripp DA, et al. Clinical and psychological parameters associated with pain pattern phenotypes in women with interstitial cystitis/bladder pain syndrome. J Urol. 2015;193(1):138–44.
8. Fry R, Crisp A, Beard R, McGuigan S. Psychosocial aspects of chronic pelvic pain, with special reference to sexual abuse: a study of 164 women. Postgrad Med J. 1993;69:566–74.
9. Krohn PL. Intermenstrual pain ("the mittelschmerz") and the time of ovulation. Br Med J. 1949;1(4609):803–5.
10. Giudice LC, Kao LC. Endometriosis. Lancet. 2004;364:1789–99.
11. Bulun SE. Endometriosis. N Engl J Med. 2009;360:268–79.
12. Malinak LR, Buttram VC Jr, Elias S, Simpson JL. Heritage aspects of endometriosis. II. Clinical characteristics of familial endometriosis. Am J Obstet Gynecol. 1980;137:332–7.
13. Fauconnier A, Chapron C, Dubuisson JB, Vieira M, Dousset B, Breart G. Relation between pain symptoms and the anatomic location of deep infiltrating endometriosis. Fertil Steril. 2002;78:719–26.
14. Mehasseb MK, Habiba MA. Adenomyosis uteri: an update. Obstet Gynaecol. 2009;11:41–7.
15. Withagen MI. Risk factors for exposure, pain, and dyspareunia after tension-free vaginal mesh procedure. Obstet Gynecol. 2011;118(3):629–36.
16. Edwards L. Vulvodynia. Clin Obstet Gynecol. 2015;58(1):143–52.
17. Magtibay PM. Ovarian remnant syndrome. Clin Obstet Gynecol. 2006;49:526–34.
18. Dubin AK. Post-ablation tubal sterilization syndrome after radiofrequency endometrial ablation: a case report and thorough review of the literature. J Minim Invasive Gynecol. 2014;21(6):s136–7.
19. Berral JE, et al. Essure and chronic pelvic pain: a population based cohort. J Obstet Gynecol. 2014;34(8):712–3.
20. Tu F, et al. Musculoskeletal causes of chronic pelvic pain: a systematic review of diagnosis. Obstet Gynecol Surv. 2005;60:379–85.
21. Rane N, et al. Pelvic congestion syndrome. Curr Probl Diagn Radiol. 2013;42(4):135–40.
22. Carnett JB. Intercostal neuralgia as a cause of abdominal pain and tenderness. Surg Gynecol Obstet. 1926;42:625–32.
23. Prendergast S. Screening for myofascial causes of pelvic pain. Clin Obstet Gynecol. 2003;46(4):773–82.
24. Albrecht K. "How-To" guide to pelvic floor muscle dysfunction. Clin Obstet Gynecol. 2015;58(3):546–50.

25. Nisenblat V, et al. Imaging modalities for the non-invasive diagnosis of endometriosis. Cochrane Database Syst Rev. 2016;2:CDOO9591.
26. Gjelsteen AC, Chimg BH, Meyermann MW, et al. CT, MRI, PET, PET/CT and ultrasound in the evaluation of obstetric and gynecologic patients. Surg Clin North Am. 2008;88:361–90.
27. Brown J, Farquhar C. Endometriosis: an overview of Cochrane reviews. Cochrane Database Syst Rev. 2014:CDOO9590.
28. Holloran-Schwartz MB. Surgical evaluation and treatment of the patient with chronic pelvic pain. Obstet Gynecol Clin NA. 2014;41(3):357–69.
29. Hirsch M, Duffy JMN, Kusznir, et al. Variation in outcome reporting in endometriosis trials: a systematic review. Am J Obstet Gynecol. 2016;214(4):452–64.
30. Milburn A, Reiter RC, Rhomberg AT. Multidisciplinary approach to chronic pelvic pain. Obstet Gynecol. 1991;77:740–4.
31. Flor H, Fyrdich T, Turk DC. Efficacy of multidisciplinary pain treatment centers: a meta-analytic review. Pain. 1992;49:221–30.
32. Stones RW, Mountfield J. Interventions for treating chronic pelvic pain in women. Cochrane Database Syst Rev. 2000;(4):CDCOOO387.
33. Reiter R. Evidence-based management of chronic pelvic pain. Clin Obstet Gynecol. 1998;41:422–35.
34. Brawn J, Morotti M, Zondervan K, et al. Central changes associated with chronic pelvic pain and endometriosis. Hum Rep Update. 2014;20(5):737–47.
35. Cheong YC, Smotra G, et al. Non-surgical interventions for the management of chronic pelvic pain. Cochrane Database Syst Rev. 2014;3.
36. Parazzini F, Mais V, Cipriani S. Adhesions and pain in women with first diagnosis of endometriosis: results from a cross-sectional study. J Minim Invasive Gynecol. 2006;13:49–54.
37. Gerner-Rasmussen J, Burcharth J, Gogenur I. The efficacy of adhesiolysis on chronic abdominal pain: a systematic review. Langenbeck's Arch Surg. 2015;400(5):567–76.
38. Daniels J, Gray R, Hills RK, et al. Laparoscopic uterine nerve ablation for alleviating chronic pelvic pain: a randomized controlled trial. JAMA. 2009;302:955–61.
39. Daniels JP, Middleton L, Xiong T, et al. Individual patient data meta-analysis of randomized evidence to assess the effectiveness of laparoscopic uterine nerve ablation in patients with chronic pelvic pain. Hum Reprod Update. 2010;16:568–76.

40. Namnoum AB, Hickman TN, Goodman SB, Gehlbach DL, Rock JA. Incidence of symptom recurrence after hysterectomy for endometriosis. Fertil Steril. 1995;64:898–902.
41. Redwine DB. Endometriosis persisting after castration: clinical characteristics and results of surgical management. Obstet Gynecol. 1994;83:405–13.
42. Gambone JC, Reiter RC. Hysterectomy: improving the patient's decision-making process. Clin Obstet Gynecol. 1997;40:868–77.
43. Pedroso J, Sigala W, et al. Pathologic findings in women undergoing hysterectomy for pelvic pain. J Minim Invasive Gynecol. 2015;22(6):S232.
44. Lamvu G. Role of hysterectomy in the treatment of chronic pelvic pain. Obstet Gynecol. 2011;117(5):117501178.
45. Goodwin SC, Spies JB, et al. Uterine artery embolization for treatment of leiomyomata: longterm outcomes from the FIBROID registry. Obstet Gynecol. 2008;111:22–33.
46. Proctor ML, Murphy PA. Herbal and dietary therapies for primary and secondary dysmenorrhea. Cochrane Database Syst Rev. 2001;(3):CDOO2124.
47. Payne C, Fitzgerald MP, Burks D, Nickel JC, Lukacz E, Kreder K, Peters K. Randomized multicenter clinical trial shows efficacy of myofascial physical therapy in women with interstitial cystitis/painful bladder syndrome (ic/pbs). J Urol. 2010;183(4):e402–3.
48. Hill K. Medical marijuana for treatment of chronic pain and other medical and psychiatric problems: a clinical review. JAMA. 2015;313(24):2474–83.
49. Fali M, Baranowski AP, Elneil S, et al. EAU guidelines on chronic pelvic pain. Eur Urol. 2010;57(1):35–48.

Chapter 7
Follow-Up of Abnormal Pelvic Ultrasound

Joseph D. Calandra and Soraya Ong

Pelvic ultrasounds (US) are commonly ordered in the outpatient setting. In premenopausal women, pelvic scans are often performed for a variety of conditions. Uterine fibroids is a common diagnosis that is followed to assess for stability and /or growth. During these exams, incidental findings are frequently identified in the adnexa. What kind of follow-up, if any, should these incidentally discovered lesions have? This chapter aims to elucidate this.

All asymptomatic ovarian and other adnexal cysts imaged at US should be followed as per the SRU (Society of Radiologists in Ultrasound) consensus guidelines [1]. The SRU convened a multidisciplinary panel of specialists from gynecology, radiology, and pathology in order to arrive at this consensus statement that was drafted in October 2009 and released in 2010. The recommendations so drafted are based on current literature and common practice strategies.

The rationale for the SRU guidelines are as follows: First, pelvic US is the primary (and in most cases preferred) imaging modality to evaluate adnexal cysts. Second, most adnexal masses (90%) can be correctly categorized based on US features alone [2]. Third, most cystic adnexal masses are benign.

J. D. Calandra, MD, FACR (✉) · S. Ong, MD, DABR, DABNM
Presence Saint Francis Hospital, Department of Radiology, Evanston, IL, USA
e-mail: jcalandra@presencehealth.org

J. V. Knaus et al. (eds.), *Ambulatory Gynecology*,
https://doi.org/10.1007/978-1-4939-7641-6_7

TABLE 7.1 Inclusion and exclusion criteria for SRU consensus guidelines

Inclusion criteria	Exclusion criteria
Asymptomatic (without clinically detectable/palpable mass)	Symptomatic (with clinically detectable/palpable mass)
Nonpregnant	Pregnant
Adult (post-menarche)	Child (premenarche)
Ovarian or adnexal CYSTIC structure(s)/lesion(s)	Ovarian or adnexal SOLID structure(s)/lesion(s)

In fact, cystic adnexal masses fall into one of three groups: definitely benign, most probably malignant, and indeterminate. The following recommendations help to determine proper management of each of the three groups.

The SRU guidelines should only be utilized in the appropriate clinical setting, with inclusion and exclusion criteria applying (Table 7.1). Inclusion criteria include that the patient be asymptomatic (i.e., no clinically detectable/palpable mass), nonpregnant, and adult (post-menarchal) and have an ovarian or other adnexal CYSTIC structure(s)/lesion(s). Exclusion criteria include symptomatic patients (i.e., those with a clinically detectable/palpable mass), pregnant patients, children/pediatric population (premenarchal), or those that have SOLID ovarian/adnexal mass(es).

When ordering pelvic US for such women, and in general, the more clinical information provided to the radiologist, the more helpful. This should include at minimum the patient's age, last menstrual period (LMP), pregnancy status, menopausal status, and of course the indication(s) for the exam. Additional helpful information would include the patient's hormonal status (if they are on any oral contraceptive pills, hormone replacement therapy, fertility drugs, etc.), personal or family history of cancer, history of prior pelvic surgery, and/or results of prior imaging studies.

One of the most important parameters that must be specified, in order to appropriately manage these women, is their menopausal status. A postmenopausal woman is defined, as per the SRU criteria, as one who has had 1 or more year(s) of amenorrhea since her last LMP. Postmenopausal women are further subcategorized to those who are in early menopause (1–5 since LMP) vs. late menopause (>5 years since LMP). The second important parameter in regard to analyzing these ovarian/adnexal masses is size. As per the SRU guidelines, the MAXIMUM size of the lesion is the relevant size to be used in the algorithm. Finally, the ovarian/adnexal lesion is analyzed in regard to its specific sonographic appearance toward the aim of defining its exact etiology (if possible) and need for further follow-up.

The SRU guidelines, then, in regard to management of asymptomatic ovarian and other adnexal cysts imaged at US are as follows [1]:

Normal and Benign Cysts

Simple Cysts (Includes Ovarian and Extra-/Para-ovarian Cysts)

Sonographic features are round or oval, thin, smooth walls, anechoic, no septation(s) or solid component(s), posterior acoustic enhancement, and no internal blood flow.

Premenopausal

Smaller than or equal to 5 cm – no follow-up needed (represent physiologic developing follicles and dominant follicles); in fact, those that are smaller than or equal to 3 cm may or may not be described in the US report, as per the discretion of the interpreting physician (Fig. 7.1).

5 cm and smaller than or equal to 7 cm – yearly US (Fig. 7.2).

+ = all figures are obtained from reference [1] unless otherwise stated.

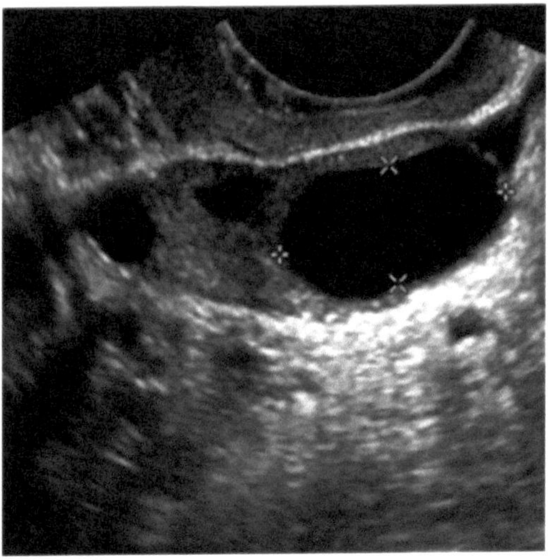

Fig. 7.1 Physiologic follicle. In premenopausal women, physiologic follicles measuring up to 5 cm in maximum size do not need US follow-up

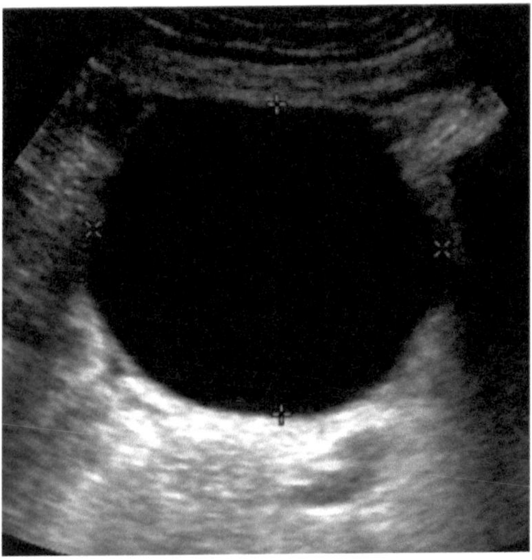

Fig. 7.2 Simple ovarian or extra-/para-ovarian cysts. Follow-up of these is based upon menopausal status and maximum size

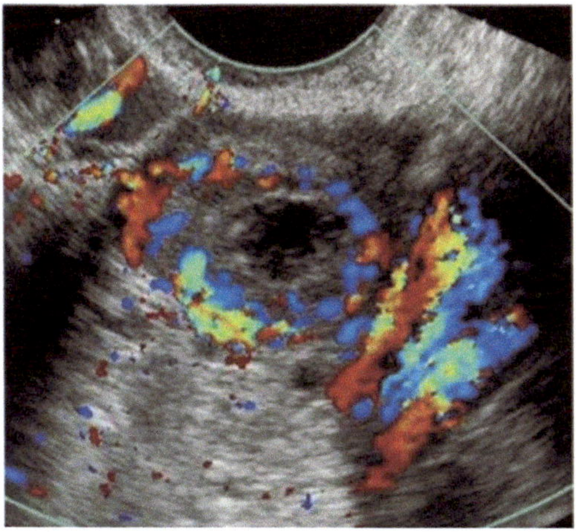

FIG. 7.3 Simple cyst smaller than or equal to 1 cm in postmenopausal woman. No US follow-up is needed as these are considered clinically insignificant

Postmenopausal

Smaller than or equal to 1 cm no follow-up needed (considered clinically insignificant) (Fig. 7.3).

Larger than 1 cm and smaller than or equal to 7 cm – yearly US* (Fig. 7.2).

* = some practices may choose a threshold size slightly higher than 1 cm before recommending yearly follow-up. Practices may choose to decrease the frequency of follow-up once stability or decrease in size has been confirmed.

Any Age

Larger than 7 cm further imaging (e.g., MRI) or surgical evaluation (Fig. 7.2)

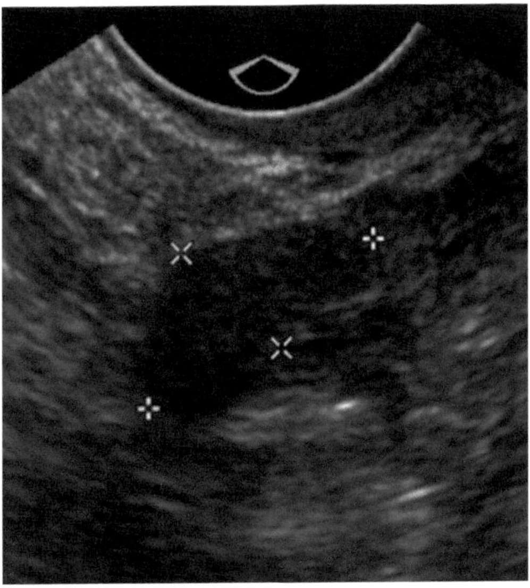

FIG. 7.4 Corpus luteum. In premenopausal women, these physiologic structures do not need US follow-up

Corpus Luteum (Fig. 7.4)

Sonographic features: size smaller than or equal to 3 cm, diffusely thick wall, ± internal echoes, ± crenulated appearance, peripheral blood flow.

Premenopausal: no follow-up needed (normal, physiologic finding).

Postmenopausal: this structure should not be seen in a postmenopausal woman and a similar appearing structure would be worrisome for malignancy. Surgical evaluation should be considered.

Postmenopausal Ovary (Fig. 7.5)

Sonographic features: small, homogeneous, without follicles

Follow-up: none needed

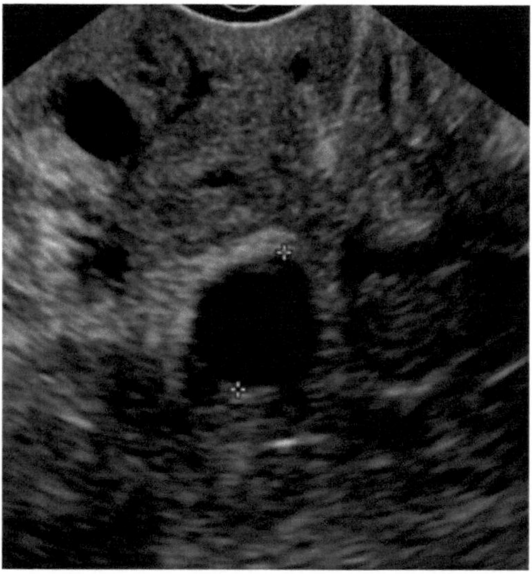

Fig. 7.5 Normal postmenopausal ovary. Normal postmenopausal ovaries are atrophic, homogeneous, and without follicles. They do not need US follow-up

Hemorrhagic Cyst (Fig. 7.6)

Sonographic features: reticular pattern of internal echoes, ± solid-appearing area with concave margins, no internal flow

Premenopausal

Smaller than or equal to 5 cm – no follow-up needed (those ≤3 cm may or may not be described in the US report, as per the discretion of the interpreting physician)

Larger than 5 cm – 6–12-week follow-up US to ensure resolution

Early Postmenopausal (1–5 Years Since LMP)

Any size: follow-up US to ensure resolution

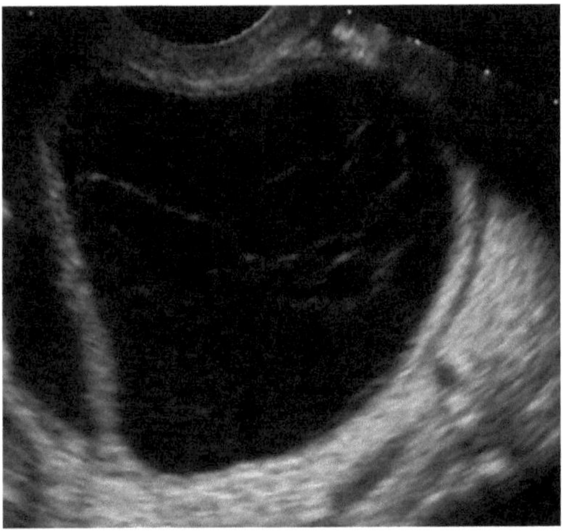

Fig. 7.6 Hemorrhagic cyst. Follow-up recommendations are based on menopausal status and maximum size

Late Postmenopausal (>5 Years Since LMP)

Consider surgical evaluation.

Endometrioma (Fig. 7.7)

Sonographic features: homogeneous low-level internal echoes, no solid component, ± tiny echogenic foci in wall

Any age: initial follow-up in 6–12 weeks, then if not surgically removed, yearly US follow-up

Dermoid (Fig. 7.8)

Sonographic features: focal or diffuse hyperechoic component, hyperechoic lines and dots, area of acoustic shadowing, no internal flow

Any age: if not surgically removed, yearly US follow-up to ensure stability

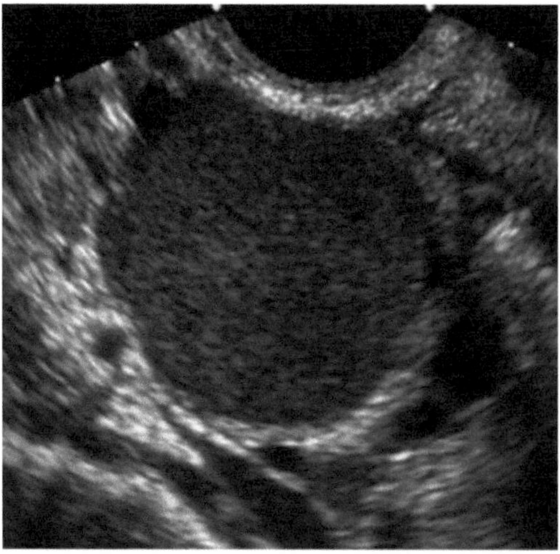

Fig. 7.7 Endometrioma. For any age, an initial follow-up US is recommended in 6–12 weeks; then if not surgically removed, yearly follow-up US

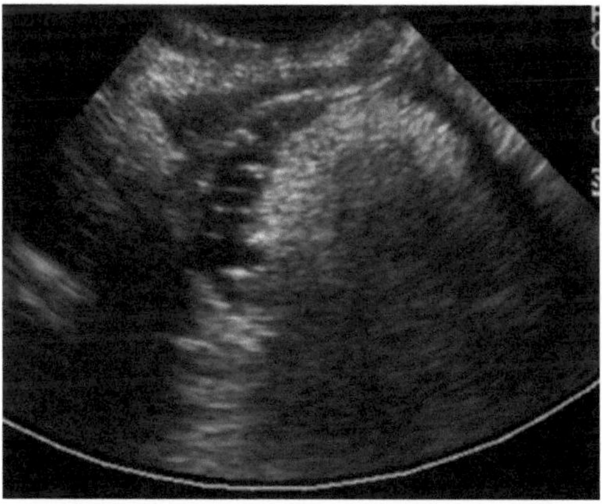

Fig. 7.8 Dermoid. For any age, if not surgically removed, yearly follow-up US is recommended to ensure stability

Hydrosalpinx (Fig. 7.9)

Sonographic features: tubular-shaped cystic mass, ± short round projections "beads on string," ± waist sign (i.e., indentations on opposite sides), ± seen separate from the ovary

Any age: as clinically indicated

Peritoneal Inclusion Cyst (Fig. 7.10)

Sonographic features: follow the contour of adjacent pelvic organs, ovary at the edge of the mass or suspended within the mass, ± septations.

Any age: as clinically indicated.

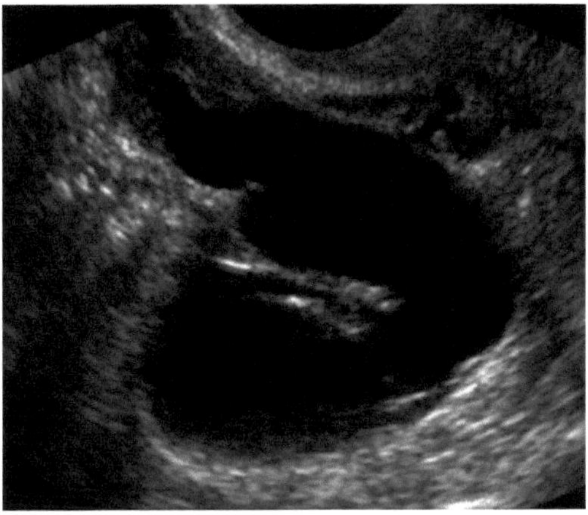

FIG. 7.9 Hydrosalpinx. For any age, follow-up is as clinically indicated

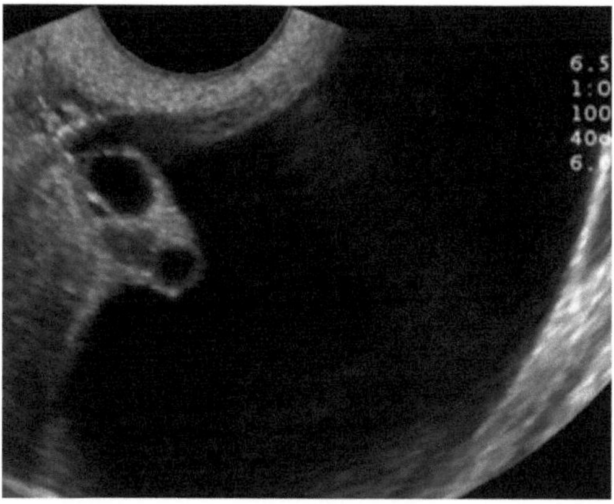

FIG. 7.10 Peritoneal inclusion cyst. For any age, follow-up is as clinically indicated

Cysts with Indeterminate, but Probably Benign, Characteristics

Findings Suggestive of, but Not Classic for, Hemorrhagic Cyst, Endometrioma, or Dermoid (Fig. 7.11)

Premenopausal: 6–12-week follow-up US to ensure resolution. If the lesion is unchanged, then hemorrhagic cyst is unlikely, and continued follow up with either US or MRI should then be considered. If these studies do not confirm an endometrioma or dermoid, then surgical evaluation should be considered.

Postmenopausal: consider surgical evaluation.

Thin-Walled Cyst with Single Thin Septation or Focal Calcification in the Wall of a Cyst (Fig. 7.12)

Management is the same as for a simple cyst, based on menopausal status and size.

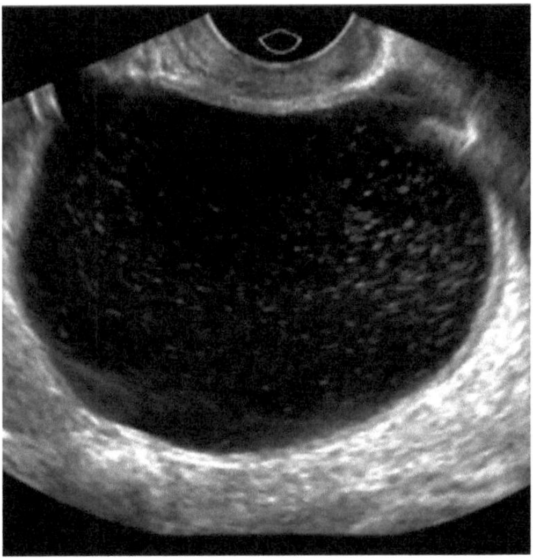

FIG. 7.11 Findings suggestive of, but not classic for, hemorrhagic cyst, endometrioma, or dermoid. For premenopausal women, 6–12-week follow-up US is recommended to ensure resolution. If the lesion is unchanged, then hemorrhagic cyst is unlikely, and continued follow-up with either US or MRI should then be considered. If these studies do not confirm an endometrioma or dermoid, then surgical evaluation should be considered. For postmenopausal women, surgical evaluation should be considered

Premenopausal

Smaller than or equal to 5 cm – no follow-up needed (represent physiologic developing follicles and dominant follicles); in fact, those that are ≤3 cm may or may not be described in the US report, as per the discretion of the interpreting physician

Larger than 5 cm and smaller than or equal to 7 cm – yearly US

Postmenopausal

Smaller than or equal to 1 cm – no follow-up needed (considered clinically insignificant).

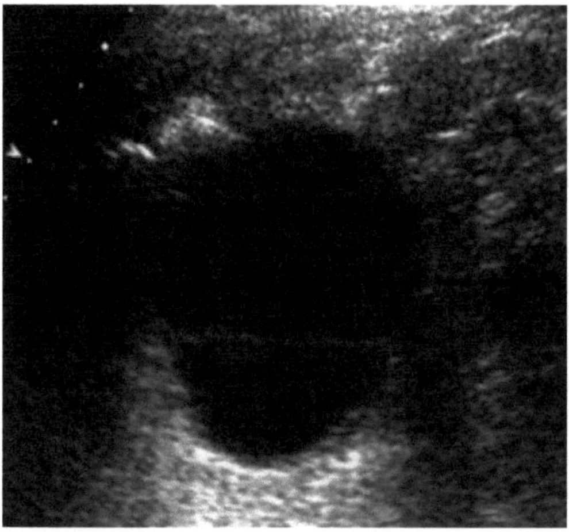

FIG. 7.12 Thin-walled cyst with single thin septation (as in this picture) or focal calcification in the wall of a cyst. The management is identical to that for simple cysts and is based upon menopausal status and maximum size of the cyst

Larger than 1 cm and smaller than or equal to 7 cm – yearly US*.

* = some practices may choose a threshold size slightly higher than 1 cm before recommending yearly follow-up. Practices may choose to decrease the frequency of follow-up once stability or decrease in size has been confirmed.

Any Age

Larger than 7 cm – further imaging (e.g., MRI) or surgical evaluation

Multiple Thin Septations (thinner than 3 mm) (Fig. 7.13)

Any age: consider surgical evaluation.

Comments: multiple septations suggest a neoplasm, but if thin, the neoplasm is likely benign.

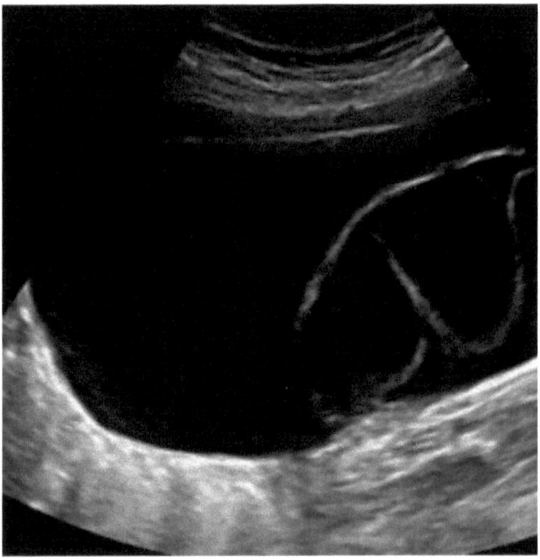

FIG. 7.13 Multiple thin septations (thinner than 3 mm). Surgical evaluation should be considered

Nodule (Non-hyperechoic) Without Flow (Fig. 7.14)

Any age: consider surgical evaluation or MRI.

Comments: solid nodule suggests neoplasm, but if no flow (and not echogenic as would be seen in a dermoid), this is likely a benign lesion such as a cystadenofibroma.

Cysts with Characteristics Worrisome for Malignancy

Thick (thicker than 3 mm), Irregular Septations (Fig. 7.15)

Any age: consider surgical evaluation.

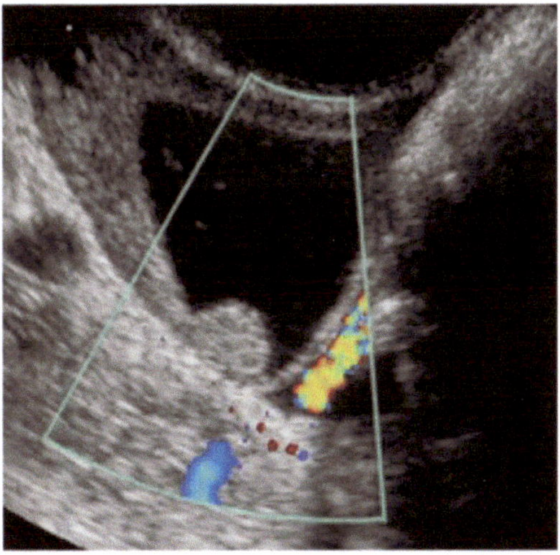

Fig. 7.14 Nodule (non-hyperechoic) without blood flow. Surgical evaluation or MRI should be considered

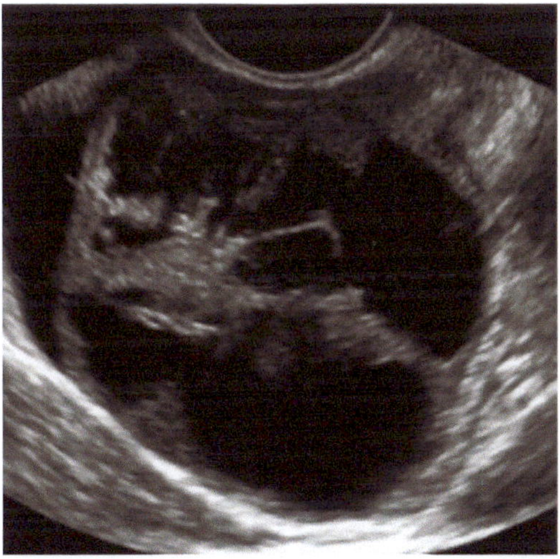

Fig. 7.15 Thick (thicker than 3 mm), irregular septations. Surgical evaluation should be considered

Nodule with Blood Flow (Fig. 7.16)

Any age: consider surgical evaluation.

A practice quality improvement (PQI) project was undertaken at our institution in an attempt to standardize the radiologists' usage of the SRU criteria in the appropriate clinical setting. Prior to introducing the SRU criteria to the diagnostic radiology residents at our program, 50 cases were reviewed that met the inclusion criteria for the SRU criteria. The US images and reports were reviewed, and their compliance with the SRU criteria determined.

Of the 50 cases reviewed, there was a compliance of only 50% with the SRU criteria initially. Of these 25 noncompliant cases, 22 cases (88%) involved overaggressive management recommendations of incidentally discovered ovarian/cysts by the radiologists, while 3 cases (12%) involved under-aggressive management recommendations. The most common entities for which overaggressive management was recommended were for physiologic simple cysts (with or without thin, single

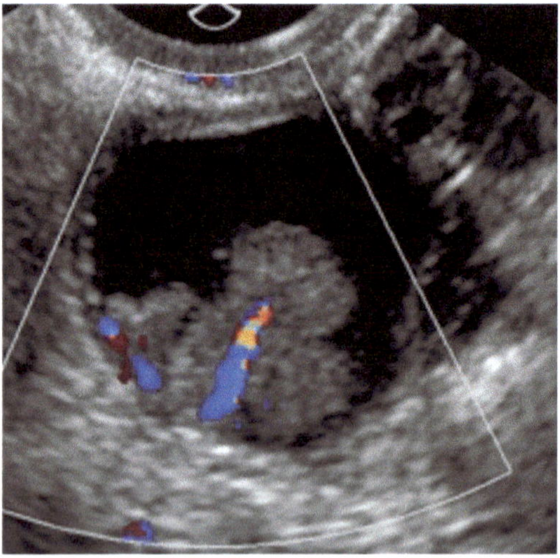

FIG. 7.16 Nodule with blood flow. Surgical evaluation should be considered

septations) in premenopausal women (13 cases), followed by hemorrhagic cysts in premenopausal women (4 cases), and corpus luteum in premenopausal women (4 cases). For all of these cases, some kind of US follow-up was recommended even though none was necessary. In the remaining case, a 3-month follow-up US was recommended for a postmenopausal woman with a cyst larger than 1 cm in size with a thin, single septation (SRU recommendation: yearly US follow-up).

Interestingly, 3 of the 25 noncompliant cases actually involved under-aggressive management recommendations by the radiologists. One of the cases involved a complex cyst with internal echoes which was not classic for either a hemorrhagic cyst, endometrioma, or dermoid in a postmenopausal woman. The radiologist recommended a 3–6-month follow-up US when in fact surgical consultation should have been recommended. In a second case, a larger than 1 cm simple cyst was found in a postmenopausal woman. The radiologist did not recommend any follow-up when in fact a yearly follow-up US should have been recommended. The final case involved a cyst that had a thick wall in a postmenopausal woman. The radiologist recommended US follow-up in 3 months. While this specific entity is not addressed in the SRU recommendations, it also does not fit into either the "normal and benign cysts" or "cysts with indeterminate, but probably benign, characteristics" categories, and therefore perhaps more aggressive management, for example, surgical consultation, should have been recommended, especially given the patient's postmenopausal status.

Following the initial pre-intervention data gathering, the SRU criteria were introduced to the diagnostic radiology residents in the format of a PQI project, and a binder made available to them that had all of the pertinent SRU recommendations in an easily available quick reference format. Again, 50 cases meeting the SRU inclusion criteria were reviewed and their compliance with the SRU criteria determined. Compliance with the SRU criteria was 60%, an improvement from 50% prior to the PQI intervention. Of the

20 noncompliant cases, 14 cases (70%) involved overaggressive management recommendations, while 6 cases (30%) involved under-aggressive management recommendations.

The 14 cases involving overaggressive management recommendations included simple cysts (seven cases), hemorrhagic cysts (four cases), and corpus luteum (three cases). In these cases, either follow-up US was recommended when none was needed, US was recommended at a greater frequency than recommended by the SRU guidelines, or MRI was recommended when it was not warranted.

The six cases involving under-aggressive management recommendations included three dermoid cysts, one endometrioma in a premenopausal woman which was being followed up, one solid para-ovarian lesion, and a cyst with a thickened, nodular septation without vascularity. For the dermoid cysts, the radiologist recommended either no follow-up (one case) or MRI follow-up (two cases). The SRU recommendation is initally for surgical removal, and if this is not done, then yearly US follow-up is recommended. For the endometrioma, either a US in 6 months or MRI was recommended. As per the SRU guidelines, endometriomas that do not resolve after initial 6–12-week follow-up should be surgically removed, and if this is not done, then annual US follow-up is recommended. For the solid para-ovarian lesion, an MRI was recommended when, as per SRU guidelines, surgical consultation should have been recommended. Finally, for the cyst with a thickened, nodular septation without vascularity, a follow-up US was recommended (with no interval specified), when in fact either MRI or surgical evaluation should have been recommended.

In analyzing the results of the PQI project, clearly the tendency is for radiologists to make over – rather than under-aggressive recommendations in regard to incidentally discovered ovarian/adnexal cystic lesions. While the percentage of overaggressive recommendations decreased post-intervention, they still made up the overwhelming majority of cases that were noncompliant with the SRU recommendations. This tendency can be attributed to the current litigious environment in which physicians, radiologists included, must practice. Many radiologists would rather err on the side of caution and be overly aggressive in their management recommendations, especially in regard to follow-up imaging, than risk "missing" something that later turns out to be an ovarian neoplasm, for example. However, as evidenced by the results of our institution's PQI project, all of the cases that were managed in an overly aggressive manner fell clearly into the category of "normal and benign cysts" and should have been managed as such.

On the other hand, sometimes radiologists also made less aggressive management recommendations than warranted by the SRU guidelines. This was especially true when the management recommendation was for either surgical consultation for, or surgical removal of, the respective lesions. Perhaps this can be accounted for by the reticence of radiologists to make clinical recommendations as it is not considered to be within their realm of expertise. While radiologists do not have an issue recommending imaging follow-up (in many cases in an overly aggressive manner as previously described), there is hesitance on many radiologists' part to tie the hands of clinicians, by committing patients to surgical management, based upon imaging findings alone. However, it must be remembered that the SRU guidelines are not made by radiologists alone but is in fact a consensus statement that involves input from gynecologists and pathologists as well. This should mitigate radiologists' fear of recommending surgical consultation or surgical removal when these are the appropriate management recommendations for indeterminate or suspicious ovarian/adnexal cystic lesions.

In conclusion, with the preponderance of pelvic US examinations that are ordered in the ambulatory gynecologic setting, the management of incidentally discovered ovarian/adnexal cysts should be based upon the 2010 SRU Consensus Statement. Every attempt should be made to encourage clinicians and radiologists alike to follow these recommendations. Along the same lines, your local radiologists should be encouraged to review the article by Brown DL et al. entitled *Adnexal Masses: US Characterization and Reporting* [2], which details distinguishing US features of benign vs. malignant ovarian/adnexal lesions. By following the SRU recommendations, both overaggressive and under-aggressive management tendencies by radiologists can be reduced. By avoiding overaggressive management, unnecessary additional imaging, patient anxiety, and healthcare costs can be reduced by appropriate categorization of the lesions as normal, benign, or indeterminate but probably benign. Similarly, by avoiding under-aggressive management, the patient can be appropriately directed toward more specific imaging techniques (e.g., MRI) or for surgical consultation/removal for sonographically suspicious lesions.

References

1. Levine D, et al. Management of asymptomatic ovarian and other adnexal cysts imaged at US: society of radiologists in ultrasound consensus conference statement. Radiology. 2010;256(3):943–54.
2. Brown DL, et al. Adnexal masses: US characterization and reporting. Radiology. 2010;254(2):342–54.

Chapter 8
Evaluation of the Adnexal Mass

John V. Knaus and Kevin Ward

Introduction

Patients found to have a pelvic adnexal mass in the ambulatory setting are most often asymptomatic or minimally symptomatic. Rather than the need for urgent surgical management common in patients with acute pelvic symptomatology, patients with an adnexal mass in the ambulatory setting more often require quantification of the risk of malignancy or a structured plan for surveillance (Table 8.1). Refinements in ultrasound diagnostics (adnexal mass morphology, color flow Doppler), serum tumor markers, multivariate index assays, and genetic testing, when appropriate, have all become useful in the assessment of an adnexal mass.

J. V. Knaus (✉)
Department of Obstetrics and Gynecology, University of Illinois at Chicago, Chicago, IL, USA

Chief, Gynecologic Oncology, Presence Saint Francis Hospital, Evanston, IL, USA
e-mail: jknaus@presencehealth.org

K. Ward
Presence Saint Francis Hospital, Department of Obstetrics and Gynecology, Evanston, IL, USA

J. V. Knaus et al. (eds.), *Ambulatory Gynecology*,
https://doi.org/10.1007/978-1-4939-7641-6_8

TABLE 8.1 Adnexal mass differential

Physiologic cysts
Follicle cyst
Corpus luteal cyst
Hemorrhagic ovarian cyst
Endometrioma
Mature cystic teratoma (dermoid)
Adnexal torsion
Ectopic pregnancy
Tubo-ovarian abscess
Hydrosalpinx
Broad ligament myoma
Ovarian/tubal malignancy
Non-gynecologic disease

Incidence, Age Distribution, and Family History

Up to 20% of women will be diagnosed with an adnexal mass during their lifetime. The majority of these adnexal masses will be ovarian in origin. Neoplastic adnexal masses in children and adolescents are uncommon. Hermans et al. [1] reported incidence rates of adnexal masses increase from 0.43 per 100,000 women per year at age 1 to 152 per 100,000 women per year by age 35. Benign cysts in girls less than a year old had an incidence of 5.70 per 100,000 girls per year. The incidence of benign tumors increased with age, from 0.34 at age 2 to 4.38 by age 12. Malignant tumors also increased with age 0.04 to 0.85 per 100,000 through age 12. In this same report of 11,595 patients from birth to age 29, histologic diagnoses were evenly distributed between surface epithelial lesions (35.1%), germ cell tumors (29.8%), and other cysts, tumors, and tumorlike lesions (32.8%). Sex cord stromal tumors were rare, representing only 2.3%. With advancing age, Koonings et al. [2] report the rate of ovarian malignancy to increase from 4% in women 20–29 years of age to 46% in women 50–59 years of age to 49% in women 60–69 years of age.

All providers of gynecologic health care are aware of the importance of hereditary cancer risk assessment. Personal and first-degree relative accurate cancer history is most important (exact histology, age, maternal/paternal, etc.). A strong family history of breast and/or ovarian cancer may indicate a familial syndrome of these cancers not a sporadic individual case. A 35-year-old woman with one ovarian cancer affected first-degree relative has her lifetime risk of ovarian cancer increase from 1.6% to 5% [3]. Women with BRCA1 or a BRCA2 mutation incur a 40–46% and 10–27% incidence of ovarian cancer by age 70, respectively. Lynch syndrome patients may incur a 10–24% lifetime risk of ovarian cancer.

Quantification of Risk of Malignancy

Refinements in imaging (primarily ultrasound, but selectively in CT and MRI), serum tumor markers, and multivariate index assays have combined to stratify most adnexal masses as to risk of malignancy with considerable accuracy. Multiple ovarian cancer screening trials [4, 5] and years of published observations have resulted in a significantly more accurate ultrasound characterization of adnexal masses primarily by tumor morphology and color flow Doppler. Currently interpretation of ovarian and adnexal abnormalities on ultrasound should rarely report a mass as indeterminate. Ultrasound reports should confidently characterize and report an ovarian mass as benign or malignant [6].

Purely unilocular ovarian cysts in postmenopausal women, even up to 10 cm in diameter, whether removed surgically or observed conservatively to spontaneous resolution, are essentially all benign [7, 8]. The risk of malignancy in septated ovarian cysts is also extremely low [9]. Serous and mucinous

cystadenomas and endometriosis are the most common histopathologies found at surgery in these patients. Patients with mixed cystic and solid masses, purely solid masses, cystic masses with internal papillary projections greater than 3mm or ascites are at high risk of having a malignancy. Serum tumor marker and/or multivariate index assay testing may further increase the suspicion of malignancy and the need for referral to a gynecologic oncologist.

Regarded as landmark, Timmerman et al. [10] in 2016 published their updated criteria for the quantification of the risk of malignancy of ovarian masses based on the *Simple Rules* described by the International Ovarian Tumor Analysis (IOTA) group. These *Simple Rules* are based on ten ultrasound characteristics (five benign, five malignant). The study is the culmination of multiple consecutive multicenter studies involving 24 centers in 10 countries from 1999 to 2012 reporting on more than 5000 patients with ovarian masses. In its most recent iteration, ovarian masses noted to be inconclusive or indeterminate by the *Simple Rules* (a major predictive flaw of many past ovarian risks of malignancy algorithms) are classified as malignant. This ultrasound method currently appears to accurately diagnose 94–97% of malignant ovarian masses. Current evidence indicates MRI is no more accurate or sensitive than a properly interpreted ultrasound [6].

The IOTA group and others (ADNEX model [11]) currently are developing risk prediction models that can differentiate ovarian tumor pathology, including borderline, early vs late stage invasive ovarian cancer and non-gynecologic ovarian metastasis.

Serum Biomarkers and Multivariate Index Assay

The multivariate index assay OVA1 (a serum tumor marker panel) and HE4 (human epididymis protein 4) have emerged as the most useful biomarkers in assessing the malignant potential of an adnexal mass. CA125, the most studied and ordered biomarker when an adnexal mass is detected, has clear limitations. CA125 is expressed in only 80% of epithelial ovarian cancers and in only 50% of stage I ovarian cancers. It is not reliably expressed in premenopausal women with ovarian cancer, particularly ovarian mucinous, clear cell, or mixed histology tumors. Additionally, CA125 may be misleadingly elevated in benign gynecologic or non-gynecologic conditions (adenomyosis, endometriosis, pelvic inflammatory disease, pancreatitis, diverticulitis, liver disease). In postmenopausal women with ovarian cancer, sensitivity, specificity, and PPV are reported as 69–87%, 81–100%, 73–100%, respectively. Adding CA125 to ultrasound diagnostics usually does not improve discrimination between benign and malignant adnexal masses [12].

Human epididymis protein 4 (HE4) is present in the sera of patients with epithelial ovarian cancer (more so serous and endometrioid histology, less so mucinous, and germ cell). The risk of malignancy algorithm (ROMA) combines HE4 and CA125. HE4 alone or within ROMA may not increase the accuracy of detection of ovarian malignancy more than CA125 alone [13].

OVA1 is a biomarker panel that incorporates five proteins: beta 2 microglobulin, transferrin, transthyretin, apolipoprotein A-1, and CA 125-II. The test has FDA approval to assess risk of malignancy in an ovarian tumor and to facilitate the appropriate referral of high-risk patients to a gynecologic oncologist. Results are reported from 0 to 10 with premenopausal and postmenopausal numeric thresholds reported for risk of malignancy.

Overall, the sensitivity of OVA1 is 99% for epithelial ovarian cancer, 82% for nonepithelial ovarian malignancies, and 75% for borderline ovarian tumors. Compared with CA 125 alone or CA 125 with physical exam, OVA1 correctly detects more ovarian cancers in premenopausal women as well as more early stage ovarian cancers. Most important in giving complete informed consent, OVA1 is associated with a negative predictive value of 98% in postmenopausal women [13]. A second-generation multivariate index assay (Overa®) has been validated [14]. Specificity and PPV are both improved in this second-generation test.

Clinical Algorithm Summary

An updated history and current physical exam are always appropriate when assessing or following an adnexal mass.

van Nagell Jr. and Miller [13] have proposed the following:

1. Unilocular and septated cystic ovarian tumors without symptoms have an extraordinarily low risk of malignancy and can be followed without surgery by periodic ultrasound examinations only. These authors recommend an initial follow-up ultrasound in 3 months. Thereafter, repeat ultrasound examinations are done annually for 5 years.
2. Complex or solid ovarian tumors should undergo secondary evaluation with serum biomarkers and tumor Doppler blood flow study. High-risk results of these tests mandate referral to a gynecologic oncologist.
3. Ovarian tumors of indeterminate character undergo ultrasound and serum biomarker retesting every 4 weeks for 3 months. Evidence of tumor progression mandates referral to a gynecologic oncologist.

Panels of biomarkers and now with validation of a second-generation multivariate index assay (Overa®) with improved specificity and PPV (unchanged sensitivity and NPV) will continue to increase the diagnostic accuracy of the risk of malignancy in patients presenting with an adnexal mass.

References

1. Herman AJ, Kluivers KB, Janssen LM, et al. Adnexal masses in children, adolescents and women of reproductive age in the Netherlands: a nationwide population-based cohort study. Gynecol Oncol. 2016;143:93–7.
2. Koonings PP, Campbell K, Mishell DR Jr, Grimes DA. Relative frequency of primary ovarian neoplasms: a 10- year review. Obstet Gynecol. 1989;74:921–6.
3. Kerlikowske K, Brown JS, Grady DR. Should women with familial ovarian cancer undergo prophylactic oophorectomy? Obstet Gynecol. 1992;80:700–7.

4. van Nagell JR Jr, Miller RW, De Simone C, Ueland FR, Podzielinski I, Goodrich S, et al. Long-term survival of women with epithelial ovarian cancer detected by ultrasoungraphic screening. Obstet Gynecol. 2011;118:1212–21.
5. Sharma A, Apostolidou S, Burnell M, Campbell S, Habib M, Gentry-Maharaj A, et al. Risk of epithelial ovarian cancer in asymptomatic women with ultrasound-detected ovarian masses: a prospective cohort study within the UK collaborative trial of ovarian cancer screening (UKCTOCS). Ultrasound Onstet Gynecol. 2012;40:338–44.
6. Benacerraf BR. Ultrasonic diagnosis of ovarian masses: can the playing field be leveled and raised at the same time? Am J Obstet Gynecol. 2016;127:419–20.
7. Baily CL, Ueland FR, Land GL, DePriest PD, Gallion HH, Kryscio RJ, van Nagell JR Jr. The malignant potential of small cystic ovarian tumors in women over 50 years of age. Gynecol Oncol. 1998;69:3–7.
8. Modesitt SC, Pavlik EJ, Ueland FR, van Nagell JR Jr. Risk of malignancy in unicocular ovarian cystic tumors less than 10 cm in diameter. Obstet Gynecol. 2003;102:594–9.
9. Saunders BA, Pidzielinski I, Ware RA, Goodrich S, DeSimone CP, Ueland FR, et al. Risk of malignancy in sonographically confirmed septated cystic ovarian tumors. Gynecl Oncol. 2010;188:278–82.
10. Timmerman D, Calster B, Testa A, et al. Predicting the risk of malignancy in adnexal masses based on the *Simple Rules* from the international ovarian tumor analysis group. Am J Obstet Gynecol. 2016;201:424–37.
11. Van Calster B, Van Hoorde K, Froyman W, et al. Practical guidance for applying the ADNEX model from the IOTA group to discriminate between different subtypes of adnexal tumors. Facts Views Vis Obgyn. 2015;7:32–41.
12. Timmerman D, Van Calster B, Jurkovic D, et al. Inclusion of CA-125 does not improve mathematical models developed to distinguish between benign and malignant adnexal tumors. J Clin Oncol. 2007;25:4194–200.
13. van Nagell JR, Miller RW Jr, et al. Evaluation and management of ultrasonographically detected ovarian tumors in asymptomatic women. Obstet Gynecol. 2016;127:848–58.
14. Coleman RL, Herzog TJ, Chan DW, et al. Validation of a second-generation multivariate index assay for malignancy risk of adnexal masses. Am J Obstet Gynecol. 2016;215:e1–11.

Chapter 9
Management of Ectopic Pregnancy

Maria B. Thomas and Jennifer Ozan

A reproductive age female presenting with pelvic pain, a positive urine pregnancy test, and an inconclusive pelvic ultrasound provokes diagnostic uncertainty and anxiety for the practicing physician. The spectrum of diagnostic possibilities ranges from a symptomatic but normally implanted pregnancy to an ectopic pregnancy implanted in the uterine tube or elsewhere outside of the uterus. While management of the patient with acute symptoms clearly calls for urgent surgical intervention, management of the asymptomatic patient whose implantation site is indeterminate requires patient follow-up with serial serum HCG levels, periodic ultrasound imaging, and repeat physical examinations. The clinician must cope with the risk of possible rupture of an ectopic pregnancy and its associated morbidities. Pregnancy of unknown location accounts for 1–2% of all gestations and 4–6% of pregnancy-related deaths worldwide [1]. This chapter will describe a current approach to the diagnosis and management of ectopic pregnancy.

M. B. Thomas (✉)
Kaiser Permanente Signal Hill Medical Offices, Department of Obstetrics and Gynecology, Signal Hill, CA, USA
e-mail: Maria.b.thomas@kp.org

J. Ozan
Women's Hospital-Cone Health, Department of Obstetrics and Gynecology, Greensboro, NC, USA

J. V. Knaus et al. (eds.), *Ambulatory Gynecology*,
https://doi.org/10.1007/978-1-4939-7641-6_9

Symptoms

The most common symptoms of an ectopic pregnancy include pelvic pain, missed menses, and vaginal spotting. Any reproductive age female who presents with abnormal vaginal bleeding must have a pregnancy test. A leaking or ruptured ectopic pregnancy may produce right upper quadrant or shoulder pain.

Physical Examination

Physical examination of the abdomen and pelvis in a patient with a suspected ectopic pregnancy may elicit variable degrees of pain. Vague, nonspecific findings are notoriously common among women with ectopic pregnancies. Rebound abdominal tenderness or cervical motion tenderness suggests peritoneal irritation from the presence of blood in the peritoneal cavity. Shock-like vital signs and acutely worsening abdominal and pelvic pain symptoms suggest rupture.

Risk Factors

Risk factors for ectopic pregnancy include prior ectopic pregnancy, history of infertility, history of sexually transmitted infection, smoking, increased age, previous miscarriage, previous pregnancy termination, prior pelvic or abdominal surgery, endometriosis, or conceiving while having an intrauterine device in place or being pregnant in spite of having a tubal ligation [1, 2].

Diagnostic Testing (See Fig. 9.1)

Serial Serum HCG

Ideally, human chorionic gonadotropin levels in a normal early pregnancy doubles every 48 h. However, this is not

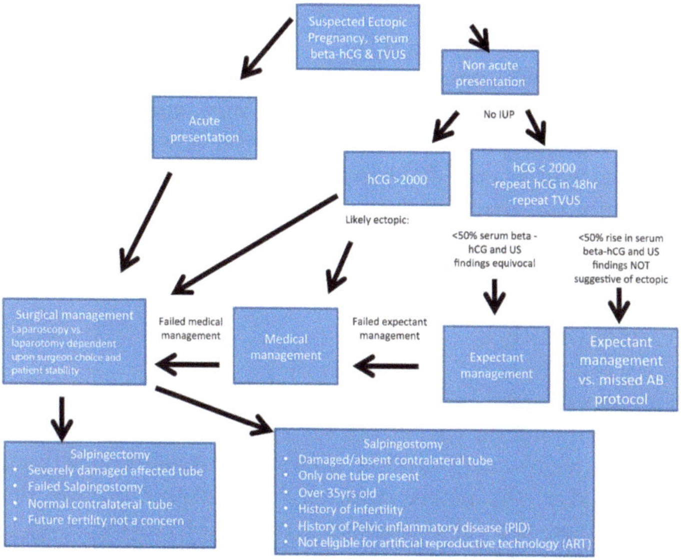

FIG. 9.1 Ectopic pregnancy management algorithm

always the case even in a normal intrauterine pregnancy, and an early ectopic pregnancy may double at this rate. HCG levels used in combination with transvaginal ultrasound comprise the gold standard for diagnosing ectopic pregnancy. A beta HCG level of greater than 1500–2000 IU/L is often referred to as the "discriminatory zone." A normally implanted pregnancy with HCG levels in this range should be visible in the uterine cavity by transvaginal sonography. However, the absence of a visible intrauterine sac on transvaginal ultrasound does not rule out the possibility of a normally implanted pregnancy but warrants further follow-up and evaluation.

Progesterone Levels

A serum progesterone level may be of some value in differentiating a normal viable pregnancy from a failing pregnancy. A serum value of 3.2–6 ng/ml has been reported as being predictive of a nonviable pregnancy [1]. In practice, the utility of serum progesterone levels in the diagnosis and management of ectopic pregnancy remains limited.

Ultrasound

Findings suggestive of an ectopic pregnancy include absence of an intrauterine gestational sac or the combination of an empty uterine cavity with an adnexal mass, with or without free fluid in the pelvis. Adnexal findings may include the appearance of a tubal ring, often referred to as the "bagel" sign or "ring of fire" sign. Visualization of an embryo with or without cardiac activity external to the uterine cavity is diagnostic of the presence of an ectopic pregnancy.

Treatment Options

Urgent surgical management is the standard of care for a hemodynamically unstable patient. Surgery is also the standard of care for the patient who has an ectopic pregnancy confirmed by ultrasound who does not meet criteria for medical or expectant management or who has failed medical management. Patients in whom noncompliance with follow-up medical management instructions is in question, should be managed surgically. The choice of surgical approach by laparoscopy or laparotomy will depend on the status of the patient and the judgment of the surgeon. (See Fig. 9.1 for surgical options of salpingostomy versus salpingectomy.)

If salpingostomy is performed, postoperative serum human chorionic gonadotropin levels should be followed to undetectable levels. Because the reported rate of persistent viable trophoblastic tissue post salpingostomy or salpingectomy has been reported to be 6.6–17.5% [1], some clinicians choose to administer one dose of methotrexate postoperatively to eliminate this risk. The patient's desire for future fertility should always be taken into account with thorough preoperative-informed consent.

Expectant Management

Asymptomatic patients with human chorionic gonadotropin levels less than 1000 mIU/ml whose pregnancy implantation site is unknown can be managed expectantly. Selected patients must meet the following criteria: ultrasound with no evidence of rupture or presence of pelvic-free fluid, stable hemoglobin, and human chorionic gonadotropin level less than 1000 mIU/ml. Patient education regarding signs and symptoms of ruptured ectopic pregnancy is critical. These patients must be instructed to immediately return to the emergency department should they experience worsening symptoms. Follow-up should be at exacting intervals and consist of serial serum human chorionic gonadotropin levels as well as serial pelvic ultrasounds and clinical examinations.

Medical Management

Like patients selected for expectant management, those selected for medical management must be clinically stable and acknowledge understanding of the importance of close monitoring. Patient compliance with prescribed examinations, testing, and follow-up visits are imperative. Medical management consists of methotrexate administration, an antifolate, antimetabolite, chemotherapy drug. Methotrexate can be used to treat ectopic pregnancy if the following criteria are met: the ectopic pregnancy is intact, measures less than 3.5 cm in greatest diameter, have no identified fetal cardiac activity, and the serum human chorionic gonadotropin level is less than 6500 mIU/ml. The clinician prescribing

MTX must be aware of the drug contraindications, interactions, and side effects. Pretreatment laboratory assessment of creatinine and liver function testing must be performed. Major contraindications to methotrexate use include alcoholism, active pulmonary disease, chronic liver or kidney disease, blood dyscrasia, peptic ulcer disease, current breast feeding, creatinine >1.3 mg/dl, and serum transaminases >50 IU/L. During treatment, the patient must discontinue taking folate, prenatal vitamins, and any nonsteroidal anti-inflammatory drugs. The patient must abstain from alcohol intake and sexual intercourse.

Several single-dose and multiple-dose MTX regimes have been proven effective in clinical studies. One common treatment regimen [3] is:

Day 1 – MTX, 50 mg/mg^2, labs: serum HCG, liver transaminases and serum creatinine, blood type, and Rh factor (with administration of $Rh_o(D)$ immune globulin if patient is Rh negative)
Day 4 – serum HCG (may increase from day 1)
Day 7 – serum HCG, CBC, serum liver transaminases, and creatinine

Patients should be counseled regarding common potential side effects of methotrexate. These include nausea, stomach upset, diarrhea, stomatitis, hair loss, fever, or rash.

Patients under treatment should be advised to expect some mild abdominal pain and vaginal spotting. Worsening or severe abdominal pain mandates immediate return to the emergency department.

Treatment is considered successful if the serum human chorionic gonadotropin level drops 15% from day 4 to day 7. If the drop is less than 15% and the patient remains stable, options include a repeat dose of methotrexate or surgical management.

The overall reported success rate for medical treatment of the ectopic pregnancy is 63–96.7% [1, 3]. Following successful treatment, the serum human chorionic gonadotropin should be serially monitored until it falls below pregnancy levels.

The progressive decrease in serum human chorionic gonadotropin to prepregnancy levels may take 35–109 days [4]. The clinician must be alert for plateauing or increasing serum human chorionic gonadotropin levels as these may indicate persistence of viable trophoblastic tissue or gestational trophoblastic disease. Upon completing therapy with methotrexate, patients are advised to wait at least 3 months to conceive due to the teratogenic potential of methrotrexate.

References

1. Odejinmi F, Huff K, Oliver R. Individualization of intervention for tubal pregnancy: historical perspectives and the modern evidence based management of ectopic pregnancy. Eur J Obstet Gynecol Reprod Biol. 2016;210:69–75.
2. ACOG patient pamphlet AP155. Ectopic pregnancy. Danvers: American College of Obstritricians and Gynecologists ISSN 1074-8601; April 2017.
3. John David Gordon MD, Jan Rydfors MD, Maurice Druzin MD, Yona Tadir MD, Yasser El-Sayed MD, John Chan MD, Dan Lebovic MD, Elizabeth Langen MD, Katherine Fuh MD. Obstetrics, gynecology and infertility, handbook for clinicians. 6th ed. p. 266–7.
4. Marrett H, Fauconnier A, Dubennard G, et al. Overview and guidelines of off-label use of methotrexate in ectopic pregnancy. Eur J Obstet Gynecol Reprod Biol. 2016;205:105–9.

Chapter 10
Screening for Cervical Cancer and Management of Its Precursor Lesions

Janice L. Johnson

Abbreviations

ACOG	American College of Obstetricians and Gynecologists
ASCCP	American Society for Colposcopy and Cervical Pathology
ASCUS	Atypical squamous cells of undetermined significance
CIN	Cervical intraepithelial neoplasia
HR HPV	High-risk human papilloma virus
HSIL	High-grade squamous intraepithelial lesion
LAST	Lower Anogenital Squamous Terminology
LEEP	Loop electrosurgical excision procedure
LSIL	Low-grade squamous intraepithelial lesion
PPV	Positive predictive value

J. L. Johnson, MD (✉)
University of Illinois at Chicago, College of Medicine,
Presence St. Francis Hospital, Department of Obstetrics
and Gynecology, Skokie, IL, USA
e-mail: Janice.Johnson@presencehealth.org

J. V. Knaus et al. (eds.), *Ambulatory Gynecology*,
https://doi.org/10.1007/978-1-4939-7641-6_10

Part I. Cervical Cancer Screening

Introduction

Cervical cytology screening of women has quite successfully led to secondary prevention of cervical cancer, primarily due to identification and treatment of cervical cancer precursors [1]. Many of us may therefore question why screening guidelines need to change. Paramount to the premise of mass screening programs, screening tests should be accurate and economical. Cytology-based cervical cancer tests have demonstrated poor reproducibility and poor sensitivity to identify precancerous lesions and are thought to be overutilized in low-risk populations [2–4]. Therefore, much interest has been generated to improve the efficiency of cervical cancer screening initiatives. One estimate of the annual cost of Pap test screening programs in women in the United States in 1992 was 6 billion dollars [5]. One can presume with rising healthcare costs, liquid-based cytology availability, and a growing population, current costs are significantly higher. Another reason to change screening programs was the realization that over-screening was potentially causing psychological and physical harm.

Human papillomavirus (HPV) studies have demonstrated that virtually all cases of cervical cancer and its precursor lesions are associated with potentially carcinogenic genotypes of HPV [6, 7]. We also now know that the vast majority of sexually active people have been exposed to HPV. Studies have shown that in most cases of healthy women, the HPV infection is transient and benign and clears within 8–24 months. Most HPV-infected women will not develop cervical cancer or even its precursors [8–11]. It is the unresolved or persistent HPV infections with carcinogenic high-risk (HR) HPV strains, in select individuals, that lead to the development of cervical cancer and its precursors [8, 12]. Studies demonstrate that the average time it takes for high-grade cervical neoplasias to progress to invasive cancer is 10 years [11]. The need to better identify who these at risk women are and provide them closer screening intervals is essential when guidelines are developed. We know that HIV-infected women are at greater risk of cervical neoplasia with high-risk HPV (HR HPV) infection and that cigarette smoking may be a cofactor for progression or persistence of HR HPV infection and cervical neoplasia [13].

The development and incorporation of testing for HR HPV, offered by liquid-based cytology specimens, have improved the efficiency and sensitivity of cervical cancer screening programs [10, 12]. In the United States, HR HPV testing has proven to be cost-effective and has improved the sensitivity for detecting cervical intraepithelial neoplasia in women with equivocal testing, such as ASCUS (atypical squamous cells of undetermined significance). HR HPV testing has also been demonstrated to be valuable for primary screening of women aged 30 and older. This is due to the fact that there is greater reproducibility of testing for the presence of HR HPV over cervical cytology. In fact, in 2014 the FDA approved the Roche Cobas test for HR HPV as an option for primary cervical cancer screening programs in women 25 and older. This assay detects the presence of 14 high risk HPV types. It specifically detects types 16 and 18 and pools the other 12 HR HPV types [14, 15] (Table 10.1). An alternate and more widely utilized screening option exists that is the method supported by the American Cancer Society, the American Society for Colposcopy and Cervical Pathology, and the American Society for Clinical Pathology. In the most recent Practice Bulletin Number 157, The American College of Obstetricians and Gynecologists recognizes both screening methods [15]. The current recommendations recognize the information that the typical progression of the incident HR HPV infection to precancer of the cervix occurs over 2–10 years and from precancer to invasive cancer over greater than or equal to 10–15 years [10, 11]. The extremely low risk of cervical cancer and the fact that most dysplasias in adolescents under 21 years of age regress spontaneously have led to the recommendation that the timing of first Pap is to be at age 21. Furthermore, it is not recommended to screen women

Table 10.1 HR HPV testing alone as a screening tool for cervical cancer

Population	
Women aged 21–24	Not specifically discussed but it is presumed cytology every 3 years
Women 25 and older	Not less often than every 3 years in women with negative screens, primary HR HPV testing should begin 3 years after the last negative cytology exam
Triage of HPV positives	HPV 16/18 genotyping and reflex cytology assist in management decisions 16/18 positive have colposcopy Positive of the other 12 pooled HR types have reflex cytology performed. If cytology is normal, repeat in 12 months. If ASCUS or worse, then colposcopy

Interim guidance utilizing Roche Cobas HR HPV assay for 14 HR strains. Specific genotyping for types 16 and 18
Modified from Huh et al. [16]

under 30 years old for HR HPV. Age 30 has been chosen in the United States because at this age, women are past the peak of self-limited transient infections, and the positive predictive value (PPV) of presence of HR HPV for cervical intraepithelial neoplasia and cancers is greater than in the younger population [12]. It is important to note that these screening guidelines do not apply to women that are HIV infected, are immunocompromised, and have a history of diethylstilbestrol (DES) exposure or history of prior cervical intraepithelial neoplasia (CIN) or cervical cancer. The age of onset of coitus is no longer a criterion that determines the need to begin Pap screenings [15]. It is also important to note that these guidelines are for screening of healthy individuals and do not apply to women with visible lesions on their cervix, post coital bleeding, or other factors associated with cervical pathology.

ACOG released new evidence-based guidelines in December 2009 and updated these in January 2016 recommending that Pap testing (cytology) begin at age 21 and be repeated every 3 years between ages 21 and 29. They did not recommend liquid-based cytology over conventional monolayer glass slides. They further stated that women over 30, whom are low risk, may have cytology-alone screening every 3 years. Preferentially, however, they recommended co-testing consisting of cytology and HR HPV testing every 5 years in low-risk women between 30 and 65. The following exclusions to this were stated: women with a history of CIN 2 or greater require cytology screens for at least 20 years after treatment and women infected with HIV present special risk, women who are immunocompromised (specifically addressed were patients that have received organ transplants), and women who had in utero DES exposure. Women whom have had a hysterectomy and have a history of CIN 2 or greater or women whom a negative history cannot be documented should continue to have Paps [13, 15]. ACOG guidelines state that "when a woman's past cervical cytology and surgical history are not available to the physician, screening recommendations may need to be modified" [13]. See Tables 10.2 and 10.3.

Controversies About Screening Intervals

Tremendous success has been achieved in decreasing cervical cancer rates in the United States. Surveillance Epidemiology and End Results (SEER) cancer data reports an incidence of 6.5/100,000 new cases of cervical cancer in US women in 2006. The same incidence in 1975 was 14.8/100,000. This represents over a 50% decline [13, 18]. As we have learned more about the biology of cervical cancer, and its requisite association with approximately 15 known HR HPV strains, we have been able to develop more accurate and efficient guidelines for detection of cervical cancer and its precursors. Evidence-based studies have demonstrated that in low-risk, well-selected women, screening intervals can be safely lengthened [18–20]. However, several recent surveys have demonstrated that the healthcare providers are reluctant to adopt the new

TABLE 10.2 Screening methods for cervical cancer for the general population: joint recommendations of the American Cancer Society, the American Society for Colposcopy and Cervical Pathology, and the American Society for Clinical Pathology

Population	Recommended screening method	Comments
Women younger than 21 years	No screening	
Women aged 21–29 years	Cytology alone every 3 years	
Women aged 30–65	Human papillomavirus and cytology Co-testing (preferred) every 5 years Cytology alone (acceptable) every 3 years	Screening by HPV testing alone is not recommended[a]
Women older than 65 years	No screening is necessary after adequate negative prior screening results Adequate negative prior testing is defined as two negative consecutive co-tests or three negative consecutive cytology results in the last 10 years. The most recent test results should have been within the last 5 years [15]	Women with a history of CIN 2, CIN 3, or adenocarcinoma in situ should continue routine age-based screening for a total of 20 years after spontaneous regression or appropriate management of CIN 2, CIN 3, or adenocarcinoma in situ
Women vaccinated against HPV	Follow age-specific recommendations (the same as unvaccinated women)	

Above table modified from Saslow et al. [17]

[a]After *The Joint Recommendations* were published, a test for screening with HPV testing alone was approved by the FDA. See Table 10.1

TABLE 10.3 Cervical cancer screens in special populations

Population	Screens
HIV infected	Commence screening at age of initiation of sexual activity and no later than age 21 years. In women under age 30 years, perform cytology at time of initial diagnosis, and repeat cytology in 12 months if normal
HIV infected 30 years–lifetime	Screens should continue through lifetime, do not stop at 65
	Can be screened with cytology alone annually and then Q 3 years if having normal three consecutive annual Paps
	May be co-tested. If normal cytology and negative HR HPV, may have testing every 3 years
DES exposure	Annual cytology is reasonable
Immunocompromised women	Annual cytology is reasonable
	Or follow the guidelines for the HIV-infected woman
Women with history of high-grade neoplasia or higher	Routine age-based screening for 20 years after regression or treatment
	Do not stop at age 65
Women with ASC-US and Neg HR HPV	Co-test in 3 years (not 5)

Modified from American College of Obstetricians and Gynecologists [15]

lengthened screening intervals. An excellent editorial exists entitled, "Identifying a 'Range of Reasonable Options' for Cervical Cancer Screening." The authors discuss the balance between too frequent screening potentially resulting in overidentification of a transient self-limited infection and maximizing early detection and treatment of significant precursors to cervical cancer [21]. A study published by Kinney et al. shared their belief that if women and their providers were given the choice of cytology and co-testing at 5-year intervals with its estimated lifetime detection rate of cervical cancer at

0.74% as compared to co-testing every 3 years of detection rate being 0.47%, most would choose the latter interval for cervical cancer screens [22]. As healthcare providers, our patients look to us for guidance in decision-making regarding their health and wellness. We are encouraged to practice evidence-based medicine. Health insurance companies have become increasingly involved in determining what tests and medical care they believe are "medically necessary" and may elect not to authorize or pay for select care and testing.

As educated and experienced providers of healthcare, we need to understand and support the care that we provide. Performing cytology testing in adolescents, in women under age 21 years old, was a means in identifying transient HPV infections and sometimes their associated cervical neoplastic changes, the majority of which clear within 1–2 years. This led to emotional difficulties, anxiety, financial concerns, and excisional procedures for dysplasia [15]. Excisional procedures for cervical dysplasia in adolescents have felt to lead to an increase in preterm births and have raised concerns regarding cervical insufficiency [23]. The American Society for Colposcopy and Cervical Pathology (ASCCP) in 2006 encouraged a conservative approach in adolescents with histology findings of less than CIN 3. ACOG endorsed these recommendations and also released new practice guidelines in 2009, moving the baseline cervical cytology exam to age 21 years. This is without regard to age of first sexual intercourse and does not negate the need for annual gynecologic exams and STI testing in sexually active adolescents [24–26]. The incidence of cervical cancer in adolescents is extremely low. 0.1% of cases of cervical cancer occur before age 21. The US Surveillance Epidemiology and End Results (SEER) data from 2002 to 2006 and the US national data from the CDC estimate an incidence rate of 1–2 cases per 1,000,000 girls aged 15–19 years old. This amounts to 14 cases on the average per year from 1998 to 2003 in that age group [14, 18]. If the new guidelines had been applied to begin cervical cytology at 21 years of age, these young women may have been diagnosed at an even more advanced stage. It is also possible that they had risk factors such as DES exposure and HIV infection or were otherwise immunocompromised. I believe this sort of data makes the healthcare provider concerned that they will miss the opportunity to identify early cervical cancers and high-grade lesions.

Despite the widespread knowledge of the new screening guidelines, healthcare providers have been slow to adopt these recommendations. Several factors may be influencing this practice. Studies have demonstrated that patients are often incorrect in remembering the timing and results of their last Pap test. Specifically, they underestimated the length of time and incorrectly reported abnormal results as normal [27, 28]. Additionally, providers need to educate women that lengthening the interval between Pap smears does not apply to all women and that annual gynecologic exams are still appropriate. Another factor that may influence healthcare providers' decision to not follow the new screening interval recommendations is their own awareness that these evidence-based guidelines also examined the cost-effectiveness and efficiency of screening programs, as described in published studies [29]. Also, the ability to identify the low-risk patient correctly may be difficult. A patient may state that she is monogamous, while in fact she is not. The patient's partner may not be monogamous. The patient or her partner may participate in high-risk sexual behavior, unknown to the provider. In a typical practice, very few healthy "low-risk" patients have HIV testing. Patients may be unaware of being infected with the HIV virus. Furthermore, documentation of prior Paps is often lacking as patients move and change clinics and healthcare providers. Providers cannot always trust the quality of the reading and the collection or even be 100% certain that the Paps were not mixed up in a busy clinic or office setting. It is also possible that the laboratories might mix up patients' specimens. Perhaps of most importance, if we perform screens every 5 years and the last result was in error, the true screening interval becomes 10 years. This is enough time for a cervical cancer to develop.

Many of us have developed what we refer to as "experience-based guidelines." In my practice I have implemented every

TABLE 10.4 "Experienced-based guidelines" for low-risk asymptomatic women

Age 21–29 years old	Age 30–65 years old
Q 3-year cytology Q 3-year cytology plus Reflex to HR HPV	Q 3-year cytology with automatic HR HPV

3 year co-testing for low-risk women aged 30 and over. I simply believe that extending the interval to every 5 years adds risk (Table 10.4). I believe we do need to stay open-minded to the new findings and recommendations. We need to realize that performing Paps on low-risk adolescents was causing more harm than being helpful. We need to develop strategies that work for us and our patients in carefully choosing who needs more frequent screens and who does not.

Part II. Management of Abnormal Pap Results

Advances in diagnosis and treatment of precursors to cervical cancer have greatly reduced the incidence of invasive cervical cancer in the United States [1]. In the past, after diagnosis of an abnormal Pap smear, women underwent random four quadrant biopsies, cervical conizations, and hysterectomies for cervical cancer precursors. In the 1970s, colposcopy was introduced, and these aggressive diagnostic and treatment choices for cervical neoplasias become less frequent. The more conservative ablative treatments of the lesions become favored and proved to be effective. Ablative methods include laser, cryotherapy, and electrocautery. Acetic acid has also been used on the cervix. In the 1990s, healthcare providers began to utilize the office-based excisional procedure, the loop electrosurgical excision procedure (LEEP). The LEEP became popular because it provided a pathologic specimen that could be examined to exclude the presence of a more advanced lesion that might be unrecognized in an ablation procedure. However, as our knowledge of the high regression rate of the cervical neoplasias grew, researchers and clinicians became concerned that we were harming women by performing unnecessary excisions on lesions that would quite often resolve on their own. These excisional procedures are associated with bleeding, scarring, and the inherent risks associated with vaginal procedures [23]. Additionally, some studies began to associate LEEPS and cervical conizations with preterm deliveries [29, 30]. The last decade has begun an ongoing investigation and series of consensus guidelines on the safest and best management for detecting, treating, and preventing cervical cancer and its precursors.

A consensus conference was held in March of 2012 entitled the LAST (Lower Anogenital Squamous Terminology) Project. The ASCCP, the College of American Pathologists, and 35 other organizations developed an updated terminology for histopathology of HPV-associated squamous lesions associated with the anogenital tract. This new terminology has simplified the nomenclature between cytology and histology. Cervical cytology, in accordance with the Bethesda system, utilizes the terms low-grade squamous intraepithelial lesion (LSIL) and high-grade squamous intraepithelial lesion (HSIL) (see Table 10.5). Cervical histopathology utilizes the three-tiered CIN (cervical intraepithelial neoplasia) terminology. Both CIN 2 and CIN 3 are considered high-grade lesions. The category of CIN 2 was found to be somewhat subjective upon review by experts. The LAST Project work group recommended adding p16 immunostaining to confirm the diagnosis of CIN 2. Positive p16 staining correlates well with the diagnosis of HSIL. They also recommended developing a two-tiered nomenclature system for histopathology. Previously named CIN 1 and p16-negative CIN 2 are now called LSIL. P16-positive CIN 2 and CIN 3 histopathology specimens are now called HSIL [32]. See Table 10.6.

Management based upon the diagnosis of high-grade or low-grade histology of the cervix correlates well with the LAST Project two-tiered nomenclature. Positive HR HPV

Table 10.5 Modification of Bethesda 2014 cervical cytology

Squamous cell abnormalities
Atypical squamous cells (ASC)
Atypical squamous cells of undetermined significance (ASC-US)
Atypical squamous cells cannot exclude a high-grade lesion (ASC-H)
Low-grade intraepithelial lesion (LSIL)
High-grade intraepithelial lesion (HSIL)
Squamous cell carcinoma
Glandular cell abnormalities
Atypical glandular cells (AGC)
Endocervical
Endometrial
Glandular cells
Atypical glandular cells, favor neoplastic
Endocervical cells, favor neoplastic
Glandular cells, favor neoplastic
Endocervical adenocarcinoma in situ (AIS)
Adenocarcinoma
Endocervical
Endometrial
Extrauterine
Not otherwise specified
Other
Benign-appearing endometrial cells. Reported only in women 45 or older
Infectious organisms
Other types of cancers. The fallopian tube, ovary, peritoneal cavity, vulva, or vagina

Modified from Nayar and Wilbur [31]

tests in women over 30 more likely represent persistent infection and are more likely to have had the opportunity to cause neoplasia. In younger women, HR HPV infection is more likely to represent the transient self-limited infection. As previously discussed, there is some concern that cervical procedures, especially the excisional methods, may lead to adverse

TABLE 10.6 Simplified management of cervical neoplasia using last project terminology

Histopathology	Management
LSIL	Observation is preferred, typically annually
HSIL	Treatment is preferred with the important age-based exceptions. Ablation or excision appropriate Women over 40 years old: excision preferred. Cryo has higher failure rates in this age group Women under 26 years old: Q 6-month colposcopy, and cytology is reasonable. This age group may be extended to include women of childbearing age up to age 30. If treatment is required, CO_2 laser or, when possible, shallow LEEPs may be safer. See discussion in text regarding when to treat

pregnancy outcomes. If one keeps these facts in mind, the treatment of abnormal cervical lesions may be simplified. Low-grade intraepithelial lesions (LSIL) should be managed by observation. With some important exceptions, high-grade intraepithelial lesions (HSIL) should be ablated or excised. Excisional procedures are typically offered for women over 40 as results from cohort studies have shown higher failure rates with cryoablation in this age group [33]. This age group is also more often done with childbearing. When we encounter HSIL lesions in adolescents and young women who have future childbearing concerns, conservative observation with semiannual colposcopy and cytology is acceptable. It is important to note that treatment is indicated, in this young group, if the lesion is large and enlarging or the entire transformation zone (inadequate colposcopy) cannot be seen. If the HSIL persists for 2 years, treatment is recommended [32].

The American Society for Colposcopy and Cervical Pathology (ASCCP) has developed extensive algorithms and a mobile "app" available for purchase at their website www.asccp.org/APP. Management guidelines can be customized for your patient by her age, pregnancy status, HR HPV, and prior testing results. These algorithms are copyright protected for publication but are available on their website.

References

1. IARC. Handbooks of cancer prevention, Cervix cancer screening, vol. 10. Lyon: IARC Press; 2005.
2. Nanda K, McCrory DC, Myers ER, et al. Accuracy of the Papanicolaou test in screening for and follow-up of cervical cytologic abnormalities: a systematic review. Ann Intern Med. 2000;132:810–9.
3. Cuzick J, Clavel C, Perry KU, et al. Overview of the European and North American studies on HPV testing in primary cervical cancer screening. Int J Cancer. 2006;119:1095–101.
4. Stoler MH, Schiffman M. Interobserver reproducibility of cervical cytologic and histologic interpretations: realistic estimates from the ASCUS-LSIL Triage Study. JAMA. 2001;285:1500–5.
5. Kurman RJ, Henson DE, Herbst AL, et al. Interim guidelines for management of abnormal cervical cytology. The 1992 National Cancer Institute Workshop. JAMA. 1994;271:1866–9.
6. Walboomers JM, Jacobs MV, Manos MM, et al. Human papillomavirus is a necessary cause of invasive cervical cancer worldwide. J Pathol. 1999;189:12–9.
7. Schiffman MH, Bauer HM, Hoover RN, et al. Epidemiologic evidence showing that human papillomavirus infection causes most cervical intraepithelial neoplasia. J Natl Cancer Inst. 1993;85:958–64.
8. Wright TC Jr, Schiffman M. Adding a test for human papillomavirus DNA to cervical-cancer screening. N Engl J Med. 2003;348:489–90.
9. Mosiccki AB, Schiffman M, Kjaer S, Villa LL. Updating the natural history of HPV and anogenital cancer. Vaccine. 2006;24(suppl 3):S3/42–51.
10. Castle PE. The potential utility of HPV genotyping in screening and clinical management. J Natl Compr Cancer Netw. 2008;6(1):83–95.
11. Baseman JG, Koutsky LA. The epidemiology of human papillomavirus infections. J Clin Virol. 2005;329(suppl (1)):S16–24.
12. Wright TC Jr, Schiffman M, Solomon D, et al. Interim guidance for the use of human papillomavirus DNA testing as an

adjunct to cervical cytology for screening. Obstet Gynecol. 2004;103:304–9.

13. Clinical Management Guidelines for Obstetrician-Gynecologists. ACOG practice bulletin no 109: cervical cytology screening. Obstet Gynecol. 2009;114(6):1409–20.
14. Silver MI, Rositch AF, Burke AE, Chang K, Viscidi R, Gravitt PE. Patient concerns about human papillomavirus testing and 5-year intervals in routine cervical cancer screening. Obstet Gynecol. 2015;125:317–29.
15. American College of Obstetricians and Gynecologists. Cervical cancer screening and prevention. Practice bulletin no. 157. Obstet Gynecol. 2016;127:e1–20.
16. WK H, Ault KA, Chlemow D, Davey DD, Goulart RA, Garcia FA, et al. Use of primary high-risk human papillomavirus testing for cervical cancer screening: interim clinical guidelines. Obstet Gynecol. 2015;125:330–7.
17. Saslow D, Solomon D, Lawson HW, Killackey M, Kulasingam SL, Cain J, et al. American Cancer Society, American Society for Colposcopy and Cervical Pathology and American Society for Clinical Pathology screening guidelines for the prevention and early detection of cervical cancer. ACS-ASCCP-ASCP Cervical Cancer Guideline Committee. CA Cancer J Clin. 2012;62:147–72.
18. Ries LA, Melbert D, Krapcho M, Stinchcomb DG, Howlader N, Horner MJ, et al. SEER cancer statistics review, 1975–2006. Bethesda: National Cancer Institute; 2009.
19. Arbyn M, Bergeron C, Klinkhamer P, Martin-Hirsch P, Siebers AG, Bulten J. Liquid, compared with conventional cervical cytology: a systematic review and meta-analysis. Obstet Gynecol. 2008;111:167–77.
20. Ronco G, Cuzick J, Pierotti P, Cariaggi MP, Dalla Palma P, Naldoni C, et al. Accuracy of liquid based versus conventional cytology: overall results of new technology for cervical cancer screening: randomized controlled trial. BMJ. 2007;335:28.
21. Sawaya GF, Kuppermann M. Identifying a "range of reasonable options" for cervical cancer screening. Obstet Gynecol. 2015;125:308–9.
22. Kinney W, Wright TC, Dinkelspiel HE, DeFrancesco M, Cox JT, Huh W. Increased cervical cancer risk associated with screening at longer intervals. Obstet Gynecol. 2015;125:311–5.
23. Khan MJ, Smith-McCune K. Treatment of cervical precancers. Back to basics. Obstet Gynecol. 2014;123:1339–42.

24. Kyrgiou M, Koliopoulos G, Martin-Hirsch P, Arbyn M, Prendiville W, Paraskevaidis E. Obstetric outcomes after conservative treatment for intraepithelial or early invasive cervical lesions: systematic review and meta-analysis. Lancet. 2006;367:489–98.
25. American College of Obstetricians and Gynecologists. Evaluation and management of abnormal cervical cytology and histology in adolescents. ACOG Committee opinion no. 436. Obstet Gynecol. 2009;113:1422–5.
26. Wright TC Jr, Massad LS, Dunton CJ, Spitzer M, Wilkinson EJ, Solomon D. 2006 guidelines for the management of women with abnormal cervical cancer screening tests. 2006 American Society for Colposcopy and Cervical Pathology-sponsored Consensus Conference. Am J Obstet Gynecol. 2007;197:346–55.
27. Mamoon H, Taylor R, Morrell S, Wain G, Moore H. Cervical screening: population-based comparisons between self-reported survey and registry-derived Pap test rates. Aus NZ J Publ Health. 2001;25:505–10.
28. Sawyer JA, Earp JA, Fletcher RH, Daye FF, Wynn TM. Accuracy of women's self-report of their last pap smear. Am J Public Health. 1989;79:1036–7.
29. Bevis KS, Biggio JR. Cervical conization and the risk of preterm delivery. Am J Obstet Gynecol. 2011;205(1):19–27.
30. Arbyn M, Kyrgiou M, Simoens C, et al. Perinatal mortality and other severe adverse pregnancy outcomes associated with treatment of cervical intraepithelial neoplasia: meta-analysis. BMJ. 2008;337:a1284.
31. Nayar R, Wilbur DS, editors. The Bethesda system for reporting cervical cytology: definitions, criteria, and explanatory notes. 3rd ed. New York: Springer; 2015.
32. Waxman AG, Chelmow D, Darragh TM, et al. Revised terminology for cervical histopathology and its implications for management of high-grade squamous intraepithelial lesions of the cervix. Obstet Gynecol. 2012;120:1465–71.
33. Melnikow J, McGahan C, Sawaya GF, Ehlen T, Coldman A. Cervical intraepithelial neoplasia outcomes after treatment: long-term follow-up from the British Columbia Cohort Study. J Natl Cancer Inst. 2009;101:721–8. 22. ASCUS-LSIL Triage Study (ALTS) G.

Chapter 11
Lower Genital Tract Disease

Elliot M. Levine

Cervicitis (Which Is Often Sexually Transmitted)

Two primary sexually transmitted pathogens that cause disease in females (and in males) include Neisseria gonorrhea (NG) and Chlamydia trachomatis (CT) [1]. They essentially infect the uterine cervix and can be identified there, typically using a Nucleic Acid Amplification Tests (NAAT), which is less costly and more effective than culturing these organisms [2]. If either of these is found with swabbing of the endocervix, the patient needs to be treated, as well as the sexual partner(s). It is not uncommon to find both of these pathogens together, which is why the treatment recommendation often includes an antimicrobial effective for treating both pathogens. When finding either of these organisms, one should treat the patient, even if she is asymptomatic at the time of presentation, since either of these pathogens can ascend the genital tract and cause pelvic inflammatory disease (PID). In fact, screening asymptomatic young women can lead to its detection in a small percentage of encounters,

E. M. Levine (✉)
Advocate Illinois Masonic Medical Center, Department of Obstetrics and Gynecology, Chicago, IL, USA

J. V. Knaus et al. (eds.), *Ambulatory Gynecology*,
https://doi.org/10.1007/978-1-4939-7641-6_11

depending on the population being screened. Table 11.1 shows the recommended medications and dosages for treatment.

Cervicitis pathogens other than GC or CT may cause sexually transmissible syndromes in women that may need to be considered for its treatment [3]. When neither GC or CT is detected in the cervix when a cervicitis is seen, this condition is referred to as a nongonococcal nonchlamydial cervicitis (NGNCC). The clinical syndrome of a cervicitis, whatever the pathogen, consists of a mucopurulent exudate arising from the cervical external os, leading to complaints of a "vaginal

TABLE 11.1 Treatment recommendations for cervicitis

Pathogen	Primary treatment	Alternative treatments	Additional information
GC	Azithromycin 1 gram orally (single dose) plus ceftriaxone 250 mg IM	Doxycycline 100 mg BID × 7 days plus ceftriaxone 250 mg IM	Will treat concomitant CT
CT	Azithromycin 1 gram orally	Doxycycline 100 mg BID × 7 days or erythromycin base 500 mg QID × 7 days or levofloxacin 500 mg once daily × 7 days	
NGNCC	Azithromycin 1 gram orally or doxycycline 100 mg BID × 7 days	Erythromycin base 500 mg QID or levofloxacin 500 mg once daily × 7 days	

GC Neisseria gonorrhea, CT Chlamydia trachomatis, NGNCC Non-gonococcal non-chlamydial cervicitis [5]

discharge." Also on examination, excessive friability of the cervix is noted as well. Naturally, this needs to be effectively treated and especially after the routine treatment that was used failed to eradicate the clinical findings and/or symptoms. In that setting, another pathogen may be the etiology. These "other" pathogens may include the Mycoplasmas (e.g., Mycoplasma hominis or genitalium) or Ureaplasma urealyticum, for which therapy may need to be specifically provided [6]. Detection of these bacteria may be unsuccessful, and empiric therapy often needs to be provided. Macrolide antibiotics are sometimes effective. It is interesting to note that the analogous syndrome in males, simply referred to as nongonococcal urethritis (NGU), behaves in this same way, sometimes requiring multiple antibiotic regimens until treatment success is obtained.

Chronic cervicitis may persist even after multiple antimicrobial therapies are unsuccessfully applied. In such cases, ablative or extirpative therapy may need to be considered, using electrocautery, or even with a loop electrical excision procedure (LEEP). However, there has been an insufficient amount of evidence provided for this [3].

Infectious Vaginitis

It should be acknowledged that many types of vaginitis can often initially present as primarily a vulvar condition, at least more prominently to the patient, relative to the specific symptoms of "vaginitis." An example of just such a vulvovaginitis is *candidiasis*, which may also be called monilia, or a "yeast infection," usually caused by candida albicans [7]. In fact, this particular fungal infection often presents with intense vulvar pruritus, which may prompt a need for immediate relief (See Table 11.2). This is more commonly identified in individuals who are diabetic, and possibly poorly controlled, and possibly those who are using hormonal contraception. Microscopy of the discharge can identify hyphae, when using potassium chloride as the medium for inspection.

Table 11.2 Treatment recommendations for vaginitis

Vaginitis	Primary treatment	Alternative treatments (or for recurrent infections)
Candidiasis	Terconazole (suppository or 0.8% cream daily × 3) or Fluconazole 150 mg orally × 1	Both may be used in combination, and may continue fluconazole q 3 days × 2–3 days or Boric acid inserts
Trichomoniasis	Metronidazole 2 g × 1 orally	Tinidazole 2 g × 1 orally
Bacterial vaginosis	Metronidazole 500 mg BID × 7 days or Metronidazole gel 0.75% apply daily × 5	Clindamycin 300 mg BID × 7 days or Clindamycin cream 2% apply daily × 7 days

Another type of vaginitis which can have a significant vulvar component includes *Trichomoniasis.* The "burning" vulvar sensation which is often described (in addition to the associated malodorous vaginal discharge) can be significant. On examination, one can usually see a frothy greenish vaginal discharge. Microscopy can identify motile flagellated organisms (Trichomonas vaginalis), when using a normal saline medium. Its effective treatment consists of the use of metronidazole 500 mg twice daily for 7 days. Alternatively, topical therapy can be provided (Table 11.2). While its sexual transmissibility has been noted in the past, the concomitant treatment of the sexual consort does not need to be provided, although evidence is mixed [8].

Bacterial vaginosis (BV), sometimes referred to as gardnerella vaginalis vaginitis (from the bacterial pathogen for which it was named), can produce a malodorous vaginal discharge. This discharge appears on speculum exam to be grayish and frothy, typically pooling in the posterior fornix. On microscopy, an abundance of "clue" cells can be seen, which can be considered as pathognomonic. These clue cells are epithelial cells covered with bacteria and seen in an unstained specimen. Though such microscopic examination can be used for its identification, there are some diagnostic kits that may be used for this, perhaps lending some greater efficiency for its clinical detection. Treatment of the sexual partner may not be necessary for a patient with bacterial vaginosis [9]. Table 11.2 shows the currently recommended treatments for these types of vaginitis [10].

Vulvar disease represents a vast array of conditions which can commonly present to the practicing gynecologist. Rather than viewing this as a single entity, however, one should consider a variety of categories in which to place it, according to its possible origins:

1. Vulvar component of Vulvovaginitis (often possibly sexually transmitted) and vulvar infectious conditions
2. Part of the continuum of neoplasia, from vulvar intraepithelial neoplasia to invasive carcinoma (of any histologic type)
3. Vulvar dystrophies, some of which can be considered to be premalignant (e.g., Lichen sclerosis)
4. Sexual pain disorder
5. Vulvodynia, general vulvar pain and discomfort, without any specific findings on examination
6. Dermatosis which can affect this area of skin, but which can also be seen elsewhere throughout the body (e.g., psoriasis)
7. Manifestation of systemic disease, but which can present as "vulvar disease" (e.g., Crohn's Disease)

Infections of the vulva which can symptomatically present include:

- Syphilis, a spirochetal infection (Treponema pallidum), can be described in primary, secondary, tertiary, or latent phases. Since the initial route of this infection is via sexual intercourse, the site of its initial presentation can typically be seen in the vulva. The primary phase of this disease appears as a chancre, which is a firm or hard, nontender ulceration, with an incubation period of 14 days from the time of first sexual contact from an infectious partner. The diagnosis is made through darkfield microscopy, though the chancre may only be present for 1–3 weeks. Serologic evidence, performed at this time, however, is often absent. Positive serology shows up in the secondary and latent phases, first with a nontreponemal screening test (e.g., RPR or VDRL) and if positive, then with a specific treponemal antibody test (e.g., FTA-Abs). Treatment in this (primary) phase is with the administration of Penicillin G benzathine 2.4 million units, though may need to be given weekly for 3 weeks, if the phase is uncertain.

- Chancroid represents a rare bacterial infection from *Hemophilus ducreyi*. Unlike a syphilitic chancre, this ulceration of the vulva that presents is typically less firm and tender to touch and is often associated with tender inguinal lymphadenopathy. Since the isolation of this bacterium can be difficult, empiric therapy may be necessary with azithromycin 1 gram.
- Herpes Simplex Virus (HSV) can cause primary (first such episode) or recurrent infections. These lesions initially present as tender vesicles (usually clustered in recurrent disease), which then proceed to ulcerations and then on to scabs. Primary disease can last as long as 3 weeks, and recurrent disease more typically lasts about 1 week. Recurrences, if they occur at all following a primary infection, can occur at varying intervals after the primary infection, though tend to cease after 5 years. Though HSV cultures are available for diagnosis, since they have less than 100% success for viral isolation, the visual diagnosis (along with history) may suffice, in order to lead to appropriate medical therapy. This can be Acyclovir or Valacyclovir, dosed differently whether it be for the treatment of primary HSV, recurrent HSV, or for suppressive therapy (i.e., prophylaxis), which can be offered for frequently recurring such infections.
- Human Papillomavirus (HPV) disease, sometimes manifesting in many verrucous lesions, appears in all areas of the vulva. This is referred to as vulvar condylomata. The spectrum of vulvar HPV disease can also include "flat"

aceto-white lesions which can be identified with the application of acetic acid. The incubation of HPV is usually seen from weeks to months, so the identification of the sexual contact from whom this originated may be often inexact. Histologic examination (from biopsy) can lead to the definitive diagnosis. Treatment can include electrocautery, cryocautery, application of trichloroacetic acid, or with imiquimod, which can be applied by the patient herself. Any possible male sexual contact should be referred to a urologist or family practitioner.

- Molluscum Contagiosum appear as mildly pruritic, erythematous umbilicated lesions, which can be biopsied for histologic diagnosis, and when the diagnosis is confirmed, be definitively treated with curetting of all lesions found. The etiologic virus is the poxvirus, "Molluscum Contagiosum Virus."

Pediculosis

Vulvar pruritus can also result from parasitic insect infestation/infection from the Phthirus pubis (or crab louse), which would be found in the hair-bearing areas (pubic hair). Use of the naked eye is possible to identify these small parasites, though microscopic magnification would reveal the recognizable ultrastructure of the pubic louse. There are a number of OTC medications available to treat this (e.g., 1% permethrin lotions and shampoos). If this is the etiology for a patient's pruritic condition, one would need to repeat use of this treatment again, to eliminate nits, or eggs that may have been laid, in addition to thoroughly cleaning towels and bed sheets. Notification of sexual partners is indicated as well.

Another parasitic infection, which can cause vulvar pruritus (as well as in other areas of the body), is referred to as scabies. In this case, the offending organism is the mite, Sarcoptes scabei, which typically burrows under the skin (in this case, in the vulva), resulting in papular or linear-appearing lesions. Diagnosis of this is more difficult than that discussed above, in that one needs to isolate this insect by scraping the skin lesions so as to isolate the mite (and then magnify it). Often though, empiric therapy with lindane shampoo, lotion, or cream may be necessary for its treatment and eradication.

Neoplasia

A continuum exists regarding vulvar neoplasia, starting with vulvar intraepithelial neoplasia (VIN) to invasive vulvar carcinoma. Though vulvar cancer and its precursors may be the least frequent of the gynecologic malignancies, its recognition, screening, prevention, and diagnosis is nonetheless important to the practicing gynecologist. This will be discussed in greater detail in the chapter on vulvar cancer.

Vulvar Dystrophy

Vulvar dystrophy includes squamous hyperplasia and lichen sclerosis, both of which can present symptomatically. Squamous hyperplasia is characterized as an often pruritic condition, being visualized as erythematous and thickened skin, sometimes appearing in large patches, and corresponding to increased acanthosis histologically [11]. The use of potent corticosteroids has been therapeutic for this [12].

Lichen Sclerosis also can be pruritic and painful as well. It usually takes on a more whitish appearance with skin that is thinner in its texture, and corresponding histologically with a thinner stratum corneum. This particular dystrophy can be considered as premalignant, making its treatment more imperative [13].

Sexual Pain Disorders

There are a variety of disorders which can be recognized as being a part of "sexual dysfunction," but which must oftentimes be considered separately from those concerns typically referring to the subjective aspects of sexual dysfunction, but rather attending to their specific gynecologic basis, which may require a more "anatomic" treatment.

While pain which can be encountered by a woman during sex (usually on penetration) as a result of a vaginitis (possibly candidiasis) or the commonly perimenopausal atrophic vaginitis, it can be more specifically a sexual pain disorder (i.e., dyspareunia). If it is determined that it is a case of dyspareunia, not related to the more common type of vaginitis, it may be categorized as either (1) vaginismus or (2) vulvar vestibulitis.

Vaginismus represents the unconscious, or involuntary, spasm of the pubococygeus muscle that is triggered by penile penetration (whether it is desired or not). The subjective feeling of this pain, which can sometimes be seen during a pelvic examination, can be diagnostic of this condition. Its successful treatment most typically involves the identification of those sometimes deep-seated thoughts and feelings that may be the route of this reaction. Of course, all gynecologists have seen this vaginismic reaction if and when a pelvic examination is performed too abruptly. However, when this condition is diagnosed as the cause of the pain which is presenting to the gynecologist as occurring during a patient's lovemaking, it most usually requires a deeper analysis, involving a lengthy discussion of all of the subjective factors that may be involved.

While the introital dyspareunia as discussed above occurs on initial penetration, if the dyspareunia is described as occurring with deep penetration, other diagnoses may need to be considered. These would include endometriosis, pelvic inflammatory disease, or ovarian cysts, to name just a few possible etiologies for this described pain. Nonetheless, such deep dyspareunia would not be a part of this particular sexual pain disorder.

Vulvar vestibulitis, which is uniquely different from vaginismus, refers to a vulvar condition in which the trigger for the perceived pain can be reproduced at the pelvic examination, most typically with a cotton tipped probe applied at the posterior fourchette. The terminology for this has varied over time in the medical literature and can be alternatively referred to as provoked vulvodynia. While some may see this as part of the spectrum of vulvodynia, which has very little in terms of pathognomonic findings on examination, this should be considered as its own distinct clinical entity.

Though there may be some controversy as to its ideal treatment, whether with physical therapy or with a surgical vestibulectomy, this may actually depend on the experience of the physical therapist (having patience using progressive dilators and relaxation techniques), or the gynecologist with the resection of sufficient vestibular tissue to have successful results. The typical histologic findings which are associated with vestibular resection and the success found in some reviews suggest the organic (or physical) cause for this condition, leading some to follow this route of therapy.

Vulvodynia

As mentioned above, this is a condition in which a woman complains of chronic vulvar discomfort, felt as sharp or aching in quality, and not necessarily precipitated by anything in particular. Specific lesions are rarely demonstrated, and there have been no associated histologic features. In many ways, nonspecific vulvodynia behaves very much like Fibromyalgia and can be similarly treated with Pregabalin (or other similar compounds). Its etiology is unclear, as well as the factors that may lead to its occurrence [14, 15].

Dermatitis

As with other areas of the body (outside of the vulva), the vulvar skin can react to allergens with contact [16]. The type of allergic reaction obviously varies between individuals, both in terms of the particular offending substance, the rapidity of the response, and the severity of the dermatologic reaction to it.

Psoriasis is a chronic dermatitis that can present in other areas of the body, most notably at extensor surfaces of the limbs, besides the vulva itself.

Some more unusual types of vulvar dermatitis include Behcet's Disease and Plasma Cell Vulvitis (vulvitis of Zoon), both of them often presenting with vesicular lesions, possibly causing confusion with the more commonly seen HSV vulvitis.

Also, less commonly seen in the vulva are pemphigus-related conditions. The bullous lesions which are seen on examination would often lead to its diagnosis for the woman presenting with such lesions.

Manifestation of Systemic Disease

Crohn's Disease represents an example of a systemic disease, or in this case, specifically a bowel disease, that can be associated with the presentation of a specific vulvar problem. This example may simply be due to the proximity of the rectum and anus to the vulvar skin. In any event, Crohn's can present with vulvar ulcerative lesions, which when accompanied by the usual associated bowel complaints can lead to the proper diagnosis especially when identified via biopsy [17]. Other systemic diseases can similarly present to the gynecologist, including Diabetes Mellitus, when persistent and/or recurring vulvar candidiasis is seen.

References

1. Smith L, Angarone MP. Sexually transmitted infections. Urol Clin N Am. 2015;42:507–18.
2. Herbst de Corina S, Bristow CC, Joseph Davey D, Klausner JD. A systematic review of point of care testing for chlamydia trachomatis, Neisseria gonorrhoeae and Trichomonas vaginalis. Infect Dis Obstet Gynecol. 2016;2016:4386127.
3. Papp JR, Schacter J, Gaydos CA, Van Der Pol B. Recommendations for the laboratory-based detection of chlamydia trachomatis and Neisseria gonorrhea – 2014. MMWR. 2014;63(2):1–18.

4. Mattson SK, Polk JP, Nvirjesy P. Chronic cervicitis: presenting features and response to therapy. J Low Genit Tract Dis. 2016;20:e30–3.
5. Workowski KA, Bolan GA. Sexually transmitted diseases treatment guidelines, 2015. MMWR. 2015;64(3):1–134.
6. Lis R, Rowhani-Rahbar A, Manhart LE. Mycoplasma genitalium infection and female reproductive tract disease: a meta-analysis. Clin Infect Dis. 2015;61(3):418–26.
7. Sobel JD. Recurrent vulvovaginal candidiasis. Am J Obstet Gynecol. 2016;214(1):15–21.
8. Van Schalkwyk J, Yudin MH, et al. Vulvovaginitis: screening for and management of Trichomoniasis, vulvovaginal candidiasis, and bacterial vaginosis. J Obstet Gynaecol Can. 2015;37:266–76.
9. Amaya-Guio J, Viveros-Carreno DA, Sierra-Barrios EM, et al. Antibiotic treatment for the sexual partners of women with bacterial vaginosis. Cochrane Database Syst Rev. 2016;10:CD011701.
10. Nyirjesy P. Management of persistent vaginitis. Obstet Gynecol. 2014;124:1135–46.
11. Reyes MC, Cooper K. An update on vulvar intraepithelial neoplasia: terminology and a practical approach to diagnosis. J Clin Pathol. 2014;67(4):290.
12. Bornstein J, Bogliatto F, Haefner HK, Stockdale CK, Preti M, Bohl TG, Reutter J. The 2015 International Society for the Study of Vulvovaginal disease (ISSVD) terminology of squamous intraepithelial lesions. J Lower Gen Tract Dis. 2016;20:11–4.
13. Fistarol SK, Itin PH. Diagnosis and treatment of lichen sclerosus: an update. Am J Clin Dermatol. 2013;14:27–47.
14. Female Sexual Dysfunction. ACOG Practice Bulletin Number 119, April 2011.
15. Wright PJ, O'Connor KM. Female sexual dysfunction. Med Clin N Am. 2015;99:607–28.
16. Hoang MP, Reuter J, Papalas JA, Edwards L, Selim MA. Vulvar inflammatory dermatoses: an update and review. Am J Dermatopathol. 2014;36:689–701.
17. Andreani SM, Ratnasingham K, Dang HH, Gravante G, Giordano P. Crohn's disease of the vulva. Int J Surg. 2010;8:2–5.

Chapter 12
The Painful Bladder

Marko J. Jachtorowycz

Every physician who provides care to female patients is regularly consulted to evaluate and treat symptoms of pelvic discomfort. These include everything from mild irritation and burning to deep visceral pain. The assessment of the undifferentiated patient with pelvic pain or discomfort calls for an organized system-by-system approach guided by the interview and physical exam findings. Women suffering from bladder pain syndrome or interstitial cystitis (IC/BPS) are frequently among patients presenting with pelvic pain or discomfort. Successful early identification of this subgroup of patients among pelvic pain sufferers is key to mitigating the adverse quality of life impact of bladder pain syndrome (formerly interstitial cystitis).

Bladder pain syndrome/interstitial cystitis (IC/BPS) is a significant quality of life disorder affecting an estimated 7.5 million [1] Americans. It is insidious, evades imaging, has no well-established serologic or urinary markers, and presents physicians with a considerable diagnostic challenge. Only infrequently does it have identifiable clinical findings. It can rarely be diagnosed on tissue biopsy. Women affected by the condition outnumber men by 5 to 1 [2]. The average sufferer

M. J. Jachtorowycz (✉)
Presence Saint Francis Hospital, Department of Medical Education, Evanston, IL, USA
e-mail: mjacht01@presencehealth.org

J. V. Knaus et al. (eds.), *Ambulatory Gynecology*,
https://doi.org/10.1007/978-1-4939-7641-6_12

sees multiple consultants before a diagnosis is made. Sufferers of IC/BPS represent a subset of patients who present with symptoms of pelvic discomfort, pelvic pain, and dyspareunia.

Bladder pain syndrome (BPS) is defined as pain in the lower abdomen or genital tract attributable to the urinary bladder. Interstitial cystitis is a subset of bladder pain syndrome. Interstitial cystitis consists of all of the symptoms of bladder pain syndrome with additional urinary symptomatology involving the lower urinary tract. It is useful for the practicing clinician to consider these points on a continuum of one clinical entity.

PBS/IC sufferers may manifest with a variety of symptoms. These often involve the urinary tract and may include frequency of urination, dysuria, and bladder overactivity. Other associated symptoms, dyspareunia, external genital pain or burning, vaginal burning, vaginal pain, and lower abdominal discomfort are among the possible clinical symptoms with which PBS/IC patient may present.

The symptoms of PBS/IC have overlap with numerous other pain conditions common in women. Included among these are endometriosis and adenomyosis, vulvar pain syndromes, and colon-rectal causes. IC/BPS must be considered in the differential diagnosis for all women who present with complaints of pelvic pain, vulvodynia, and dyspareunia. IC/BPS should also be included as part of the comprehensive assessment of any patient presenting with complaints of vague lower abdominal pain or discomfort.

The key to successful identification diagnosis and management of the IC/BPS patient among patient presenting with pelvic symptoms is vigilance for it on the part of the clinician. It must be considered as an element in the overall differential diagnosis of lower abdominal and pelvic pain etiologies.

Common presentations include women who have a long-term history of "frequent urinary tract infections." Further inquiry and examination of such cases will identify a pattern of improvement (albeit temporary) with empiric antibiotics for lower urinary tract infection and an absence of culture-proven infections. Most of these "bladder infections" are reported as having been diagnosed on office urine dipstick urinalysis.

TABLE 12.1 Pelvic pain etiologies

Musculoskeletal, cutaneous	**Visceral**
Peripheral neuropathy	Uterine
Infectious and dermatologic lesions	Interstitial cystitis/painful bladder syndrome
Myofascial	Colorectal

Other common scenarios include prolonged or recurrent vaginal or vulvar burning. Such patients are frequently treated empirically for vaginal candidiasis or bacterial vaginosis. Examination during an acute episode frequently reveals an absence of the characteristic clinical signs of discharge associated with the diagnosis of bacterial vaginosis or vaginal candidiasis. Examination may reveal normal physiologic discharge with negative wet mount evaluation. Vaginosis screening tests are frequently negative or equivocal.

Lower abdominal pain is a common presenting sign of IC/PBS. It characteristically is described by the sufferer as suprapubic but may radiate laterally. It is often described as vague and has no trigger points on abdominal examination.

Because of the clinically variable nature of IC/BPS, it must be considered in the differential diagnosis of any female patient who presents with pelvic pain of any type, including genital burning and dyspareunia. It must be actively considered by all clinicians who treat women (Table 12.1).

Evaluation

Because of the overlap between the symptoms of IC/BPS and other etiologies of pelvic pain, the evaluation of the IC/BPS patient has considerable overlap with the general evaluation for pelvic pain, dysuria, and dyspareunia. Important in the initial evaluation is a careful survey and assessment of urinary symptoms. Complaints of urinary urgency, frequency, nocturia, or dysuria raise the possibility of IC/BPS.

In the undifferentiated patient, a meaningful assessment can be undertaken in two visits.

Interview and Physical Exam: The Initial Assessment

On initial evaluation, the patient interview can provide a considerable guidance regarding the underlying etiology (-ies) of the discomfort or pain. The standard information regarding the location, duration, and severity of symptoms should always be elicited. The addition of specific organ system-focused inquiries may provide benefit in identifying an etiology.

These inquiries should include the presence or absence of urinary frequency, dysuria, dyspareunia, vaginal discharge, and exacerbation with certain activities. Specific attention should be paid to any history of loose or bloody stools as these may be indicators for inflammatory bowel disease or irritable bowel syndrome. Additional elements in the history which are not part of the customary review of systems but which can suggest IC/BPS include exacerbation with intake of certain foods or variation in severity with stress. Specifically, intake of spicy or high potassium-containing foods [3] may exacerbate symptoms of IC/BPS.

A careful, focused pelvic exam can provide considerable guidance in the diagnosis of IC/BPS. Prior to examination the patient should be asked to void. A clean catch spontaneously voided specimen should be collected and sent for cytology.

Abdominal examination should be performed. Any tenderness on any of the abdominal quadrants should be noted. Particular focus should be directed toward the suprapubic region.

Attention should also be focused on the bony portions of the lower abdomen. The ischium should be palpated from the anterior superior ischial spine to the symphysis pubis. Any trigger point tenderness should be noted.

The pelvic examination in the patient presenting with extended duration pelvic pain should be comprehensive and should assess not only the genital organs but also the portions of musculoskeletal, alimentary, and urinary tracts which are located in the pelvis. Findings in these areas can provide guidance in further evaluation (Fig. 12.1). Pelvic examination should begin with a careful and comprehensive examination of the external genital skin for any signs of vulvar skin disease. Vulvar skin lesions if identified should be assessed appropriately as vulvar dystrophy, and other associated skin conditions of the vulvar skin may manifest with burning and pain and can guide the evaluation. In some circumstances, contact of the affected skin

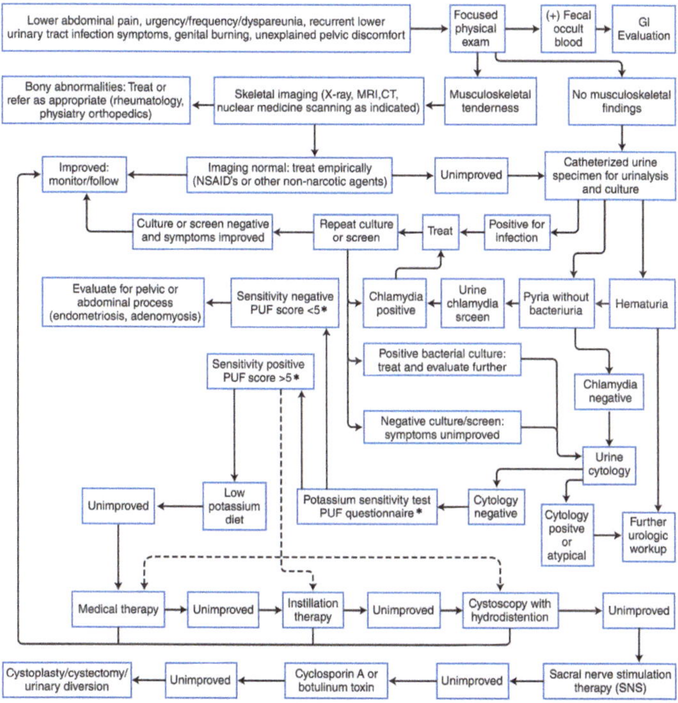

*originally described as a diagnostic test for IC/PBS the potassium sensitivity test is no longer routinely recommended as instillation of potassium may trigger significant pain and the test may not add significantly to information which can be gleaned from a validated symptom questionnaire

Fig. 12.1 *Dotted lines*: optional pathways within the algorithm for patients with more severe symptoms or symptoms of longer duration

with urine, either from splash associated with voiding or with soaking related to continuous leakage of urine in patients suffering from urinary incontinence, can be subjectively misinterpreted as dysuria. Biopsy of any abnormal appearing areas is indicated. Empiric treatment, as clinically appropriate for vulvar skin conditions, can provide early relief and can guide the evaluation.

The vaginal vestibule should be assessed in the course of the examination. The vaginal vestibule is the mucosal region on the external genitalia which is immediately distal to the hymen or hymenal remnant. Any visible changes in the mucosa of that region should be noted and assessed appropriately. Pain mapping of the region should be performed with a sterile cotton-tipped swab. The periurethral regions should be gently palpated with the swab, and any discomfort in disproportion to that anticipated from contact with a cotton-tipped swab should be noted. Trigger point pain in this region can be associated with IC/BPS or vulvar vestibulitis syndrome.

Sterile urethral catheterization should be performed to collect a specimen for urinalysis and culture and sensitivity. This will also provide a measurement of the urinary post-void residual volume. Significantly elevated residual volumes suggest the need for additional evaluation of voiding function, urinary storage, and neurologic disorders.

The degree of discomfort associated with "in and out" catheterization should be noted. Nominal discomfort is anticipated. Severe, sharp, stabbing, or lingering pain is abnormal and should be noted. For pateint with severe genital burning or suprapubic pain the clinician may choose to skip bladder catheterization as it may result in exacerbation of the pain.

Examination with a speculum should follow. The entire lower genital tract should be assessed for atrophy (estrogen status), visible lesions, inflammation, friability, or other anatomical alteration.

Bimanual examination should begin with the "360 degree" pelvic examination. This includes palpation of all bony and muscular structures which can be palpated on vaginal examination and should be performed prior to palpation of the uterus and adnexa. Any trigger point tenderness should be noted. Assessment should begin with palpation of the anterior surfaces of the sacrum and coccyx. Similarly any tenderness of the sacroiliac joints should be noted. The sacrospinous ligaments should be palpated. The ischial spines should also be assessed for trigger point pain. The anterior surface of the levator ani muscle should be assessed for trigger point tenderness or pain. The patient should be asked to perform a pelvic floor contraction (Kegel exercise) in order to facilitate evaluation of levator muscle strength and any symptoms of pelvic pain associated with activity of the pelvic floor.

The lateral pelvic sidewalls should also be assessed. Palpation of the posterior surface of the pubic rami should be performed. The palpable posterior portions of the symphysis pubis should be assessed for trigger point pain. Finally, the anterior vaginal wall should be assessed along its entire length, from the suburethral region to the anterior fornix with careful notation of any trigger point tenderness in this region. IC/BPS patients will commonly show tenderness at the bladder trigone and urethra.

Any musculoskeletal pain trigger points should be assessed in aggregate and appropriate additional workup or therapy prescribed.

Assessment of the uterus, cervix, parametrium, and adnexa follows. It is helpful to begin with a palpation of the uterosacral ligaments. Nodularity or trigger point tenderness (with faithful reproduction of presenting symptoms) in these structures can suggest the presence of endometriosis on the premenopausal female. Similarly, thickening or tenderness in the parametria may also be indicative of endometriosis of the pelvic peritoneum.

Examination of the uterus should include assessment of its size and position. Trigger point tenderness of the uterus can suggest the presence of adenomyosis. The uterosacral ligaments should be assessed and any trigger point pain noted.

Bimanual evaluation of the adnexa should include not only an assessment for palpable masses but also for the presence of any tenderness on palpation.

Rectovaginal examination should be performed with vigilance for any nodularity palpable between the rectum and vagina. Fecal occult blood testing should be performed in patients who provide a history of bloody or repeatedly loose stools.

Additional Diagnostic Steps

Findings on the initial assessment should be evaluated further as indicated by their location and severity.

Any significant finding of tenderness in the bony, tendinous, or muscular structures palpable on pelvic examination calls for further evaluation.

Bony or muscular trigger point findings should be further evaluated with appropriate guided testing. Plain film imaging studies can provide meaningful additional data in the assessment of bone and joint disorders, including diastasis pubis, fracture, arthritic changes, as well as lytic lesions. Empiric pharmacologic therapy with non-steroidal anti-inflammatory agents may be appropriate if the imaging studies do not uncover any abnormalities.

Adnexal tenderness and/or uterine tenderness can be further assessed with transvaginal imaging. The presence of adenomyosis can be elucidated by flow study.

Tenderness on palpation of the anterior vaginal compartment suggests bladder pain syndrome.

After initial assessment is complete, appropriate initial management of pelvic pain and urinary symptoms can be undertaken.

Atrophic changes of the lower genital mucosa should be addressed with local estrogen cream for those whose supplemental estrogen is not contraindicated and the patient reassessed for resolution.

Any findings of hematuria or cytologic atypia on urinary testing should be followed appropriately. This may require cystoscopy and, if indicated, biopsy. Imaging studies may be required to assess the upper collecting system.

Cystitis as diagnosed on urine culture should be treated and the patient reassessed for resolution of symptoms.

Patients with dysuria whose urinary testing exhibits pyuria with no bacteriuria should be evaluated for chlamydial urethritis.

Positive fecal occult blood findings should prompt additional gastrointestinal evaluation. Inflammatory bowel disease must be considered as a possible underlying etiology of pelvic discomfort or pain [4].

Pathophysiology of Interstitial Cystitis

The urinary bladder mucosa is protected by a glycosaminoglycan (GAG) layer. Beneath the GAG layer lies the bladder mucosa. Beneath the mucosa is the submucosa, the bladder interstitial tissue. Within the interstitial tissue are unmyelinated C-fibers which carry afferent sensory traffic via the autonomic nervous system to the CNS [5].

Though the exact pathophysiology of IC/BPS is not known, two theories have been put forth to explain the evolution of symptoms: the "leaky epithelium" theory and the "neurogenic upregulation" theory.

The "leaky epithelium" theory suggests that in IC/BPS defects occur in the protective GAG layer. These defects allow inspissation of potassium cations (and other substances) from the excreted urine through the bladder mucosal epithelium into the interstitial space of the urinary bladder. Once there, irritating substances facilitate ongoing inflammatory changes [6]. Further release of substance P, histamines, and prostaglandin from mast cells within the detrusor muscle potentiates inflammation and stimulates nociception via bladder C-fibers. "Neurogenic upregulation" occurs in C-fibers. As the process progresses more and more, low-grade inflammatory tissue response evolves and afferent C-fiber traffic increases. When nociceptive afferent traffic reaches threshold, symptoms of pain appear. There is data which suggests that affected bladders have a higher density of C-fibers [5].

Preganglionic autonomic afferents distribute to numerous anatomic locations and have evolved to signal visceral pain. They are not efficient pinpoint pain indicators. As such nociceptive impulses carried on these fibers may be perceived as arising from sources elsewhere along the distribution of sacral afferents. Stimuli may thus be perceived as pain arising from the vulva, vagina, urethra, or lower abdomen.

Clinical Features of IC/BPS

IC/BPS is commonly diagnosed in the fourth decade of life or later [7]. Eighty percent of patients with IC/BPS report dyspareunia, both superficial and deep. Pain often persists after intercourse. Sixty-five percent of patient with IC/BPS report urinary urgency and frequency (without incontinence) [8].

Many patients see multiple consultants before the diagnosis is considered. Analysis of claims data in IC/PBS patients indicates that the average sufferer sees seven consultants over a 7-year period before diagnosis.

The Follow-Up Visit

Sufferers of IC/BPS will have what can be termed "frustratingly negative" test results. Urinalysis, culture, and cytology are very frequently negative. In the absence of any other findings on initial evaluation and follow-up investigation, a urinary tract etiology should be pursued.

Diagnostic Testing

Several valuable instruments are available. The PUF questionnaire [10] is a validated instrument which can be administered on the follow-up visit. The questionnaire assesses symptoms related to IC/BPS by several symptom categories.

It is an eight-item inventory which assesses the symptom and bother score related to symptoms of urinary frequency, urgency, and dyspareunia. The patient is asked to rate her severity in each category. The inventories when totaled generate a "symptom score," a "bother score," and a total score (which represents the sum of the symptom and bother scores). A score of 5 or greater in the symptom list suggests the diagnosis of interstitial cystitis [1].

Another available diagnostic test for interstitial cystitis is the potassium sensitivity test.

Originally described as a diagnostic physiologic test for interstitial cystitis [2], the value of the potassium sensitivity test (PST) centers on the pain response to infusion of a potassium solution. The theory underlying the test's validity is the reaction of the bladder interstices to potassium [9]. Physiologically excreted potassium ions in the urine inspissate into the bladder interstices through the defects in the mucosal glycosaminoglycan (GAG) layer of the bladder to produce a local inflammatory result. C-fibers in the interstices carry pain sensation via afferent autonomics [3]. Any pain response to the solution is considered a positive result.

The test can be performed during an office visit. Two solutions are instilled, one (the first) being sterile water and the second a dilute potassium solution. The patient is blinded as to which is which.

The patient is asked to void and is placed in lithotomy. A seven Fr. catheter (a sterile pediatric feeding catheter can be used) is introduced into the bladder. The patient is provided with a questionnaire. The questionnaire addresses the baseline level or urinary urge or pain.

The test begins with the instillation of "solution A" (60 ml or sterile water over a 4–5-min period). The patient is asked to rate symptoms of pain and urgency in response to the instillation. The sterile water is drained. "Solution B" (60 ml of a 0.4 M potassium chloride solution) is then instilled. The patient is asked to rate her pain and urgency symptoms. If there is no initial response, the test can be extended for an additional 5 min. If there is a strong reaction and the patient feels significant discomfort, the potassium solution should be drained, the bladder irrigated with sterile water, and a "rescue" solution (containing lidocaine, heparin, and hydrocortisone) can be instilled. The final two questions on the accompanying questionnaire to be answered address which solution induced more discomfort and how significant the difference in induced pain or urgency between solutions was. Any response to the instillation of dilute potassium is considered positive, whether it induces pain or burning.

The test is simple, straightforward, and easily incorporated into a clinical practice. Among its limitations, however, is a high false-positive rate. The test may also unnecessarily produce pain and discomfort in IC/BPS patients. The utility of the potassium sensitivity test as a diagnostic tool has been questioned in that its outcome may not ultimately affect the management or treatment approach if the diagnosis is suggested by other validated instruments [4].

The PUF questionnaire has been identified as having the same sensitivity as the PST without the associated risk of pain exacerbation. The PST has largely fallen out of use in most facilities.

Another tool useful in the assessment and follow-up of the IC/BPS patient is the O'Leary Sant Questionnaire [11]. It divides responses into a symptom index and problem index. This symptoms inventory can discriminate between IC/BPS and other urologic diagnoses. The questionnaire is useful in establishing a baseline degree of symptom severity for comparison after intervention.

Once diagnosed, IC/BPS can be treated with multiple measures.

Therapy

Therapeutic options for IC/BPS are available and should be employed after thorough evaluation and appropriate diagnostic testing. Therapeutic options for the IC/BPS patient should focus on relief of pain and amelioration of symptoms of urinary frequency.

Cystoscopy with Hydrodistention

Cystoscopy with hydrodistention is both diagnostic and therapeutic for IC/BPS. Under general anesthesia the bladder epithelium is examined cystoscopically (with appropriate tissue sampling of suspicious appearing areas). The urinary bladder is then filled to 70–80 cm H_2O pressure and held at that pressure for 5 min. With the release of the distention fluid (decompression), the mucosa is monitored for the appearance of vascular glomerulations in the bladder mucosa.

Fulguration of Hunner's ulcers (if identified) has also been associated with relief of pain symptoms. Injection of triamcinolone into Hunner's ulcers has also been associated with relief of bladder pain.

Instillation Therapy

Dimethylsulfoxide (DMSO) is FDA approved for use in the treatment of IC/BPS. It is typically instilled on a weekly basis for a total of six treatments [12, 13].

Other agents can be used to manage symptom flares. These include heparin, corticosteroids, lidocaine, and sodium bicarbonate.

Medical Therapy

One FDA-approved agent for the treatment of symptoms related to interstitial cystitis, pentosan polysulfate sodium (Elmiron®) ([14–17]) is available in the United States.

Pentosan polysulfate sodium (PPS, Elmiron®) is an oral agent whose structure is similar to that of the GAG layer. It works to stimulate a regeneration of the glycosaminoglycan layer of the urinary bladder. This re-establishes the natural protection of the bladder interstices from the contents of excreted urine. The drug is generally well tolerated and leads to improvement or resolution of symptoms in 60% of sufferers [18]. Duration of therapy is typically 3–6 months.

The addition of other agents enhances the symptom relief provided by PPS alone. Hydroxyzine, an antihistamine, is thought to reduce the inflammatory response within the bladder interstitial spaces by stabilizing mast cells. Antihistamines also have a sedative effect which improves sleep and exerts mild anticholinergic properties which may reduce urinary frequency and overactive bladder symptoms. All of these act in concert to reduce symptoms in IC/BPS sufferers [19].

H2 blockers may also prove useful (cimetidine).

Tricyclic antidepressants (amitriptyline, nortriptyline, etc.) are believed to reduce the transmission of pain along non-myelinated C-fibers in the lower urinary tract. Their anticholinergic effect may also reduce urinary frequency, while their sedative effect may improve sleep quality and reduce nocturnal bladder urgency [20].

The addition of other anticholinergic agents may further reduce the degree of urinary frequency with further improvement of quality of life. Additional agents which have been reported as useful in the management of IC/BPS syndrome symptoms in refractory cases are cyclosporin A [10] and injectable botulinum toxin A. These agents do not have FDA approval for use in IC/BPS patients but can be used by experienced practitioners who have experience with them and are willing to provide long-term care to IC/BPS patients.

Adjunctive Measures

The adverse effect on quality of life brought on by the pain and urinary frequency cause by IC/BPS accompanied by dyspareunia can have significant detriment on quality of life.

Patients identified with IC/BPS should be encouraged to seek information on self-help to develop strategies to manage and cope with the symptoms of IC/BPS. Support groups are organized and available on a local and regional basis.

Acupuncture is described as providing relief by many sufferers of IC/BPS. Though definitive data on acupuncture is lacking, anecdotal evidence suggests that as an adjunctive measure acupuncture may provide episodic relief and help sufferers cope with the syndrome's symptoms.

Certain over-the-counter agents (chondroitin sulfate/glucosamine, L-arginine) have also been described as helpful in providing symptomatic relief, though no supportive research data is available to support their use.

Dietary Measures

Intake of certain food substances in the diet can contribute to symptoms related to IC/BPS. These include foods which are high in potassium. Among such foods are many items which are considered a good part of a healthy diet and include citrus fruits, tomatoes, strawberries, and grapes. Ironically, foods recommended for genital and bladder health, like yogurt and cranberries/cranberry juice, have high potassium content which can exacerbate symptoms of IC/BPS. In addition, spicy and acidic foods are generally best avoided.

Sacral Nerve Stimulation

Sacral nerve stimulation (SNS) therapy is indicated for the treatment of urinary frequency associated with overactive bladder. Given the overlap of symptoms between urge frequency syndrome (overactive bladder) and IC, there is utility for SNS therapy in IC patients [23].

The patient is asked to keep a urinary symptom diary (3–7 days). Once the baseline data is gathered, the first step of two is undertaken. Under fluoroscopic guidance, an electrode is placed transcutaneously into the third sacral foramen (S3). It is tunneled under the skin, and an exit point for the electrode lead is developed to the right or left of the midline ipsilateral to the foramen into which the contact equipped lead end was placed. The lead is connected to an external signal generator which the patient uses and carries with her on a belt. The test period consists of wearing an external generator for a trial period. Stimulation of inhibitory fibers carried along the S3 nerve root can lead to a reduction in bladder activity (reduction in urinary frequency). The patient keeps a urinary diary. After a 14-day test trial, the data from the urinary log are reviewed. If an improvement over baseline is noted and demonstrable relief is identified, the system is internalized (in a manner similar to that of a cardiac pacemaker). The signal generator is implanted beneath the skin of the upper outer buttock. The signal generator can be programmed via a remote which is placed over the skin which covers it. There is evidence which suggests that improvement in pain related to IC is also attained from SNS therapy. The signal generator may require periodic reprogramming in order to maintain its efficacy.

Cystectomy/Augmentation Cystoplasty

Surgical removal of the bladder or interposition of intestinal tissue to increase bladder volume is considered the end-stage procedure for IC. These therapies are generally reserved for patients with severe symptoms who have not responded to other therapies, though this therapy may only be necessary in a small number of patients.

Long-Term Care and Follow-Up of IC/BPS

Sufferers of the IC/BPS syndrome will require ongoing care. There may be episodic flares of pain related to dietary factors, seasonal allergies, or interim episodes of cystitis. It is important for the physician caring for affected patients to maintain vigilance for recurring symptoms and to appropriately evaluate each episode of exacerbation to rule out other interim lower urinary tract pathology.

Ordering and Prioritizing Therapy

In its 2011 clinical guideline on management of IC/BPS, the American Urological Association put forth a suggested hierarchy of therapies for management of the patient with IC/BPS [10].

First-Line Therapy

Initial therapy should include an assessment of the patient's understanding and knowledge of the condition. Therapy begins with education regarding the condition and the available treatments. It should also include behavior modification(s) to improve symptoms and manage exacerbation associated with stress. This may include dietary modification, relaxation techniques, and pain management. The potential need for multiple treatments (multimodal therapy) should be introduced.

Second Line

If relief goals are not met with first-line therapies, additional treatment steps include trigger point massage or myofascial release (if appropriate consultants are available). Pharmacologic therapy, either oral (pentosan sulfate, hydroxyzine, amitriptyline, cimetidine) or instillation (DMSO, lidocaine, heparin), is an appropriate second-line treatment.

Third Line

Cystoscopy with hydrodistention (and fulguration of Hunner's ulcers, if present) represents a third-line therapy for patients who have not attained meaningful or targeted relief of symptoms. Injection of corticosteroid (triamcinolone) into Hunner's ulcers may provide relief from bladder pain [21].

Fourth Line

Sacral neuromodulation should be considered in patients who continue to have symptoms adversely affecting quality of life after behavioral and pharmacologic therapies have been attempted [23]. Sacral neuromodulation has FDA approval for urinary frequency and bladder overactivity but not directly for management of pain related to IC/BPS. IC/BPS sufferers should undergo the appropriate initial trial period. Relief with the initial trial should prompt permanent implantation.

Fifth Line

Oral cyclosporine A administered orally can be considered if other treatments have failed. Limited data on the effectiveness of this anti-rejection drug suggests that its use may provide relief of IC-/BPS-related pain. Its use should be limited to those clinicians who have experience with its use and who are willing to provide long-term ongoing treatment for IC/BPS patients.

Intradetrusor injections of on a botulinum toxin A can also be used to control symptoms of frequency and pain [22]. Currently this agent (Botox®) is approved for detrusor overactivity in patients with upper motor neuron disease.

Sixth Line

Major surgical intervention should be reserved for patients who are refractory to all treatments and whose quality of life is adversely affected by IC/BPS symptoms. Surgical options may include augmentation cystoplasty, substitution cystoplasty, and urinary diversion with or without cystectomy.

As investigative efforts proceed, additional therapies will likely emerge. In managing the IC/BPS patient, therapy should be individualized to meet the goals of each patient.

Multiple, simultaneous treatments may be necessary to provide meaningful relief. Ineffective therapies should be discontinued. The treating physician should maintain regular follow-up with IC/BPS patients and appropriately assess exacerbations and advance therapy if needed.

References

1. Parsons CL, Dell J, et al. Increased prevalence of interstitial cystitis: previously unrecognized urologic and gynecologic cases identified using a new symptom questionnaire and intravesical potassium sensitivity. Urology. 2002;60:573–8.
2. Clemens JQ, Joyce GF, Wise M, Payne C. Interstitial cystitis and painful bladder syndrome. In: Litwin MS, Saigal CS, editors.

Urologic diseases in America. Washington: US Department of Health and Human Services, Public Health Service, National Institutes of Health, National Institute of Diabetes and Digestive and Kidney Diseases; 2007. p. 123.

3. Friedlander JI, Shorter B, Moldwin RM. Diet and its role in interstitial cystitis/bladder pain syndrome (IC/BPS) and comorbid conditions. BJU Int. 2012;109:1584–91.
4. Stowe SP, Redmond SR, Stormont JM, Shah AN, Chessin LN, Segal HL, Chey WY. Gastroenterology. An epidemiologic study of inflammatory bowel disease in Rochester, New York. Hosp Incidence. 1990;98(1):104–10.
5. Hohenfellner M, Nunes L, et al. Interstitial cystitis: increased sympathetic innervation and related neuropeptide synthesis. J Urol. 1992;147:587–91.
6. Parsons CL, Greenberger M, et al. The role of urinary potassium in the pathogenesis and diagnosis of interstitial cystitis. J Urol. 1998;159:1862–7.
7. Simon LJ, Landis JR, Erickson DR, Nyberg LM. The interstitial cystitis data base study: concepts and preliminary baseline descriptive statistics. Urology. 1997;49(5A Suppl):64–75.
8. Minaglia S, Ozel B, Bizhang R, Mishell DR Jr. Interstitial cystitis in women with detrusor overactivity refractory to anticholinergic therapy. Division of Female Pelvic Medicine and Reconstructive Surgery, Department of Obstetrics and Gynecology, University of Southern California Keck School of Medicine, Los Angeles, California. Urology. 2005;66:702–6.
9. Parsons CL. Argument for the use of the potassium sensitivity test in the diagnosis of interstitial cystitis. For. Int Urogynecol J Pelvic Floor Dysfunct. 2005;16(6):430–1.
10. Hanno PM, Burks DA, Clemens JQ, Dmochowski RR, Erickson D, Fitzgerald MP, Forrest JB, Gordon B, Gray M, Mayer RD, Newman D, Nyberg L Jr, Payne CK, Wesselmann U, Faraday MM. Interstitial Cystitis Guidelines Panel of the American Urological Association Education and Research, Inc., AUA guideline for the diagnosis and treatment of interstitial cystitis/bladder pain syndrome. J Urol. 2011;185(6):2162–70.
11. Kushner L, Moldwin RM. Efficiency of questionnaires used to screen for interstitial cystitis. J Urol. 2006;176:587–92.
12. Rossberger MF, Peeker R. Critical appraisal of dimethyl sulfoxide treatment for interstitial cystitis: discomfort, side-effects and treatment outcome J. Department of Urology, Sahlgrenska University Hospital, Goteborg, Sweden. Scand J Urol Nephrol. 2005;39:73–7.

13. Peeker R, Haghsheno MA, Holmang S, et al. Intravesical bacillus Calmette-Guerin and dimethyl sulfoxide for treatment of classic and nonulcer interstitial cystitis:a prospective, randomized double-blind study. J Urol. 2000;164:1912–6.
14. Mulholland SG, Hanno P, Parsons CL, Sant GR, Staskin DR. Pentosanpolysulfate sodium for therapy of interstitial cystitis: a double-blind placebo-controlled clinical study. Urology. 1990;35:552–8.
15. Parsons CL, Benson G, Childs SJ, Hanna P, Sant GR, Webster G. A quantitatively controlled method to study prospectively interstitial cystitis and demonstrate the efficacy of pentosanpolysulfate. J Urol. 1993;150:845–8.
16. Holm-Bentzen M, Jacobsen F, Nerstrom B, Lose G, Kristensen JK, Pedersen RH. A prospective double blind clinically controlled multicentre trial of sodium pentosan polysulfate in the treatment of interstitial cystitis and related painful bladder disease. J Urol. 1987;138:503–7.
17. Philip M. Analysis of long-term Elmiron therapy for interstitial cystitis. Hanno Urol. 1997;49(5, Supplement 1):93–9.
18. Hanno PM. Analysis of long-term Elmiron therapy for interstitial cystitis. Urology. 1997;49 (5A suppl):93–9.
19. Theoharides TC, Sant GR. Hydroxyzine therapy for interstitial cystitis. Urology. 1997;49(5A Suppl):108–10.
20. van Ophoven A, Pokupic S, et al. A prospective, randomized, placebo controlled, double-blind study of amitriptyline for the treatment of interstitial cystitis. J Urol. 2004;172:533–6.
21. Cox M, Klutke JJ, Klutke CG. Assessment of patient outcomes following submucosal injection of triamcinolone for treatment of Hunner's ulcer subtype interstitial cystitis. Can J Urol. 2009; 16:4536.
22. Pinto R, Lopes T, Frias B, Silva A, Silva JA, Silva CM, Cruz C, Cruz F, Dinis P. Trigonal injection of botulinum toxin A in patients with refractory bladder pain syndrome/interstitial cystitis. Eur Urol. 2010;58(3):360–5. Epub 2010 Mar 6.
23. Comiter CV. Sacral neuromodulation for the symptomatic treatment of refractory interstitial cystitis: a prospective study. J Urol. 2003;169:1369–73.

Chapter 13
Office Management of Female Pelvic Floor Dysfunction

Sara Kostant and Michael D. Moen

Introduction

Pelvic floor dysfunction, including urinary incontinence and pelvic organ prolapse, affects millions of American women. These problems are more common than most healthcare providers realize. About 24% of all women have at least one symptom of pelvic floor dysfunction [1]. The lifetime risk of undergoing surgery for pelvic organ prolapse or incontinence is 20% [2], which does not take into account women who undergo medical management of their symptoms or do not seek treatment at all.

The prevalence of pelvic floor disorders is set to increase significantly over the next few decades. One study estimates that by 2050, the number of women with urinary incontinence will increase 55% to 28.4 million, and the number of women with pelvic organ prolapse will increase 46% to 4.9 million [3].

S. Kostant
Hackensack University Medical Center, Department of Obstetrics and Gynecology, Hackensack, NJ, USA

M. D. Moen (✉)
Rosalind Franklin University Chicago Medical School, Advocate Lutheran General Hospital, Department of Obstetrics and Gynecology, Park Ridge, IL, USA
e-mail: Michael.moen@advocatehealth.com

J. V. Knaus et al. (eds.), *Ambulatory Gynecology*,
https://doi.org/10.1007/978-1-4939-7641-6_13

Increasing age is a risk factor for pelvic floor dysfunction, and the number of women over age 65 will have doubled between 2008 and 2050 [4].

A general gynecologist is often the first provider to see patients with pelvic floor dysfunction, as most women do not seek out a specialist when these symptoms initially occur. General gynecologists can expect to see an increase in women presenting with urinary incontinence, pelvic organ prolapse, and voiding dysfunction to his or her office over the next decades. Management of these issues might seem daunting to many gynecologists. Graduating OB/GYN residents have less experience managing issues related to pelvic floor dysfunction than obstetric and benign gynecological issues common to the premenopausal patient.

The general gynecologist will have a growing responsibility to manage urinary incontinence, pelvic organ prolapse, and voiding dysfunction. The purpose of this chapter is to provide a framework for the evaluation and management of these issues. Voiding dysfunction, for the purposes of this chapter, refers to patient complaints of changes in her urine flow and ability to empty her bladder.

Pelvic Floor Dysfunction Terminology

Standardized terminology for female pelvic floor dysfunction eases communication between providers and patients. The following definitions are taken from the most recent *International Urogynecological Association (IUGA)/International Continence Society (ICS)* guidelines [5].

Stress incontinence

The complaint of the involuntary loss of urine on effort or physical exertion

Urgency

The complaint of a sudden, compelling desire to pass urine which is difficult to defer

Urgency incontinence

The complaint of the involuntary loss of urine associated with urgency

Mixed incontinence

The complaint of involuntary loss of urine associated with urgency and also with effort or physical exertion or on sneezing or coughing

Frequency

The complaint that urination occurs more frequently during waking hours than previously deemed normal by the woman

Nocturia

The complaint of the interruption of sleep one or more times because of the need to urinate

Overactive bladder (OAB, urgency) syndrome

Urinary urgency, usually accompanied by frequency and nocturia, with or without urgency urinary incontinence, in the absence of urinary tract infection or obvious pathology

Feeling of incomplete (bladder) emptying

The complaint that the bladder does not feel empty after urination

This symptom may or may not actually correlate with an elevated post-void residual on exam. Patients presenting with this complaint may mention a need to strain or change position in order to feel like she is emptying her bladder.

Pelvic Organ Prolapse

The descent of one or more of the anterior vaginal wall, posterior vaginal wall, the uterus (cervix), or the apex of the vagina (vaginal vault or cuff scar after hysterectomy)

A patient with this finding would likely be presenting with a complaint of a "bulge" sensation in the vagina.

Evaluation

A complete medical, surgical, and gynecological history should be obtained from the patient. The patient's non-gynecological medical history may explain a patient's symptoms. Patients with neurologic disorders may experience both overactive bladder and incomplete emptying. Frequently used medications for hypertension, such as diuretics and acetylcholinesterase inhibitors, can increase urinary frequency. Sleep apnea can often be responsible for nocturia, and the introduction of CPAP therapy may resolve the patient's symptoms. The patient's medical history may also guide treatment. If a patient reports a history of closed-angle glaucoma or bowel obstructions due to constipation, anticholinergic medications will be contraindicated.

Increased gravidity and parity can predispose patients to pelvic floor disorders. A history of a third- or fourth-degree episiotomy should be noted as fecal incontinence is more common in these patients, but women are often embarrassed to reveal this symptom. Prior pelvic surgery can contribute to denervation injury, which may contribute to overactive bladder or incomplete emptying. Pelvic radiation for gynecological cancer can lead to a loss of compliance of the bladder wall and urethra. This can lead to stress incontinence due to the scarring of the bladder neck and urethral sphincter muscles and urinary urgency and frequency due to reduced bladder capacity.

The healthcare provider should thoroughly review the patient's current symptoms. The onset and duration of the patient's symptoms is important. If incontinence is the main complaint, it is critical to differentiate between stress and urge incontinence, recognizing that more than a third of women will have components of both (mixed incontinence) [6].

The abdominal and pelvic examination is key to the assessment of women with pelvic floor dysfunction. The vulva and vagina should be examined for signs of urogenital atrophy. Loss of rugations and thin, pale vaginal mucosa may be noted in this circumstance. The patient is asked to cough, and the mobility of the urethra and leakage of urine is noted. A change in the angle of the urethra of more than 30 degrees indicates a hypermobile urethra. The neuromuscular exam includes an assessment of perineal and vulvar sensation, pelvic floor resting tone, and pelvic floor muscle strength. Perineal sensation can be assessed with a q-tip or by direct light palpation. The patient can then be instructed to contract her pelvic floor muscles as if she is trying to stop the flow of urine or trying to hold gas in the rectum. Pelvic floor contraction strength can be graded according to a modified Oxford scale as shown in Table 13.1.

Prolapse of the anterior and posterior vaginal walls, uterus, and vaginal apex are measured in the supine position with the patient performing a Valsalva maneuver. A half speculum is useful for examination of the anterior and posterior walls separately.

Many providers are confused by the appropriate documentation of the stage of prolapse. The Pelvic Organ Prolapse Quantification System (POP-Q), describes the measurement of nine points of vaginal support. A newer, abbreviated system focuses on the evaluation of four points – the anterior and posterior vaginal walls, the vaginal apex, and the cervix. In women who have had a hysterectomy, the cervix is left out and only three points are documented. This system has been noted to have good inter-observer and inter-system reliability [7]. Table 13.2 describes the points in the vagina that are used for measurement of each compartment, and Table 13.3 shows how each point corresponds to staging.

Multichannel urodynamic testing is not necessary in the initial evaluation of most patients with incontinence. Simple cystometry, or a "bladder fill", is a quick, inexpensive tool for bladder function assessment. After the urethral meatus is swabbed with iodine, a red rubber catheter is placed in the bladder using sterile technique. The end of the catheter is connected to a 50–60 ml funnel syringe. The bladder is then

Table 13.1 Modified Oxford scale for pelvic muscle contraction strength

Grade	Definition
0	No contraction
1	Flicker
2	Weak
3	Moderate
4	Good (with lift)
5	Strong (with lift)

Laycock [26]

Table 13.2 Simplified pelvic organ prolapse quantification (POP-Q) system

Vaginal compartment	Area of measurement
Anterior wall	A point 3 cm proximal to the urethral meatus
Cervix	Most distal aspect of the cervix
Apex/cuff	Posterior fornix; if post-hysterectomy, then most distal aspect of the cuff
Posterior wall	A point 3 cm proximal to the hymenal remnants

Swift et al. [7]

filled with sterile water or saline. The patient is asked to report when she feels the following sensations: first sensation of fluid in the bladder, first urge to urinate, strong urge to urinate, and her maximum bladder capacity. Sensations of urgency during bladder filling may be indicative of an overactive bladder. After the maximum capacity is reached, the catheter is removed, and a cough stress test can be performed. The physician can also re-catheterize the patient after she voids to check a post-void residual if there is a concern for incomplete emptying.

Table 13.3 POP-Q staging system

Stage	Location of area of measurement at Valsalva
I	More than 1 cm proximal to the hymenal remnants
II	Between 1 cm proximal and 1 cm distal to the hymenal remnants
III	More than 1 cm distal to the hymenal remnants but without complete vaginal eversion
IV	Vaginal mucosa is completely everted

Swift et al. [7]

Treatment

Therapies Useful for All Pelvic Floor Disorders

Fluid and Diet Management

Unless otherwise medically indicated, fluid restriction is not recommended as a means to decrease urinary frequency. Likewise, excessive hydration is not helpful or necessary. Concentrated urine can further irritate the bladder, actually increasing urgency and frequency. Women should be encouraged to drink enough to satisfy their thirst and counseled that this may result in a transient exacerbation of their overactive bladder symptoms.

Timed Voiding/Bladder Training

Timed voiding can help women manage both overactive bladder symptoms and incomplete emptying. Women with frequency are encouraged to slowly increase the intervals between their voids. For example, if a woman normally feels the urge to void every hour, she is encouraged to increase this interval by an additional 15 min for 1 week. If she is able to wait 1 h and 15 min between voids without leakage, she should increase the interval the next week to an hour and a half, and so forth. Each woman should be encouraged to proceed at her own pace; some women may need to wait 2 or 3 weeks before increasing their voiding intervals. Timed voiding can be used in conjunction with anticholinergic therapy in women with frequent leakage.

Patients with incomplete bladder emptying are advised to void every 3 h, whether or not they feel the urge to void at that time. "Double voiding" – having the patient stand up from the commode and then sit down again – may allow the patient to begin or continue emptying her bladder. Running water from a tap can also be useful cue to help a patient start voiding. Emptying the bladder more frequently may increase bladder sensitivity in women who have become accustomed to waiting several hours between voids. For patients who continue to have elevated post-void residual volumes despite timed voiding, intermittent self-catheterization may be necessary.

Topical Estrogen

Postmenopausal women with urogenital atrophy may have increased irritation of the urethra, leading to dysuria and urgency, even in the absence of a urinary tract infection. Topical estrogen may be a useful adjunct to timed voiding and anticholinergic medication in these women, especially if vaginal dryness, dyspareunia, and recurrent urinary tract infections are also present.

Topical estrogen may be delivered by a vaginal cream (Estrace or Premarin cream), ring (Estring 2 mg/3 months), or tablet (Vagifem 10 mcg). All forms of topical estrogen are equally effective in treating vaginal atrophy. A patient should use the form of delivery that most appeals to her and will increase her compliance. Use of the tablet, ring, or low dose (1–2 g twice weekly) cream preparations do not raise systemic serum estradiol levels to premenopausal levels [8]. Traditionally, hormone replacement therapy, including topical estrogen, has been avoided in patients with a history of breast cancer. There is evidence that breast cancer recurrence may not be associated with either oral or vaginal hormone therapy use [9].

Supplemental progesterone is not routinely recommended in women using topical estrogen who still have a uterus. The endometrial safety of the estrogen ring and tablet have been shown for use up to 12 months and for low doses of estrogen cream for use up to 6 months [10]. As there is a lack of data regarding topical estrogen use in these patients after 12 months of use, consideration may be given to providing supplemental progesterone in women who have been using topical estrogen for over a year; however, this is not routine in our practice.

Pessary users with atrophy may have less vaginal abrasions and therefore a greater likelihood of continuing pessary use, if they use topical estrogen [11].

Pelvic Floor Exercises

Since Dr. Arnold Kegel first discussed the benefits of pelvic floor exercises, [12] multiple studies have shown they can improve symptoms of pelvic floor disorders.

Pelvic floor exercises, even when done correctly and regularly, will likely provide more of an improvement of incontinence and prolapse symptoms, rather than a cure.

Most women presenting to a gynecologist's office with pelvic floor dysfunction have heard of "Kegel exercises" through the popular media. However, less than half of patients have been taught how to properly perform pelvic floor muscle contractions, and most patients who have been taught received verbal training only [13]. Verbal training and reading instructions on pelvic floor exercises do not seem to be sufficient, as less than 25% of patients are able to perform a pelvic floor contraction with a strength rating of 3, 4, or 5 on the Oxford scale [14]. The ideal teaching of pelvic floor contractions occurs during the pelvic exam. The healthcare provider should demonstrate the pelvic floor muscles by palpation and instruct the patient to contract these muscles around the provider's examining finger. The patient should be counseled to avoid performing a Valsalva maneuver or using her abdominal and gluteal muscles during the pelvic floor contraction.

Treatment Options Specific to Different Types of Pelvic Floor Dysfunction

Pelvic Organ Prolapse

Pessaries in general have been underutilized in recent years due to misconceptions about the difficulties of pessary fitting and management. Younger patients, in particular, may have a misconception that pessaries are only an option for "elderly" women or believe that they will not be able to be sexually active if they wear a pessary. In fact, pessary use is an excellent option for women of all ages, especially premenopausal women who desire future pregnancies. Most women can be taught to remove, clean, and replace their pessaries so that sexual activity is not precluded. All women presenting with symptomatic pelvic organ prolapse should be offered a trial of a pessary.

A properly fitted pessary is comfortable and is not felt at all by the patient. Advanced stages of prolapse should not discourage a physician from offering a pessary. Successful continuation of pessary use has not been found to be related to the severity of prolapse or location of the pelvic defect (i.e., cystocele vs rectocele) [15]. Pessaries come in a number of different shapes and sizes, which may seem intimidating to gynecologists unfamiliar with their use. However, most patients can be fitted successfully with a ring with support pessary. Ring pessaries have the longest continuation rate due to their ease of use and are the least likely to cause bothersome vaginal abrasions and vaginal discharge [16]. In addition to standard ring pessaries, there are also ring pessaries with knobs, which can be used in patients with stress incontinence

(Fig. 13.1). Gellhorn pessaries and cube pessaries (Fig. 13.2) are used when a ring pessary cannot stay in the vagina due to the severity of the prolapse. The cube pessary is more likely to cause vaginal abrasions and discharge if not removed on a regular basis [17]. A patient who cannot be managed with a ring pessary may benefit from a referral to a specialist.

After initial pessary placement, the patient returns within 1–2 weeks to assess the comfort and effect of the pessary. If the patient can remove the pessary herself, she should be encouraged to do so at least weekly and leave the pessary out overnight after its cleaning. These women do not need any additional special follow-up and can be seen again at the time of their annual exams. Women who cannot or are not willing to remove the pessary on their own should return at 2–3-month intervals for pessary removal and cleaning. At these follow-up visits, a speculum exam is performed to assess for abrasions, ulcerations, foul-smelling vaginal discharge, and granulation tissue. The vagina may be cleaned at this time with hydrogen peroxide, but there is no evidence to support that this prevents infections. The pessary can be replaced after cleaning if only superficial, hemostatic abrasions are

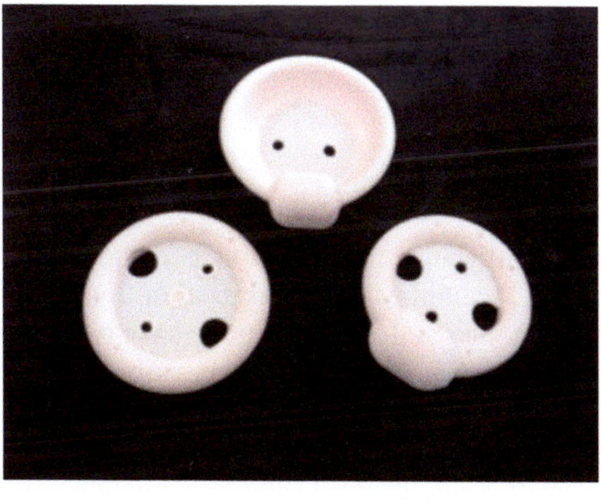

FIG. 13.1 Ring with support, ring with knob, and incontinence dish pessaries

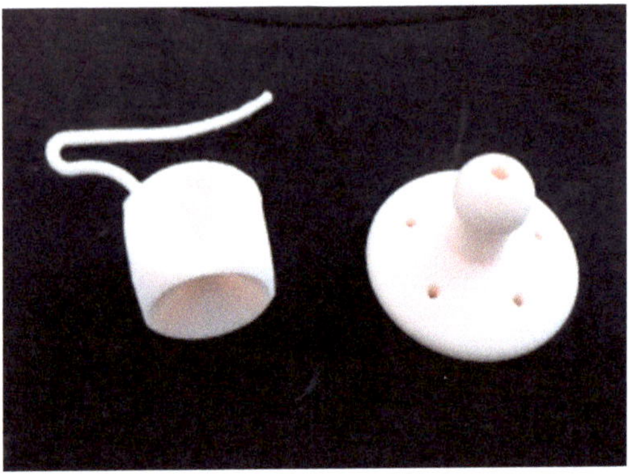

FIG. 13.2 Cube and Gellhorn pessaries

present. Small areas of granulation tissue can be removed with applications of silver nitrate. Bacterial vaginosis can be treated with a 5-day intravaginal course of metronidazole gel. If bleeding ulcerations are noted, the pessary is left out for 2 weeks and topical estrogen is started to assist with healing and is continued after the pessary is replaced.

Not all patients who use pessaries require the use of topical estrogen. As frequent abrasions and vaginitis may discourage pessary use, patients with these findings may benefit from treatment of the atrophy. If a postmenopausal patient has atrophy but no bothersome discharge or abrasions, topical estrogen use can be deferred.

Stress Urinary Incontinence

The midurethral sling procedure has become standard treatment for SUI. A number of nonsurgical options, however, are available to manage SUI, although none have been shown to be as effective as the sling procedure. In our office, we offer every patient presenting with SUI the opportunity to try conservative therapy first, although it is not mandatory for patients who wish to proceed with a midurethral sling immediately. Conservative therapies are useful in patients who have relatively mild stress incontinence, are ambivalent about surgery, poor surgical candidates, pregnant, or planning a future pregnancy.

Incontinence pessaries have been shown to improve incontinence symptoms in 40–50% of women [17, 18]. The combination of pessary use and pelvic floor exercises has not been found to be more effective than either treatment alone [17], but may be useful in women with mixed incontinence symptoms. The advantage of an incontinence pessary over pelvic floor exercises is that it can decrease stress incontinence as soon as it is placed. Incontinence pessaries come in two types: A ring pessary with a knob (with or without a diaphragm) or an incontinence dish (Fig. 13.1). Incontinence pessaries can be fitted during a pelvic exam, using the same guidelines described above for general pessary fitting. In order for the pessary to be effective, the knob of the incontinence ring or dish should rest approximately underneath the midurethra. The patient is taught to remove, clean, and replace the pessary on her own.

Midurethral sling procedures are typically not recommended until a patient has completed childbearing, as to minimize the risk of recurrence of SUI after the surgery. There are, however, case reports of pregnancy and vaginal delivery after undergoing a midurethral sling procedure with maintenance of continence [19].

Overactive Bladder

In addition to timed voiding, pelvic floor exercises, and pelvic floor physical therapy, anticholinergic medications can be used as first-line treatment for overactive bladder. Patients with more bothersome OAB symptoms may want to start these medications immediately rather than go through a trial of behavioral modification and pelvic floor exercises first.

Table 13.4 shows the anticholinergic medications available today that are used to treat OAB. Several studies have shown the efficacy of these medications in reducing frequency and urge incontinence episodes [20–24]. The mechanism of action of these medications is well known. The neurotransmitter acetylcholine stimulates detrusor muscle contraction. Anticholinergic medications work by blocking acetylcholine from attaching to muscarinic receptors on the bladder. Common side effects of

TABLE 13.4 Anticholinergic medications used to treat overactive bladder

Generic name	Brand name	Dosage
Oxybutynin	Ditropan	5 mg bid-tid
	Ditropan XL	5–15 mg daily
	Oxytrol (patch)	3.9 mg twice weekly
	Gelnique (3% topical gel)	84 mg to skin daily
Tolterodine	Detrol	2–4 mg bid
	Detrol LA	4 mg daily
Trospium	Sanctura	20 mg bid
	Sanctura XR	60 mg daily
Solifenacin	Vesicare	5–10 mg daily
Darifenacin	Enablex	7.5–15 mg daily
Fesoterodine	Toviaz	4–8 mg daily

anticholinergic medications include dry eyes, dry mouth, and constipation. Absolute contraindications to anticholinergic medications include closed-angle glaucoma, obstipation, and pre-existing urinary retention (unless the patient is already catheterized), and these medications should be used with caution in the elderly and patients with dementia.

No single anticholinergic medication has been shown to be significantly more effective than another. Generic forms of several of these medications are available if cost is an issue for a patient.

We see patients for follow-up 4 weeks after starting an anticholinergic medication to assess efficacy and side effects. The post-void residual is rechecked if the patient does not feel she is emptying her bladder. If the patient has had a sub-optimal response, the dose will be increased or another anti-cholinergic will be tried. Once the optimal anticholinergic medication and dose has been found, the patient continues the medication for about 6 months. When the patient is able to comfortably maintain a voiding schedule of every 2–3 h, she may attempt to wean from the medication. Typically, this involves decreasing the medication to every other day and then eventually discontinuing the medication.

Voiding Dysfunction

Any of the following patient complaints can fall under the category of voiding dysfunction: hesitancy, slow stream, intermittency, straining to void, feeling of incomplete (bladder) emptying, and postmicturition leakage. All of these symptoms can occur with true incomplete emptying but can also occur as a sensation of incomplete emptying without significant residual urine volumes. The priority for the general gynecology or primary care physician is to ensure the patient is emptying her bladder. This can be accomplished with a simple post-void residual. Most women have a post-void residual less than 50 ml; a value over 200 ml indicates inadequate emptying [25].

If the patient is unable to void at all, or is in pain due to incomplete emptying, a Foley catheter should be placed in the office and the patient given a leg bag for drainage, while she awaits consultation with a specialist. If the patient has incomplete emptying but is not uncomfortable, a catheter should not be placed at this visit. The patient should perform timed voiding at home to decrease the residual until she sees a specialist. Decisions regarding intermittent catheterization in these patients can be left to the specialist.

Conclusion

As the population ages, healthcare providers in the general gynecology field will find themselves caring for an increasing number of women with incontinence, prolapse, and voiding dysfunction. The initial evaluation of these concerns can be intimidating even to a healthcare provider who is familiar with gynecology. Many providers do not encounter these issues frequently in training. The above outlined approaches will help guide the initial evaluation and management of patients with pelvic floor disorders. A patient should be referred to a specialist if she has any of the following: unsatisfactory results from the above treatment options, a desire for surgery for incontinence or prolapse, incomplete emptying with elevated post-void residual volume, and evidence of vaginal mesh exposure on exam from a prior surgery (or any suspicion that the above symptoms could be related to a prior surgery or ongoing pathologic process).

References

1. Nygaard I, Barber MD, Burgio KL, Kenton K, Meikle S, Schaffer J, et al. Prevalence of symptomatic pelvic floor disorders in US women. JAMA. 2008;300:1311–6.
2. Wu JM, Matthews CA, Conover MM, Pate V, Funk MJ. Lifetime risk of stress incontinence or pelvic organ prolapse surgery. Obstet Gynecol. 2014;123:1201–6.
3. Wu JM, Hundley AF, Fulton RG, Myers ER. Forecasting the prevalence of pelvic floor disorders in U.S women: 2010 to 2050. Obstet Gynecol. 2009;114:1278–83.
4. United States Census Bureau [homepage on the Internet]. 2012 National population projections: summary tables. Table 2. Projections of the population by selected age groups and sex for the United States: 2015 to 2060. Available from : http://www.census.gov/population/projections/data/national/2012/summarytables.html. Accessed 27 Mar 2013.
5. Haylen BT, de Ridder D, Freeman RM, Swift SE, Berghmans B, Lee J, Monga A, Petri E, Rizk DE, Sand PK, Schaer GN, International Urogynecological Association, International Continence Society. An international Urogynecological association (IUGA)/international continence society (ICS) joint report on the terminology for female pelvic floor dysfunction. Neurourol Urodyn. 2010;29(1):4–20.
6. Stewart WF, Van Rooyen JB, Cundiff GW, Abrams P, Herzog AR, Corey R, et al. Prevalence and burden of overactive bladder in the United States. World J Urol. 2003;20:327–36.

7. Swift S, Morris S, McKinnie V, Freeman R, Petri E, Scotti RJ, et al. Validation of a simplified technique for using the POPQ pelvic organ prolapse classification system. Int Urogynecol J Pelvic Floor Dysfunct. 2006;17(6):615–20.
8. Mandel FP, Geola FL, Meldrum DR, Lu JH, Eggena P, Sambhi MP, et al. Biological effects of various doses of vaginally administered conjugated equine estrogens in postmenopausal women. J Clin Endocrinol Metab. 1983;57(1):133–9.
9. O'Meara ES, Rossing MA, Daling JR, Elmore JG, Barlow WE, Weiss NS. Hormone replacement therapy after a diagnosis of breast cancer in relation to recurrence and mortality. J Natl Cancer Inst. 2001;93(10):754–62.
10. Handa VL, Bachus KE, Johnston WW, Robboy SJ, Hammond CB. Vaginal administration of low-dose conjugated estrogens: systemic absorption and effects on the endometrium. Obstet Gynecol. 1994;84:215.
11. Hanson LA, Schulz JA, Flood CG, Cooley B, Tam F. Vaginal pessaries in managing women with pelvic organ prolapse and urinary incontinence: patient characteristics and factors contributing to success. Int Urogynecol J Pelvic Floor Dysfunct. 2006;17:155–9.
12. Kegel AH. Progressive resistance exercise in the functional restoration of the perineal muscles. Am J Obstet Gynecol. 1948;56:238–48.
13. Moen MD, Noone MB, Vassallo BJ, Lopata R, Nash M, Sum B. Knowledge and performance of pelvic muscles exercises in women. J Pelvic Med Surg. 2007;13:113–7.
14. Moen MD, Noone MB, Vassallo BJ, Elser DM. Pelvic floor muscle function in women presenting with pelvic floor disorders. Int Urogynecol J. 2009;20:843–6.
15. Wu V, Farrell SA, Baskett TF, Flowerdew G. A simplified protocol for pessary management. Obstet Gynecol. 1997;90:990–4.
16. Culligan PJ. Nonsurgical management of pelvic organ prolapse. Obstet Gynecol. 2012;119:852–60.
17. Richter HE, Burgio KL, Brubaker L, Nygaard IE, Ye W, Weidner A, Bradley C, Handa VL, Borello-France D, Goode PS, Zyczynski H, Lukacz ES, Schaffer J, Barber M, Meikle S, Spino C. For the pelvic floor disorders network. A trial of continence pessary vs. behavioral therapy vs. combined therapy for stress incontinence. Obstet Gynecol. 2010;115:609–17.
18. Robert M, Ross S. Conservative management of urinary incontinence. J Obstet Gynaecol Can. 2006;28:1113–8.

19. Lewis CM, Salamon C, Culligan P. Uncomplicated vaginal delivery following midurethral sling. Female Pelvic Med Reconstr Surg. 2011;17:147–8.
20. Van Kerrebroeck P, Kreder K, Jonas U, Zinner N, Wein A, Tolteridine Study Group. Tolterodine once-daily: superior efficacy and tolerability in the treatment of the overactive bladder. Urology. 2001;57:414–21.
21. Dmochowski RR, Sand PK, Zinner NR, Transdermal Oxybutynin Study Group, et al. Comparative efficacy and safety of transdermal oxybutynin and oral tolterodine versus placebo in previously treated patients with urge and mixed urinary incontinence. Urology. 2003;62:237–42.
22. Foote J, Glavind K, Kralidis G, Wyndaele JJ. Treatment of overactive bladder in the older patient: pooled analysis of three phase III studies of darifenacin, an M3 selective receptor antagonist. Eur Urol. 2005;48:471–7.
23. Nitti VW, Dmochowski R, Sand PK, et al. Efficacy, safety, and tolerability of fesoterodine for overactive bladder syndrome. J Urol. 2007;178:2488–94.
24. Appel RA, Sand P, Dmochowski R, Overactive Bladder: Judging Effective Control and Treatment Study Group, et al. Prospective randomized control trial of extended-release formulations of oxybutynin and tolterodine for overactive bladder: results of the OPERA trial. Mayo Clin Proc. 2003;78:687–95.
25. Gehrich A, Stany MP, Fischer JR, Buller J, Zahn CM. Establishing a mean postvoid residual volume in asymptomatic perimenopausal and postmenopausal women. Obstet Gynecol. 2007;110:827–32.
26. Laycock J. Clinical evaluation of the pelvic floor. In: Schussler B, Laycock J, Norton P, Stanton SL, editors. Pelvic floor re-education. London: Springer-Verlag; 1994. p. 42–8.

Chapter 14
Osteopenia and Osteoporosis

Sharon Beth Rosenberg

Osteoporosis is a term that means "porous bones." It is a skeletal disease affecting both women and men. Osteoporosis is a condition in which bones have lost minerals especially calcium, making them weaker, more brittle, and susceptible to fractures. Any bone in the body can be affected by osteoporosis, but the most common places where fractures occur are the back (spine), hips, and wrists.

Osteoporosis is becoming a healthcare crisis in the USA. There were over 1.5 million osteoporotic fractures in women in the USA in 2010, more than all the incidences of heart attack, strokes, and breast cancer combined. The economic burden of these fractures is more than $18 billion dollars per year, and that cost is expected to rise to $25.3 billion by 2025. Worse, for the individual patient, the odds of returning to full and normal functioning after a major osteoporotic fracture are very poor. Only 20% of patients who sustain an osteoporotic hip fracture will return to full and normal functioning. Approximately 20% will actually die from complications directly related to the hip fracture, and, scarier for most patients, 20% will end up needing to reside in a nursing home for the rest of their lives [1–6].

S. B. Rosenberg, MD (✉)
Saint Francis Hospital Evanston, Department of Internal Medicine, Evanston, IL, USA

J. V. Knaus et al. (eds.), *Ambulatory Gynecology*,
https://doi.org/10.1007/978-1-4939-7641-6_14

There is so much we can do to prevent and treat osteoporosis prior to it reaching crisis stage for our patients. The key is in knowing who to screen and who to treat.

In approaching the screening, diagnosis, and treatment of osteoporosis and low bone mass (previously known as osteopenia), we first need to identify the patients that are at risk and refer them for bone mineral densitometry (BMD or DEXA testing). These patients are:

1. Women age 65 and older
2. Postmenopausal women 50–65 who have risk factors (see risk factor assessment)
3. Anyone over 50 who has suffered a potential fragility-based fracture (hip, spine, pelvis, or wrist)

There are a tremendous number of risk factors for the development of osteoporosis. These are listed in the table below. Any woman with two or more of these risk factors should be DEXA tested at menopause or before if they have already a fracture. As you can see by this list, almost every patient will need a baseline DEXA at menopause (Figs. 14.1 and 14.2, Table 14.1)!

Now that we've decided which patients need to be scanned, the next step is to understand the results of the scan and figure out who needs treatment.

DEXA scanning gives two pieces of information:

1. The actual bone mineral density (BMD) expressed in absolute terms of grams of mineral per centimeter scanned (g/cm^2).
2. A comparison to "young normal" adults of the same sex (*T*-scores). This is expressed as standard deviations above or below the mean. Usually one standard deviation is equal to a loss of 10–15% BMD.

From this data we can get definitions for and diagnosis of osteoporosis and low bone mass (formerly called osteopenia):

WHO definitions: [8]

Normal – *T*-score – 1.0 or above

Low bone mass (formerly osteopenia) – *T*-score between −1.0 and −2.5

Osteoporosis – *T*-score – 2.5 and below

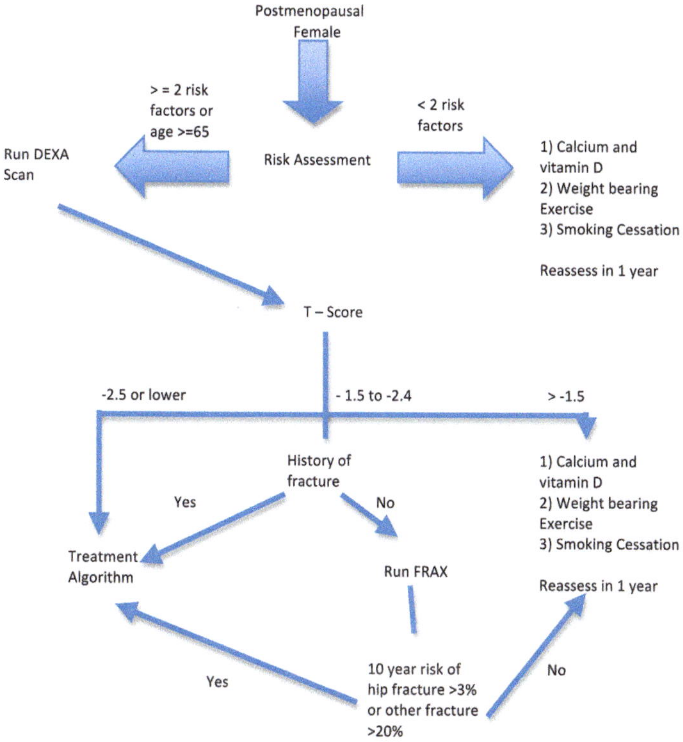

FIG. 14.1 Osteoporosis and low bone mass screening algorithm

Please note that patients who have already had a fragility fracture are deemed to have osteoporosis even if their *T*-score is in the low bone mass range.

Interpreting DEXA Testing

When easy and effective medical treatment became available for osteoporosis, physicians jumped on the bandwagon in droves, putting thousands of women with only minimal decreases in bone mass on medication in the name of osteoporosis prevention. We have since learned that this is

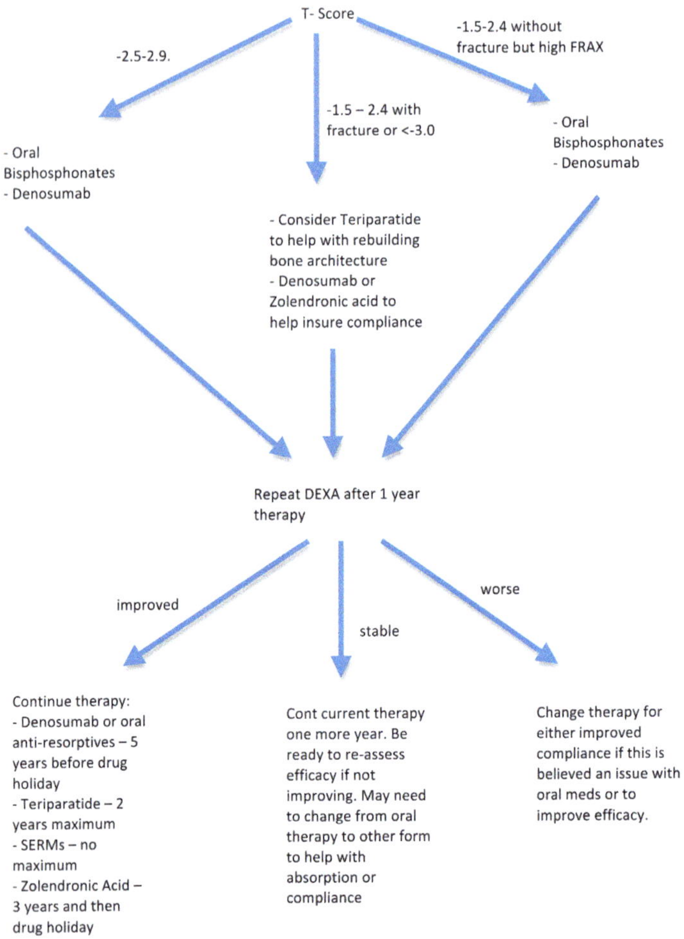

FIG. 14.2 Osteoporosis treatment algorithm

probably overkill, and with the new data on risk of abnormal fractures in patients on long-term bisphosphonates 9 or even possible increases in esophageal cancer, [10] may even be risky. The question becomes who is really at risk?

The best answer to this is to use the FRAX algorithm. What is FRAX?

Table 14.1 Conditions, diseases, and medications that cause or contribute to osteoporosis and fractures

Lifestyle factors		
Low calcium intake, high caffeine intake, alcohol (3 or more/day), smoking	Vitamin D deficiency High salt intake Inadequate physical activity	Falls Excess vitamin A, aluminum (antacids), small frame
Genetic factors		
Cystic fibrosis, Ehlers-Danlos syndrome, Gaucher's disease, glycogen storage diseases, Hemochromatosis	Homocystinuria, hypophosphatasia, idiopathic hypercalciuria Marfan syndrome, Menkes steely hair	Osteogenesis imperfecta, parental history of hip fracture Porphyria Riley-Day syndrome
Hypogonadism		
Androgen insensitivity, anorexia and bulimia, athletic amenorrhea	Hyperprolactinemia, panhypopituitarism, premature ovarian failure	Turner's syndrome, Klinefelter's syndrome
Endocrine		
Adrenal insufficiency, Cushing's syndrome	Diabetes mellitus I and II, hyperparathyroidism	Thyrotoxicosis
Gastrointestinal		
Celiac disease, gastric bypass GI surgery	Inflammatory bowel disease Malabsorption	Primary biliary cirrhosis Pancreatic disease
Hematologic		
Hemophilia Leukemia and lymphoma	Multiple myeloma, sickle cell disease	Systemic mastocytosis, thalassemia
Rheumatologic		
Ankylosing spondylitis	Lupus	Rheumatoid arthritis

(continued)

TABLE 14.1 (continued)

Miscellaneous		
Alcoholism amyloidosis	Emphysema	Muscular dystrophy, parenteral nutrition
Chronic metabolic acidosis, congestive heart failure, depression	Chronic kidney disease epilepsy Idiopathic scoliosis multiple sclerosis	Posttransplant bone disease, prior fracture as an adult, sarcoidosis
Medications		
Anticoagulants, anticonvulsants, aromatase inhibitors, barbiturates	Chemotherapeutics, cyclosporine and tacrolimus Depo-medroxyprogesterone	Glucocorticoids (≥5 mg prednisone for ≥3 months) GnRH Lithium

From: The Surgeon General's Report with modifications [7]

The WHO FRAX algorithm was designed to calculate the 10-year risk of osteoporotic fracture in patients who had never been on medical therapy. It is a very simple program to use, and many DEXA scanners now have the algorithm built into the system. The website location for the FRAX calculation tool is http://www.shef.ac.uk/FRAX/.

You only need to answer 12 questions:

1. Patient age
2. Sex
3. Weight
4. Height
5. Previous fractures
6. Parental hip fracture
7. Current smoker
8. Steroid use (equivalent of 5 mg daily prednisone for more than 3 months in the past 1 year)
9. Rheumatoid arthritis

10. Secondary osteoporosis risk (any of the conditions listed in the prior table)
11. Alcohol use three or more drinks per day
12. Femoral neck BMD/*T*-score

The calculator will then give you the 10-year risk of hip fracture and other major osteoporotic fracture. Patients who have a 10-year risk of hip fracture greater than 3% or a 10-year risk of other major osteoporotic fracture greater than 20% should be started on preventative medical therapy. Patients who fall outside of this risk group may be managed non-pharmacologically.

Non-pharmacologic Therapy

As more and more of our patients are drug adverse or seeking "natural" ways of dealing with chronic health issues, we need to become better informed about what works in lifestyle modification and vitamin supplementation and what does not. Though we always encourage our patients to eat a balanced diet, get enough calcium and vitamin D, exercise regularly, and stop smoking, we may not realize how much these issues impact their health when it comes to osteoporosis.

Nutrition

Women over the age of 65 who lose weight, purposefully or not, have accelerated bone loss and are at higher risk for hip fractures [11]. Due to fears of skin cancer, sun exposure in most parts of the USA is way down, and consequently Vitamin D levels are down as well.

Calcium levels in food in western diets are low, and as we age, our intestines do not allow for good calcium absorption, either. Confounding the problem is that many women are now concerned about calcium supplementation due to a recent study published about calcium supplements and coronary artery disease [12]. What do we know is fact?

Good Evidence

Calcium: 1200–1500 mg elemental calcium intake daily [13]
Vitamin D: 800–1000 IU of vitamin D daily [14]

In Need of More Study

Vitamin C: positive effect in smokers to help increase BMD [15]

Exercise

We all know that weight-bearing exercise and strength training are beneficial to bone development and maintenance [16–18], but extreme exercise is not necessary to have benefit. Mild exercise, like walking, works well, and there are positive results in applying passive stress to bone via whole-body high-frequency vibration systems [19]. Muscle strengthening and balance exercises in women 75 and older have been shown to reduce falls and fall-related injuries by 75% [20] showing that we can't just strengthen the bone, but we need to emphasize stability as our patients age.

Smoking Cessation

Women smokers lose bone more rapidly, have lower bone mass, and reach menopause 2 years earlier than non-smokers. [21]. For postmenopausal women who smoke, there is disturbing data that shows higher fracture rates than non-smokers [22]. So, as with a host of other medical issues, quitting smoking is one of the best things you can get your patients to do for their bone health.

Pharmacologic Therapy

There has been a wealth of new data just in 2010 about pharmacologic therapy for osteoporosis, and it has left both physicians and patients rather confused. With recent studies implying increased rates of esophageal cancer in oral bisphosphonate users, ten concerns about odd fractures in long-term antiresorptive therapy, and newer drugs coming to market, it can be very difficult not only figuring out what to prescribe but also getting patients to take the prescribed medications. Even prior to 2010, studies of adherence to therapy at the 6–12 month mark ranged from less than 25% to 81% depending on the medication [23]. Here we will review drugs by class, and tables will follow to help guide individual selections.

Please remember that for any of these drugs to be at their most effective, patients must have adequate levels of calcium and vitamin D. Please make sure to check at minimum calcium, renal functions, and vitamin D 25-0H levels prior to starting medication.

Bisphosphonates

The first class of drugs in widespread use for osteoporosis, bisphosphonates treat osteoporosis by shutting down osteoclastic activity in the bones to prevent resorption of bone matrix and allowing for further mineralization of the bone matrix. In women with osteoporosis, these drugs reduce the risk of vertebral fractures by 40–70% and non-vertebral fractures, including the hip, by half that amount [24]. They are available in a host of dosing forms and regimens, oral and IV dosed anywhere form daily to once per year. Because osteoblastic activity is triggered by osteoclastic activity, the inhibition of osteoclastic activity causes a significant decrease in osteoblastic activity. This may be the mechanism by which issues of osteonecrosis of the jaw and unusual femur fractures develop in people on long-term bisphosphonates therapy (Table 14.2).

TABLE 14.2 Bisphosphonate therapies

Drug name/ BMD changes	Dosage/ forms	Indications	Cautions
Alendronate	Prevention: 35 mg/week	Prevention and treatment postmenopausal osteoporosis	Esophageal
4% increase at L-S spine and femoral neck	Treatment: 70 mg/week Oral only		Irritation/ question of increased cancer, odd fractures with use greater than 5 years, osteonecrosis of the jaw
Risedronate 3.5% increase at L-S spine	35 mg/week or 150 mg/m for both prevention and treatment, oral only	Prevention and treatment of osteoporosis in both men and women	Esophageal irritation/ question of increased cancer, odd fractures with use greater than 5 years
Ibandronate 6.4% increase L-S spine at 3 years	150 mg/ month oral 3 mg IV every 3 mo.	Prevention and treatment postmenopausal osteoporosis	As above Also, fracture reduction significant only at 3-year mark
Zoledronic acid 6.7% increase at L-S spine at 3 years	5 mg IV annually	Treatment of postmenopausal osteoporosis	Use with caution in patients with reduced kidney function

References for this table: [9, 10, 25–32]

Because none of these drugs have any anabolic effect on new bone growth, they are best for patients that have *T*-scores better than –3.0, where bone microarchitecture is still significantly preserved, and for patients that meet the FRAX criteria for preventative therapy. These patients also need to be able to comply with the regimen for taking the drugs (for the oral medications, on an empty stomach with a full 8 oz. of water, waiting 30 min before taking any other medications or eating, and not lying down for 30 min after taking the pill). For patients with *T*-scores –3.0 or worse, an anabolic agent like teriparatide is preferred.

PTH Analogues: Teriparatide

Teriparatide is recombinant human PTH 1–34. While antiresorptives inhibit osteoclastic activity, teriparatide stimulates osteoblastic activity, actively promoting the laying down of new bone matrix. This allows for a buildup of both cortical and trabecular bone, increasing the density of the microarchitecture. This increases bone density and gives new stability to bone weakened by osteoporosis. Because of its unique mechanism of action, it has the best increases in BMD over the shortest period of time, as high as 11.8% in 18 months time [33–35].

Teriparatide is given for 2 years, after which the patient will need another osteoporosis medication to help preserve the gains in bone density. Teriparatide is a daily subcutaneous injection, which is probably the biggest stumbling block to patients using the medication. It was shown to have an increased of osteosarcoma in rats who were given supertherapeutic doses, but the risk in human beings is only theoretical.

Teriparatide is an excellent choice for patients who cannot tolerate bisphosphonates, patients who have a *T*-score –3.0 or less, or patients who have already had an osteoporotic fracture. It also has a specific indication for patients with glucocorticoid-induced osteoporosis.

Teriparatide should not be used in patients with active cancer and Paget's disease or those who have received prior skeletal radiation.

SERMS

Selective estrogen receptor modulators, or SERMs, raloxifene being the only one approved in the USA, are molecules that act like estrogen in the bones but act like antiestrogens in the breast and other tissues. They treat osteoporosis by restoring the balance between estrogen-like actions and interleukin-6 on osteoclast activity, resulting in bone turnover that more closely resembles premenopausal patterns. BMD increases are most significant in the lumbar spine, 2.6%, but are also seen in the femoral neck, 2.1% [36]. Raloxifene also has the added indication of decreasing the risk of invasive breast cancer in high-risk patients, decreasing the overall incidence of invasive breast cancer by more than 70% [37].

Estrogens

You will note that I have not addressed true estrogen-replacement therapy as treatment for osteoporosis. Though this was used extensively in the past, after the Women's Health Initiative showed increased rates of cardiovascular disease with long-term estrogen usage, the use of estrogen specifically for osteoporosis prevention and treatment is no longer recommended.

RANK-Ligand Antibody

Approved by the FDA in June of 2010, denosumab is a human IgG2 monoclonal antibody with affinity and specificity for human RANKL (receptor activator of nuclear factor kappa-B ligand). RANKL is expressed on osteoclasts, and inhibition of this receptor causes decreased osteoclastic activity. Denosumab increases BMD in the L-S spine by 8.8% at the 3-year mark [38].

Just like with bisphosphonates, inhibiting osteoclastic activity leads to inhibition of osteoblastic activity as well, and this drug also carries a warning about osteonecrosis of the jaw. In addition, because RANKL is expressed on cells in the immune system, there is a higher rate of serious skin infections with this drug.

Denosumab is the only osteoporosis medication that is dosed subcutaneously every 6 months, and because it is given in a physician's office, it helps significantly with compliance. It is also the only medication that does not need to be altered in dosing or withheld in renal failure patients.

Following Up

So now that you have identified who needs medication, have answered all their questions, allayed all their fears, and gotten them started on their medications, how do you follow up? There is no clear consensus right now, and what opinions that are out there right now are changing. As of the time of publication, here are the best practice guidelines:

1. Repeat DEXA at 1 year after beginning therapy to assess response. If the *T*-scores continue to decline while on therapy, consider changing to a different form of antiresorptive or teriparatide.
2. Drug holiday at the 5-year mark for antiresorptive therapies to allow for a return of normal bone remodeling and to minimize the risks of esophageal irritation and risk of esophageal cancer for oral medications.
3. While on drug holiday, repeat DEXA yearly. If BMD drops 5% or more, consider restarting therapy or changing to another drug class.

References

1. Cooper C, Atkinson EJ, Jacobsen SJ, et al. Population-based study of survival after osteoporotic fractures. Am J Epidemiol. 1993;137:1001.
2. Leibson CL, Tosteson AN, Gabriel SE, et al. Mortality, disability, and nursing home use for persons with and without hip fracture: a population-based study. J Am Geriatr Soc. 2002;50:1644.
3. Magaziner J, Lydick E, Hawkes W, et al. Excess mortality attributable to hip fracture in white women aged 70 years and older. Am J Public Health. 1997;87:1630.
4. Magaziner J, Simonsick EM, Kashner TM, et al. Predictors of functional recovery one year following hospital discharge for hip fracture: a prospective study. J Gerontol. 1990:45. MlOl
5. Riggs BL, Melton LJ 3rd. The worldwide problem of osteoporosis: insights afforded by epidemiology. Bone. 1995;17:505S.
6. Kannus P, Parkkari J, Niemi S, Palvanen M. Epidemiology of osteoporotic ankle fractures in elderly persons in Finland. Ann Intern Med. 1996;25:975.
7. US Department of Health and Human Services. Bone health and osteoporosis: a report of the surgeon general. Rockville: US Department of Health and Human Services, Office of the Surgeon General; 2004.
8. Kanis JA, Melton LJ III, Christiansen C, Johnston CC, Khaltaev N. The diagnosis of osteoporosis. J Bone Miner Res. 1994;9(8):1137–41.
9. Nieves JW, Cosman F. Atypical subtrochanteric and femoral shaft fractures and possible association with bisphosphonates. Curr Osteoporos Rep. 2010;8:34–9.
10. Green J, Czanner G, Reeves G, Watson J, Wise L, Beral V. Oral bisphosphonates and risk of cancer of the oesophagus, stomach and colorectum: case-control analysis within a UK primary case cohort. BMJ. 2010;341:c4444.
11. Ensrud KE, Ewing SK, Stone KL, Cauley JA, Bowman PJ, Cummings SR. For the study of osteoporotic fractures research group. Intentional and unintentional weight loss increases bone loss and hip fracture risk in older women. J Am Geriatr Soc. 2003;51:1740–7.
12. Bolland MJ, Avenell A, Baron JA, et al. Effect of calcium supplements on risk of myocardial infarction and cardiovascular events: meta-analysis. BMJ. 2010. https://doi.org/10.1136/bmj.c3691.

13. Prince RL, Devine A, Dhaliwal SS, Dick IM. Effects of calcium supplementation on clinical fracture and bone structure: results of a 5-year, double-blind, placebo-controlled trial in elderly women. Arch Intern Med. 2006;166:869–75.
14. Dawson-Hughes B, Dallal GE, Krall EA, et al. A controlled trial of the effects of calcium supplementation on bone density in postmenopausal women. N Engl J Med. 1990;23:878–83.
15. Sahni S, Hannan MT, Gagnon D, Blumberg J, Cupples LA, Kiel DP, Tucker KL. Protective effect of total and supplemental vitamin C intake on the risk of hip fracture-a 17-year follow-up from the Framingham osteoporosis study. Osteoporos Int. 2009;20:1853–61.
16. Lunt M, Masaryk P, Scheidt-Nave C, et al. The effects of lifestyle, dietary dairy intake and diabetes on bone density and vertebral deformity prevalence: the EVOS study. Osteoporos Int. 2001;12:688–98.
17. Wilsgaard T, Emaus N, Ahmed LA, et al. Lifestyle impact on lifetime bone loss in women and men: the Tromso study. Am J Epidemiol. 2009;169:877–86.
18. Dook JE, James C, Henderson NK, Price RI. Exercise and bone mineral density in mature female athletes. Med Sci Sports Exerc. 1997;29:291–6.
19. Verschueren SM, Roelants M, Delecluse C, Swinnen S, Vanderscheren D, Boonen S. Effect of 6-month whole body vibration training on hip density, muscle strength, and postural control in post-menopausal women: a randomized controlled pilot study. J Bone Miner Res. 2004;19:343–51.
20. Robertson MC, Campbell AJ, Gardner MM, Devlin N. Preventing injuries in older people by preventing falls: a meta-analysis of individual-level data. J Am Geriatr Soc. 2002;50:905–11.
21. Krall EA, Dawson-Huges B. Smoking and bone loss among post-menopausal women. J Bone Miner Res. 1991;6:331–8.
22. Baron JA, Johnell O, Oden A, et al. Smoking and fracture risk: a meta-analysis. Osteoporos Int. 2005;16:155–62.
23. Tosteson ANA, Grove MR, Hammond CS, et al. Early discontinuation of treatment for osteoporosis. Am J Med. 2003;115:209–16.
24. McClung M. Bisphosphonates. Endocrinol Metab Clin N Am. 2003;32:253–71.
25. Black DM, Cummings SR, David B, Karpf DB, et al. Randomised trial of effect of alendronate on risk of fracture in women with existing vertebral fractures. Lancet. 1996;348:1535–41. [FITI trial]

26. Cummings SR, MD, Black DM, Thompson DE, et al. Effect of alendronate on risk of fracture in women with low bone density but without vertebral fractures: results from the fracture intervention trial. JAMA. 1998;280:2077–2082. [FIT2 trial].
27. Harris ST, Watts NB, Genant HK, et al. Effects of risedronate treatment on vertebral and non-vertebral fractures in women with post-menopausal osteoporosis: a randomized controlled trial. JAMA. 1999;282:1344–52.
28. Reginster J, Minne HW, Sorenson OH, et al. Randomized trial of the effects of risedronate on vertebral fractures in women with established postmenopausal osteoporosis. Vertebral Efficacy with Risedronate Therapy (VERT) study group. Osteoporos Int. 2000;11:83–91.
29. Reginster JY, Adami S, Lakatos P, et al. Efficacy and tolerability of once-monthly oral ibandronate in postmenopausal osteoporosis: 2 year results from the MOBILE study. Ann Rheum Dis. 2006;65(5):654–61. [MOBILE trial]
30. Delmas PD, Adami S, Strugala C, et al. Intravenous ibandronate injections in postmenopausal women with osteoporosis: one-year results from the dosing intravenous administration study. Arthritis Rheum. 2006;54(6):1838–46. [DIVA trial]
31. Black DM, Delmas PD, Eastell R, et al. Once-yearly zoledronic acid for treatment of postmenopausal osteoporosis. NEJM. 2007;356(18):1809–22. [HORIZON Pivotal Fracture trial]
32. Lyles KW, Colon-Emeric CS, Magaziner JS, et al. Zoledronic acid and clinical fractures and mortality after hip fracture. N Engl J Med. 2007;357:1799–809. [HORIZON Recurrent Fracture trial]
33. Neer R, Arnaud C, Zanchetta JR, et al. Recombinant human PTH [rhPTH(l-34)] reduces the risk of spine and non-spine fractures in postmenopausal osteoporosis. NEJM. 2001;344:1434–41. [Fracture Prevential trial]
34. Lindsay R, Scheele WH, Neer R, et al. Sustained vertebral fracture risk reduction after withdrawal of teriparatide in postmenopausal women with osteoporosis. Arch Intern Med. 2004;164:2024–30. [Fracture Prevential trial follow-up]
35. Gallagher JC, Genant HK, Crans GG, Vargas SJ, Krege JH. Teriparatide reduces the fracture risk associated with increasing number and severity of osteoporotic fractures. J Clin Endocrinol Metab. 2005;90:1583–7.
36. Ettinger B, Black DM, Bruce H, Mitlak BH, et al. Reduction of vertebral fracture risk in postmenopausal women with osteoporosis

treated with raloxifene: results from a 3-year randomized clinical trial. JAMA. 1999;282:637–45. [MORE trial]

37. Cummings SR, Eckert S, Krueger KA, et al. The effect of raloxifene on risk of breat cancer in postmenopausal women: results from the MORE randomized trial. Multiple outcomes of raloxifene evaluation. JAMA. 1999;281:2189–97.
38. Cummings SR, Martin JS, McClung MR, et al. For the FREEDOM trial. Denosumab for the prevention of fractures in postmenopausal women with osteoporosis. N Engl J Med. 2009;361:756–65.

Chapter 15
Hormone Replacement Therapy in Menopause

Edward S. Linn and Lara Weyl

Introduction

Vasomotor and vaginal symptoms are the hallmark symptoms of menopause. The reported prevalence of vasomotor symptoms is 50–82% in women who experience natural menopause [1]. The occurrence of symptoms increases during perimenopause and usually peaks at the actual onset of menopause [1].

However, moderate to severe symptoms often last for a decade or longer [8].

While originally most studies of vasomotor symptoms were done with Caucasian women, results from a recent study, the Study of Women's Health Across the Nation

E. S. Linn (✉)
Cook County Health and Hospitals System, Northwestern University Feinberg School of Medicine, Department of OB/GYN, Chicago, IL, USA
e-mail: elinn@cookcountyhhs.org

L. Weyl
Saint Francis Hospital Evanston, Department of OB/GYN, Evanston, IL, USA

J. V. Knaus et al. (eds.), *Ambulatory Gynecology*,
https://doi.org/10.1007/978-1-4939-7641-6_15

(SWAN), showed that African-American women reported the most vasomotor symptoms and Asian women reported the least [1].

Vasomotor symptoms (VMS) include hot flushes, which consist of the sensation of extreme heat in the upper body (face, neck, and chest). Hot flushes usually last 1–5 min and are characterized by sweating, chills, clamminess, anxiety, and palpitations. They can also cause sleep disturbances [1].

Vaginal changes following menopause can include vaginal atrophy which can present as vaginal pain, itching, discharge, or dyspareunia. This is now known as genitourinary syndrome of menopause, formerly known as vulvovaginal atrophy [9]. The symptoms associated with vaginal atrophy are due to a loss of superficial epithelial cells, which causes a thinning of tissue. A loss of vaginal rugae and elasticity causes a narrowing and shortening of the vagina [1].

Hormone therapy (HT) is considered the most effective therapy for vasomotor and vaginal symptoms of menopause. Hormone therapy includes estrogen alone (ET) or estrogen plus progestin (EPT) [1].

Hormone Therapy Overview

The Women's Health Initiative (WHI) trials had a major impact on the world of HT. Prior to 2002, HT was recommended routinely to postmenopausal women for the prevention of osteoporosis and coronary heart disease. The WHI trials, which began in the early 1990s and its results published in 2002, were initiated with the intent to look at the benefits and risks of HT when taken for chronic disease prevention, specifically cardiovascular disease, in postmenopausal women [1]. The trial of estrogen plus progestin was stopped early because of a numerical increase in events of breast cancer, coronary heart disease, stroke, and pulmonary embolism. Later, in 2004, an estrogen-alone trial was stopped because of an increased number of stroke events. These observations changed the landscape of hormone therapy.

Women started receiving reduced exposure of HT, in lower-dose systemic forms, such as transdermal or vaginal, and only for treatment of vasomotor symptoms. Many women were, and continue to be, denied hormone therapy all together. The use of systemic hormone therapy has decreased by as much as 80% among US women since the initial findings of the WHI trials [8].

Women in the WHI trials were on average 63 years old, and its results have been used inappropriately in making decisions about treatment for women in their 40s and 50s [8].

One of the major criticisms of the WHI studies is that a single type and dose of ET and EPT formulations were used (conjugated equine estrogen and medroxyprogesterone acetate) creating difficulty in extrapolating that data to different formulations of ET and EPT used today.

In recent years, the data from the WHI trials have been revaluated, and the benefits of HT for the bone, brain, heart, and overall mortality are being reexamined.

Post-intervention follow-up (median 8.2 years) from the WHI trials found differences in the benefit-to-risk profile for estrogen plus progestin (EPT) versus estrogen alone (ET). For example, in the ET group, no increase was found in the risk of coronary heart disease or increased risk of breast cancer [9].

It also was determined that the role of age and time since menopause onset affected the outcome. One study found that overall, the WHI findings suggested that HT has an increased effect on CHD risk among older women, whereas the results in younger women were inconclusive [5].

This post-intervention reanalysis of the WHI data has given way to the "timing hypothesis." This hypothesis suggests that HT may be used relatively safely for the management of menopausal symptoms in healthy postmenopausal women younger than 60 years and within 10 years of the final menstrual period [9].

More recent trials have been conducted, such as the Kronos Early Estrogen Prevention Study (KEEPS), which have validated the timing hypothesis showing that EPT started soon after menopause appears to be safe, relieves many of the symptoms of menopause, and improves mood, bone density, and several markers of cardiovascular disease [7].

Benefits of Hormone Therapy

The natural estrogen deficiency that takes place during menopause leads to bone loss and osteoporosis in women. Current research has shown that HT is effective and appropriate for the prevention of osteoporosis-related fractures. Low-dose HT effectively maintains or improves bone mineral density.

Observational studies have shown that ET may decrease coronary heart disease [1]. A study of 42–58-year-old women, 6–36 months from last menses, showed that 4 years of early HT did not affect the progression of atherosclerosis despite improving some markers of CVD risk [10].

One study found that ET at time of surgical menopause benefits verbal memory over the short term [4]. In the KEEPS cognitive study, they found that women who received oral conjugated equine estrogen improved significantly on measures of depression-dejection and anxiety-tension as compared to placebo [7].

The Endocrine Society Scientific Statement reports that HT is associated with 40% reduction in mortality in women <60 years old and within 10 years of menopause [4].

Current Recommendations

The North American Menopause Society (NAMS)

The North American Menopause Society, along with the American Society for Reproductive Medicine, the Asia Pacific Menopause Federation, the Endocrine Society, the European Menopause and Andropause Society, the

International Menopause Society, and the International Osteoporosis Foundation, released a global consensus statement on menopausal hormone therapy in 2013:

1. HT is the most effective treatment for vasomotor symptoms associated with menopause at any age, but benefits are more likely to outweigh risks for symptomatic women before the age of 60 years old or within 10 years after menopause.
2. HT is effective and appropriate for the prevention of osteoporosis-related fractures in at risk women before age 60 years old or within 10 years after menopause.
3. Standardized clinical trials and observational data as well as meta-analyses provide evidence that standard dose ET may decrease coronary heart disease.

The American College of Obstetricians and Gynecologists (ACOG)

The American College of Obstetricians and Gynecologists (ACOG) released a Practice Bulletin titled Management of Menopausal Symptoms in January 2014 with the following recommendations:

1. Systemic hormone therapy (HT), with estrogen alone (ET) or in combination with progestin (EPT), is the most effective therapy for vasomotor symptoms related to menopause [1].
2. The use of the lowest effective dose for the shortest duration that is needed to relieve vasomotor symptoms is recommended [1].

Special Populations

Women with breast cancer present a unique challenge when it comes to HT. The NAMS 2012 position statement stated that although ET did not increase breast cancer risk in the WHI trials, there is a lack of safety data supporting the use of ET in breast cancer survivors [1]. In March 2016, ACOG reported in Committee Opinion #659, The Use of Vaginal Estrogen in Women with a History of Estrogen-Dependent Breast Cancer, that the data did not show an increased risk of cancer reoccurrence among women currently undergoing treatment for breast cancer or those with a personal history of breast cancer who use vaginal estrogen to relieve urogenital symptoms [11]. However, nonhormonal approaches are the first-line choices for managing urogenital symptoms as well as VMS in women during or after treatment for breast cancer.

Controversies in Hormone Therapy

Venous Thromboembolism and Cerebrovascular Accidents

Venous thromboembolism (VTE) and cerebrovascular accidents (CVA) are two major concerns surrounding the use of HT. This is mostly because the WHI EPT and ET trials demonstrated an increased risk of ischemic stroke [1]. Data from other studies have also consistently demonstrated an increased risk of VTE with oral HT [1]. However, it is important to remember that the risks of VTE and CVA have been found specifically with oral HT. Transdermal ET has been found to have little or no effect in elevating prothrombic substances and therefore likely does not carry the same risks that oral HT carries [6]. Also, different types of EPT carry different risks. For example, a combination of estrogen plus medroxyprogesterone acetate carries a higher risk of coronary heart disease and VTE, while combinations of estrogen plus micronized progesterone do not [12].

Breast Cancer

The use of HT and its link to increased risk of breast cancer diagnoses has been controversial. Studies have shown, however, that the increased risk of breast cancer diagnosis is primarily associated with the addition of a progestin to estrogen therapy (EPT) as opposed to estrogen alone (ET) and is also related to the duration of use [3]. In the WHI trials, women who were receiving ET did not have an increased risk of breast cancer diagnoses [1]. In fact, there was noted to be a significant reduction in breast cancer diagnoses seen with the estrogen with no concomitant MPA (ET) patients [5].

Endometrial Cancer

It is well known that unopposed estrogen exposure in a woman with an intact uterus is a risk factor for endometrial cancer. Therefore, the recommendation from NAMS 2017 position statement is that all women with an intact uterus who use systemic ET should also be prescribed adequate progestin to negate the increased risk of endometrial cancer from systemic ET use [3]. However, the use of local ET, such as vaginal estrogen, has not been found to be associated with an increased risk of endometrial hyperplasia, and therefore, the addition of progestin for endometrial protection is not needed [1].

Bioidentical Hormones/Compounded Hormones

"Bioidentical hormones" is a term that has been recently popularized and generally refers to custom, compounded hormone regimens that may be dose adjusted based on hormone level monitoring.

This practice has become popular in large part due to the fear of practitioners and patients in prescribing and using conventional hormone preparations, mainly due to the potential adverse effects as described above.

The problem with "bioidentical hormones" or compounded HT is that most are not FDA-approved. The purity, potency, and quality of these products are a serious concern [2]. Many times these compounded substances are marketed to the general public as "natural" and "safe." The estrogens and progestins used in these compounded formulations can be the same with that used in conventional HT; therefore they are no more "natural" than conventional HT. As far as safety, the manufacturers of conventional HT have had to go through rigorous testing and oversight to meet the very high standards set by the FDA. Conventional HT has also been accepted by ACOG, NAMS, and the Endocrine Society specifically for treatment of VMS of menopause. Producers of compounded HT do not undergo similar scrutiny and oversight.

Monitoring for hormone levels in blood and urine can vary greatly or, in the case of saliva, be completely unreliable. Therefore, monitoring of these levels is not recommended.

Routes of administration such as subdermal, rectal, and sublingual have not been approved by the FDA.

Both ACOG and NAMS do not recommend compounded HT or "bioidentical hormones" [1].

There are some rare circumstances in which a specific patient (e.g., with an allergy to a product used in conventional HT, like sesame oil) may need a compounded HT. Otherwise, compounded HT is not recommended for treatment of VMS in postmenopausal women.

Testosterone

Testosterone alone is currently not FDA-approved for use in women [1].

Management

The management of each patient and their VMS and vaginal symptoms is individualized. The North American Menopause Society (NAMS) has released a free mobile app, MenoPro, (available on iOS and Android devices) to assist clinicians in decision-making.

MenoPro employs the following algorithm (Fig. 15.1), published in Fertility and Sterility in 2014 by Dr. JoAnn Mason. The algorithm provides an easy-to-follow, step-by-step guide on how to individualize HT for patients with VMS.

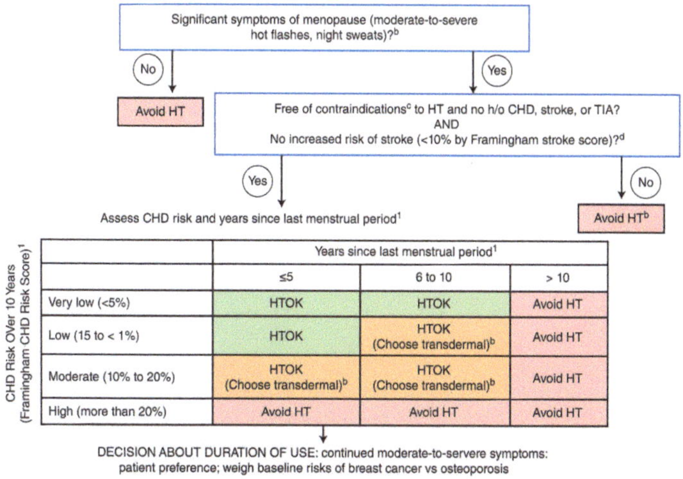

Fig. 15.1 Algorithm to individualize HT for patients with VMS (Modified from Current recommendations, JoAnn E. Manson, MD: Fertility and Sterility, Vol 101, April 2014)

Types of Estrogens and Progestins

There are many types of estrogens that are available. Most of the oral preparations are plant derived, and all have similar efficacy [12]. The available types include:

- Conjugated estrogen
  - Equine: extracted from pregnant mares' urine
  - Plant-based synthetic formulations
- Micronized 17-beta estradiol: identical to main product of premenopausal ovary
- Esterified estrogen
- Estropipate
- Ethinyl estradiol: used in all combined oral contraceptives

The types of progestins include:

- Medroxyprogesterone acetate
- Natural progesterone (micronized progesterone)

- Drospirenone
- Levonorgestrel
- 19-Nortestosterone derivatives:
  - Norethindrone
  - Norethindrone acetate-ß

Route of Administration

There are several common routes of administration for FDA-approved products including oral, transdermal (aka systemic), and local.

Systemic

Systemic ET is often administered orally or transdermally [13]. Oral ET has been shown to cause a 75% reduction in weekly hot flush frequency [1]. However, transdermal forms, including patches, gels, and sprays, have also been shown to relieve vasomotor symptoms as well [1]. In addition, transdermal ET appears to have little or no effect in elevating prothrombic substances [6]. Therefore, the practitioner should take into consideration the possible thrombosis sparing properties of transdermal ET [6].

Local

Vaginal ET is considered the mainstay of local HT. FDA-approved cream, ring, and tablet formulations are effective in treating atrophic vaginitis [1]. Also, products with higher vaginal doses can achieve systemic blood levels in order to treat VMS. It is important that with these higher doses, a progestin should be considered for women with a uterus [14].

Dosing (Tables 15.1 and 15.2)

TABLE 15.1 Menopausal hormone therapy preparations

Preparation	Starting dose	Comments
Estrogen		
Oral		
17 β-Estradiol	0.5 mg/day	1 tablet/day
Ethinyl estradiol	2.5 mcg/day	1 tablet/day
Conjugated estrogen	0.3–0.45 mg/day	1 tablet/day
Transdermal		
17 β-Estradiol patch	0.014–0.0375 mg/day	1 patch twice/week
17 β-Estradiol gel	0.25 or 0.75 mg/day	0.25 g gel daily, 1.25 g gel daily
17 β-Estradiol spray	1.53 mg/day	1 spray daily
17 β-Estradiol emulsion	8.7 mg/day	2 foil-laminated pouches/day
Vaginal		
17 β-Estradiol vaginal cream	0.2 mg (2 g of cream)/day	2 g-4 g daily for 2 weeks, then taper to maintenance dose of 1 g twice/week
Conjugated estrogen vaginal cream	0.3125 mg (0.5 g of cream)/day	0.5 g daily for 21 days on and 7 days off or twice/week
17 β-Estradiol vaginal tablet	10 mcg/day	1 tablet/day for 2 weeks, then 1 tablet twice/week
17 β-Estradiol vaginal ring	2 mg/ring (7.5 mcg/day) or 12.4 mg/ring (50 mcg/day)	1 ring/90 day

(continued)

Table 15.1 (continued)

Preparation	Starting dose	Comments
Progestogen		
Oral		
Medroxyprogesterone acetate	1.5–2.5 mg/day	Daily in combination preparations or 14 day/month; 1.5 mg with 0.3 mg of conjugated estrogen combination
Norethindrone acetate	0.1 mg/day	Daily in combination preparations or 14 day/month
Drospirenone	0.25 mg/day	Daily
Micronized progesterone	100–200 mg/day	100 mg/day continuously or 200 mg/day for 12 days/month
Transdermal		
Norethindrone acetate	0.14 mg/day	1 patch twice/week
Levonorgestrel	0.015 mg/day	1 patch/week

Table 15.2 Treatment options for menopausal vaginal symptoms

Treatment	Dosage	Evidence of benefit[a]	FDA approved
Hormonal			
Estrogen			
Systemic			
Standard dose	Conjugated estrogen 0.625 mg/day	Yes	Yes
	Micronized estradiol-17β 1 mg/day	Yes	Yes
	Transdermal estradiol-17β 0.0375–0.05 mg/day	Yes	Yes

(continued)

TABLE 15.2 (continued)

Treatment	Dosage	Evidence of benefit[a]	FDA approved
Low dose	Conjugated estrogen 0.3–0.45 mg/day	Yes	Yes
	Micronized estradiol-17β 0.5 mg/day	Yes	Yes
	Transdermal estradiol-17β 0.025 mg/day	Yes	Yes
Ultralow dose	Micronized estradiol-17β 0.25 mg/day	Mixed	No
	Transdermal estradiol-17β 0.014 mg/day	Mixed	No
Vaginal/local	Estradiol-17β ring 75 μg/day	Yes	Yes
	Estradiol vaginal tablet 10 μg/day	Yes	Yes
	Estradiol ring 0.05mg/day	Yes	
	Estradiol-17β cream 2g/day	Yes	
	Conjugated estrogen cream 0.5–2 g/day	Yes	
Nonhormonal			
Estrogen agonists-antagonists			
Raloxifene and tamoxifen		No	
Ospemifene	60 mg/day	Yes	
Vaginal lubricants	as needed	Yes	

(continued)

Table 15.2 (continued)

Treatment	Dosage	Evidence of benefit[a]	FDA approved
Vaginal moisturizers	per manufacturers recommendation	Yes	
Herbal remedies and soy products		No	

[a]Compared with placebo
Abbreviation: *FDA* U.S. Food and Drug Administration.

In Summary

- Hormone therapy is the most effective treatment of vasomotor symptoms of menopause.
- It can be safely used for the alleviation of VMS, especially in younger women.
- Transdermal forms may be associated with less risk of VTE.
- While HT is not currently recommended for prevention of CVD and osteoporosis, studies have shown it to have beneficial effects on both. It has also been associated with decreased mortality and risk of dementia in younger women (within 10 years of menopause).
- Further studies need to be done on hormone therapy for primary disease prevention, but at this time, it is not recommended.

References

1. ACOG Practice Bulletin 141, January 2014 (Reaffirmed 2016): Management of menopausal symptoms.
2. ACOG Practice Bulletin 126, March 2012: Management of gynecological issues in women with breast cancer.
3. Position Statement: The 2017 Hormone Therapy Position Statement of the North American Menopause Society.
4. ACOG Committee Opinion, August 2012: Compounded bioidentical menopausal hormone therapy.

5. Global Consensus on Menopausal Hormone Therapy, 2013: International menopause society and the European menopause and andropause society.
6. Executive Summary: Postmenopausal Hormone Therapy: An Endocrine Society Scientific Statement 2010.
7. Manson J, et al. Menopausal hormone therapy and health outcomes during the intervention and extended post stopping phases of the women's health initiative randomized trials. JAMA. 2013;310(13):1353–68. https://doi.org/10.1001/jama.2013.278040.
8. ACOG Committee Opinion 2013 (Reaffirmed 2015): postmenopausal estrogen therapy: route of administration and risk of VTE.
9. KEEPS Report, NAMS 2012 Meeting. www.menopause.org.
10. Manson, Kaunitz NEJM 2016 Menopause management-getting clinical care back on track.
11. Hormone Therapy and Alternative Therapies for Menopause, ACOG: Clinical Updates in Women's Health Care. Volume XIV, Number 4., October 2015
12. Harman, American College of Physicians et al. 2014 Arterial imaging outcome and cardiovascular risk factors in recently menopausal women: a randomized trial.
13. Uptodate.com, Preparations for menopausal hormone therapy.
14. ACOG Committee Opinion 2016, The use of vaginal estrogen in women with a history of estrogen dependent breast cancer.

Chapter 16
Basic Infertility Evaluation

Migdalia Cortina and Jennifer Ozan

Infertility for women younger than 35 years old is defined as 1 year of unprotected intercourse without conception. However, for women who are older than 35, this time frame decreases to 6 months. As women pursue careers and put family planning on hold, childbearing and infertility have become rising issues. The ASRM has published a committee opinion reviewing the decline of fecundity in women starting at the age of 32 [1], and according to the National Survey of Family Growth in 2013, approximately 11% (6.9 million) of reproductive age women have utilized fertility services in their lifetime [2]. While most couples who present to your office may not meet the strict definition of infertility, the likelihood of success without treatment declines by approximately 5% for each additional year of the female partner's age and by 15–25% for each added year of infertility [3]. Therefore, all patients who present with concern of family planning or infertility should be counseled regarding the

M. Cortina (✉)
St. Francis Hospital, Department of Obstetrics and Gynecology, Evanston, IL, USA

J. Ozan
Women's Hospital-Cone Health, Department of Obstetrics and Gynecology, Greensboro, NC, USA

J. V. Knaus et al. (eds.), *Ambulatory Gynecology*,
https://doi.org/10.1007/978-1-4939-7641-6_16

reproductive process and the relationship of age and fertility. Additionally, a history and physical exam tailored to addressing infertility are warranted to ensure further evaluation is not indicated. This chapter on infertility will help guide you through this process.

First, check with both the patient and patient's partner to see if a prior workup with another physician has already been conducted. Reviewing these results will save valuable time and resources. If no prior workup has been done, starting with both the patient and her partner's history is of utmost importance in not only discovering underlying common infertility etiologies but determining which couples need further evaluation.

History

Female

Menstrual History

Determine cycle length and characteristics including any pelvic pain, bloating, or breast tenderness. This will help to determine if the patient is ovulating. A woman who reports cycles every 28–30 days with breast tenderness and cramping is likely to be ovulating, whereas a woman who reports oligomenorrhea suggests concern of ovulatory dysfunction. Additionally, if she reports significant dysmenorrhea or bowel complaints, one may consider endometriosis.

Gynecologic History

Determine history of sexually transmitted infections, pelvic inflammatory disease (PID), abnormal PAP smears and related treatment, prior contraception use, and previous intrauterine devices. The strong association between pelvic infection and infertility is undeniable and would warrant immediate infertility workup. Depo-Provera shots may cause irregularity in a woman's cycle for up to 1 year and may explain her inability to conceive.

Obstetrical History

Determine previous pregnancy outcomes and pregnancy complications. Though uncommon, a patient may have needed a uterine curettage following a postpartum hemorrhage.

Medical History

This includes chronic medical problems, such as diabetes that may alter the hypothalamic-pituitary axis. Also, inquire regarding a history of any cancer and organ failure specifically liver or renal failure.

Surgical History

Inquire regarding both abdominal and pelvic surgeries. Due to the emotional hardship of a miscarriage, patients may often forget about surgical management with a dilation and curettage.

Sexual History

Determine the frequency of coitus, history of dyspareunia, or any sexual dysfunction.

Social History

Inquire regarding age, smoking, exercise, stress, diet/change in weight, occupation, DES, or other occupational exposure. These social factors may shed light on a factor that was unknown to the couple. For example, the ASRM published a committee opinion supporting the association between infertility and smoking [4].

Family History

Inquire regarding infertility in the family, genetic mutations, birth defects, mental retardation, and hereditary conditions (e.g., fragile X). A strong family history of early menopause may place a patient at increased risk of fertility problems.

Review of Symptoms

Addressing symptoms pertaining to thyroid, adrenal, and pituitary dysfunction will also aid in ruling out possible etiologies. (e.g., galactorrhea, hirsutism, and weight changes).

Male

Even if the male has fathered a pregnancy in the past, this does not mean male factor infertility should be discounted. Highlights of the male's history should include the following information:

Medical History

Inquire regarding childhood illnesses (mumps or orchitis), previous genital trauma, developmental defects (undescended testes), and systemic diseases (diabetes or chronic respiratory infections) which should all be assessed.

Medication Exposure

Ask about both current medications and any anabolic steroid use, prior chemotherapy, or radiation.

Sexual History

Verify any prior sexually transmitted diseases or any sexual dysfunction.

Social History

Age, smoking, exercise, stress, diet, changes in weight, occupation, and exposure to any gonadotoxins should also be discussed.

Physical Examination of the Female

A thorough physical exam is an essential step, and while some may focus on the pelvic organs, there are other fundamental features that may be useful.

General

Calculate the BMI: Both obese and underweight patients are at risk for infertility. Look for signs of incomplete development of secondary sexual characteristic including breast development, body hair, and body habitus. Assess for endocrinopathies: goiter, hirsutism, acne, virilization, and male-pattern baldness.

HEENT

Check for thyroid enlargement, nodules, or tenderness. Note any signs of androgen excess such as acanthosis nigricans or acne.

Pelvic Exam

Palpate for uterine size and shape that may suggest leiomyomas or other anomalies. Check for any vaginal or cervical abnormalities including abnormal discharge, cervical motion tenderness, or masses that may suggest chronic pelvic inflammatory disease or endometriosis.

Based on the above information, couples requiring further evaluation include:

1. A patient that meets criteria for infertility. Either a woman younger than 35 with regular unprotected intercourse for 1 year or a woman older than 35 unable to conceive after 6 months. Additionally, due to substantial decrease in fecundity, a woman over 40 should also have a full infertility evaluation.
2. Patients with irregular or infrequent menses, history of pelvic infection, endometriosis, or reproductive tract malformations warrant immediate infertility workup.
3. If there is any question as to whether a further evaluation is warranted, consider consultation with an infertility specialist.

The following algorithm may be used to help identify the potential cause of infertility:

Determine if Male Factor Is Contributing

Semen Analysis

To guarantee optimal results, be sure to include the following instructions:

- Abstinence for 24–72 h. A decrease in sperm count is associated with frequent ejaculations; however, no optimal period of abstinence has been determined.
- The specimen should be submitted to the laboratory within 1 h of collection and should be kept at room temperature.
- The specimen should be obtained by masturbation without using lubricant and placed in a clean container.

The WHO criteria have set lower limits of normal, and should any of the values be found to be abnormal, referral should be made to urology for further evaluation:

Sperm volume: Normal ejaculate is typically 1.5–5 mL.

Sperm concentration: Lower limit of normal is 20 million sperm per milliliter. Sperm motility: Lower limit varies according to laboratory but is usually >50%.

Sperm morphology: Greater than or equal to 4% is considered normal Morphology: Greater than 14% normal morphology is associated with normal rates of fertilization using in vitro fertilization (IVF).

Confirm Ovulation

Many tests are available to confirm ovulation; however, there is no "gold standard" or best test available. The following tests are all possible options to confirm ovulation.

Menstrual History

A woman with regular, predictable cycles is consistent with ovulation. Consequently, irregular, infrequent cycles with inconsistent duration is suggestive of oligo or anovulation.

LH Monitoring

Also known as "ovulation test kits," these tests document the LH surge, which occurs 34–46 h prior to ovulation. LH is rapidly cleared through the urine and can be detected when a threshold LH level is reached. For this test to be a plausible option, the overall cycle length must be known as the test requires daily LH checking starting 2 to 3 days before the expected surge. Only one positive test is needed to confirm ovulation.

The positive and negative predictive values of these kits are 90% and 96%, respectively. While a positive test is reassuring for ovulation, a negative test does not guarantee anovulation as 5–10% of women may yield a false-positive or false-negative result. In this scenario, consider testing for serum LH.

Basal Body Temperature (BBT) Recording

The patient should measure temperature each morning before getting out of bed. Normal BBT ranges from 97.0 to 98.0 during the follicular phase. Since progesterone is thermogenic and the level rises after ovulation, an elevation of temperature by 0.5 above baseline can be observed. A graph of the BBT recordings will produce a biphasic pattern indicating ovulation. While this test is inexpensive, it can be extremely time-consuming on the patient, and near 10% of women may not exhibit this classic biphasic pattern.

Midluteal Progesterone

A serum progesterone level greater than 3 ng/mL verifies ovulation [5]. The best time to obtain this test is day 21 (of 28-day cycle) or in a longer cycle approximately 1 week prior to menses. Rather than considering a level greater than 3 normal, any woman with a progesterone level less than 3 ng/mL necessitates workup for anovulation.

Ultrasound Monitoring

Documentation of a primary follicle using serial ultrasound has not been shown to be a financially effective method and would not be recommended at this time.

If, in fact, the absence of ovulation has been established, the focus turns to identifying the etiology of the ovulatory dysfunction. Collection of cycle day 3 labs should be performed, which include FSH, LH, and estradiol as well as testing for other endocrine disorders via TSH, T3 and T4, prolactin, total testosterone, and cortisol. From this information, specific endocrine or ovulation disorders can be identified.

Thyroid Disease

Specifically, hypothyroidism has been linked to irregular cycles, infertility, and early miscarriage.

Hypothalamic-Pituitary Axis Disorders

Disturbance along any level of this axis may lead to anovulation. The first domain to consider is suppression of the hypothalamus due to the patient's lifestyle. This includes anorexia nervosa, the female athlete triad, and stress.

Other hypothalamic-related causes are hypogonadotropic hypogonadism or Kallmann's syndrome and will present with low FSH, LH, and estradiol. If these conditions are suspected, further workup is warranted including a referral to an endocrinologist.

Problems of the pituitary gland that may lead to anovulation include hyperprolactinemia and panhypopituitarism. Each of these disorders will present with unique clinical symptoms that should be ascertained from the H&P and confirmed by the laboratory tests mentioned above.

Ovulatory Dysfunction

Polycystic ovarian syndrome (PCOS): The most common cause among women with oligo-ovulation and anovulation who present for infertility is PCOS. According to the revised Rotterdam 2003 criteria, a patient must have two of the three conditions present:

1. Oligo and/or anovulation.
2. Clinical and/or biochemical signs of hyperandrogenism: Clinically, this would include male-pattern hair loss, hirsutism, or acne. Biochemically, this would include elevated testosterone level.
3. Polycystic ovaries noted on ultrasound and exclusion of other etiologies (congenital adrenal hyperplasia, androgen-secreting tumors, Cushing's syndrome).

Women with PCOS who desire a pregnancy often require ovulation induction and should be seen by a specialist for this management.

Decreased Ovarian Reserve

Unfortunately, a woman's fecundability decreases with age as the amount of viable oocytes steadily declines. The cycle day 3 lab values will be useful in distinguishing if decreased ovarian reserve is a factor. An FSH value greater than 10–15 IU/mL as well as an elevated estradiol (greater than 80 pg/ml) implies a significant decline in ovarian reserve [5]. Serum mulerian-inhibiting substance (MIS) also called anti-mullerian hormone (AMH) is a test for ovarian reserve and reflects remaining follicles. This test can be measured on any day of the woman's cycle. A value 1.0–1.5 ng/ml is considered low normal range and less than 1.0 ng/ml is low. Other screening tests may include serum inhibin B and clomiphene citrate challenge test. Should ovarian failure be identified as a probable cause of anovulation, referral to an fertility specialist is warranted.

Establish Tubal Patency

Tubal and peritoneal pathology is the primary diagnosis of 30–35% of infertile couples. Tubal damage or peritoneal factors stem from prior pelvic inflammatory disease (PID), pelvic or tubal surgery, or endometriosis that may have caused significant adhesions. While PID is classically associated with tubal infertility, nearly half of women with tubal damage have no risk factors. Every infertility workup should include a check for tubal patency with one of the following:

Hysterosalpingogram (HSG)

This procedure is the most common way to observe tubal patency and has a sensitivity of 85–100% in identifying tubal occlusion [6]. The test is performed between days 6 and 11 of cycle. To avoid HSG-associated pelvic infection, a prophylactic regimen of doxycycline 100 mg twice daily should be started the day before the procedure and continued for

5 days. Additionally, a nonsteroidal anti-inflammatory should be taken 30 min prior to the procedure to minimize the discomfort of uterine cramping.

To perform the procedure, the vaginal area should be cleaned. An acorn (Jarcho) cannula or other injection device should be placed through the cervix. Careful and slow injection of 3–4 mL of contrast media will fill the uterine cavity, and an additional 5–10 mL will demonstrate tubal patency. The options for contrast include a water-soluble or a low viscosity oil-based dye.

Considerations

- A proximal tubal occlusion often represents testing artifact from tubal spasm or catheter positioning. Tubal spasms may be alleviated by giving diazepam 30 min prior to the start of the procedure. If tubal spasm is suspected, options include terbutaline 0.25 mg subcutaneous during the procedure or repeating the HSG, fluoroscopic or hysteroscopic selective tubal perfusion, or laparoscopic chromotubation.
- If endometriosis or pelvic adhesions are suspected, HSG should not be the initial test. Consider instead performing a diagnostic laparoscopy and chromotubation, which will allow for treatment as well as diagnosis.
- Any abnormalities seen on HSG (tubal obstruction, uterine cavity abnormalities) require further testing and referral to a reproductive endocrinologist.

Hysterosalpingo-Contrast Sonography (HyCoSy)

This test captures ultrasound images of the uterus, tubes, and adnexa both before and after transcervical injection of contrast media.

Research is still being performed to assess the reliability of this test.

Laparoscopy

Allows for direct visualization of all pelvic organs as well as assessing tubal patency. Chromotubation involves injections of transcervical dye and direct visualization of tubal patency. Laparoscopy may be considered if other factors such as endometriosis are expected.

Uterine Factors

Along with tubal patency, establishing a normal uterine cavity confirms that the patient's anatomy will support a viable pregnancy. Abnormalities that may negatively impact the uterine cavity include endometrial polyps, submucosal fibroids, intrauterine adhesions, mullerian anomalies and DES exposure. Hysterosalpingography, transvaginal ultrasound or sonohysterography, and hysteroscopy may all be considered for the evaluation of the uterine cavity.

Cervical Factors

The postcoital test is an examination to evaluate the quality of cervical mucus and the presence of sperm. After many years of scrutiny, it has been determined that there is no clinical significance to this exam as the results do not contribute to a couple's treatment course.

Unexplained

Up to 30% of women may not have an identifiable etiology [6]. For these women, referral to a specialist is the best option.

Conclusion

A key component to infertility is making patients aware of their personal risk and counseling them regarding the decline in fecundity with age. Recognizing that infertility is a disorder of the couple is strategic in identifying underlying etiologies and throughout the infertility workup. Due to the time sensitivity and emotional weight infertility has on a couple's livelihood, if there are any questions or uncertainty regarding the evaluation, referral to a reproductive endocrinology and fertility specialist is recommended.

References

1. The American College of Obstetricians and Gynecologists Committee on Gynecologic Practice and The Practice Committee of the American Society for Reproductive Medicine. Committee opinion no. 589. Fertil Steril. 2014;101:633.
2. http://www.cdc.gov/nchs/nsfg/key_statistics/i.htm#infertility. Accessed Nov 2015.
3. Berek JS. Berek & Novak's gynecology. 14th ed. Philadelphia: Lippincott Williams & Wilkins; 2007.
4. The American College of Obstetricians and Gynecologists Committee on Gynecologic Practice and The Practice Committee of the American Society for Reproductive Medicine. Smoking and infertility: a committee opinion. Fertil Steril. 2012;98:14006.
5. Kuohung W, Hornstein MD. Evaluation of female infertility. In: UpToDate, Waltham, MA. Accessed Jan 2016.
6. Speroff L, Fritz MA. Clinical gynecologic endocrinology and infertility. 7th ed. Philadelphia: Lippincott William & Wilkins; 2005.

Chapter 17
Recurrent Pregnancy Loss

Carolyn B. Coulam and Melissa J. Miller

Although many advances in reproductive medicine have been made during the past 25 years, miscarriages remain the most common complication of pregnancy. While most miscarriages are sporadic and not repetitive, there is a subset of couples that suffer recurrent miscarriage. In the past, the definition of recurrent pregnancy loss was considered to be three or more miscarriages. A short time ago, the American Society for Reproductive Medicine published a change of definition of recurrent pregnancy loss: "Recurrent pregnancy loss is a disease distinct from infertility, defined by 2 or more failed pregnancies" [1]. Historically, the cause of recurrent pregnancy loss was unknown in most couples. More recently, however, much progress has been made in understanding the mechanisms involved. Two major reasons for recurrent pregnancy loss exist. One is that there is a problem with the pregnancy itself that prohibits the pregnancy from growing properly. The other reason is a problem within the uterine environment that does not allow an otherwise normal embryo to grow properly.

C. B. Coulam
Reproductive Medicine Institute, Evanston, IL, USA

M. J. Miller (✉)
Advocate Sherman Hospital, Elgin, IL, USA
e-mail: Melissajmiller1981@yahoo.com

J. V. Knaus et al. (eds.), *Ambulatory Gynecology*,
https://doi.org/10.1007/978-1-4939-7641-6_17

Problems with the Pregnancy

Problems with the pregnancy are usually characterized by the presence of an abnormal chromosome of the conceptus. Abnormal chromosome complement comprises the most common cause for all miscarriages including recurrent miscarriages. When products of conception from over 200 miscarriages of women with repeat pregnancy loss were tested with chromosomal analysis, 55% were abnormal. Of interest, only 35% of women experiencing recurrent pregnancy loss after a live birth were chromosomally abnormal [2]. Some pregnancy losses associated with abnormal chromosomes such as trisomy have been reported to have a high risk of a repeating. However, if such chromosomal "accidents" explained all of recurrent miscarriage, the probability of two or more miscarriages in a row resulting from "accidents" would account for 5% or less of the observed incidence of losses. Therefore, while chromosomal abnormalities play a major role in early pregnancy losses, other causes account for approximately 40% of all miscarriages.

Problems Within the Uterine Environment

Problems within the uterine environment have been classified as *anatomic, hormonal, immunologic, and thrombophilic.* While anatomic and hormonal abnormalities have been associated with preimplantation pregnancy losses, their roles in post-implantation pregnancy loss have been controversial. Several uterine *anatomic factors* including congenital uterine anomalies, uterine synechiae, and fibroids have been reported as associated with recurrent pregnancy loss, although there is not always proof of a causative role. Congenital anomalies of the uterus are the result of lack of unification of the Mullerian ducts during embryologic development. Included in Mullerian duct abnormalities are uterine septa, bicornuate uterus, and uterus didelphys. Of the various congenital structural anomalies, the septate uterus is the most common. While all of the uterine anomalies have been associated with late pregnancy loss, their role in early pregnancy loss has been questioned and remains controversial [3].

Hormonal disorders including luteal phase defect, thyroid disease, and diabetes mellitus have in the past been associated with recurrent pregnancy loss. While hormonal imbalances such as luteal phase defect have been associated with occult pregnancy loss, they do not play a role in clinically recognized pregnancy loss [4]. For some years, hyper- or hypothyroidism has been thought to be associated with recurrent pregnancy loss. Current evidence suggests that treated thyroid dysfunction is not associated with recurrent pregnancy loss, although antithyroid antibodies can represent a risk factor [5]. Similarly, well-controlled diabetes mellitus is not associated with recurrent pregnancy loss [6]. Insulin resistance is more frequent among women with a history of recurrent pregnancy loss when compared with age-, race-, and body mass index-matched controls [7].

Immunologic mechanisms have recently been recognized as a major cause of recurrent pregnancy loss associated with the loss of chromosomally normal pregnancies. Forty-five percent of miscarriages and 95% of late pregnancy losses from women experiencing recurrent pregnancy loss are chromosomally normal. Literature is developing which suggests a role of the immune system in the majority of these losses [8].

The end result of the immunologic processes that leads to loss of the pregnancy involves interference of the blood supply to the pregnancy. The mechanism of the losses in post-implantation pregnancy failures seems to involve clotting off the small placental vessels so that the pregnancy "withers on the vine." Clotting of these vessels is mediated through activation of thrombin. Thrombin activation stimulates both coagulation and fibrinolysis so that paradoxical bleeding (subchorionic bleeding) can also be a clinical manifestation of thrombin activation. Thrombin activation can result from the activity of pro-inflammatory cytokines that are produced by immunologic cells within the lining of the uterus or from complement activated by antiphospholipid antibodies.

Thrombophilias are inherited or acquired conditions that predispose an individual to thromboembolism. The most common thrombophilia is acquired and is manifested by elevated circulating antiphospholipid antibodies [9]. About 30% of obstetrical complications are associated with inherited thrombophilia [10]. The most widely reported inherited thrombophilias are factor V von Leiden, prothrombin, and methylenetetrahydrofolate reductase (MTHFR) mutations. When the prevalence of polymorphisms of genes for prothrombin, MTHFR, and factor V von Leiden were compared among women experiencing recurrent pregnancy loss and women without miscarriage, the results were conflicting. When ten thrombophilic genes were investigated, three correlated significantly with recurrent pregnancy loss compared with controls [11]. These three inherited thrombophilias included PAI- I 4G/5G ($P = 0.0037$), Factor XIII V34L ($P < 0.0001$), and homozygous MTHFR C667T ($P = 0.04$) [11, 12]. Furthermore, more than three gene mutations among the ten genes studied were observed in 68% of women with recurrent miscarriage and 21% of controls ($P < 0.0001$). Thus, the association of thrombophilias with recurrent pregnancy loss was manifested by total number of mutations as well as the specific genes involved [12].

Diagnosis of Recurrent Pregnancy Loss

There are a number of tests that can identify risk factors mentioned in the above description of the cause of recurrent pregnancy loss that are available for diagnosis; however, there is a moderate proportion within the population of couples suffering from recurrent pregnancy loss that will remain unexplained.

Problems with the Pregnancy

Abnormal chromosome complement comprises the most common cause for all miscarriages including recurrent miscarriages resulting from problems within the conceptus itself.

Karyotypes of previous pregnancy losses are the best way to diagnose pregnancies lost because of abnormal chromosomes. Frequently that information is not available, and karyotypes of both male and female partners can identify those who have balanced translocations. Low ovarian reserve can be a risk factor for embryonic aneuploidy. The most accurate test to predict low ovarian reserve is serum measurement of *anti-Mullerian hormone* [13]. Besides advancing maternal age, the most common causes of ovarian failure are autoimmune problems diagnosed by autoantibodies including *anti-ovarian antibodies, antiphospholipid antibodies, anti-nuclear antibodies, and antithyroid antibodies* and genetic abnormalities including CGG repeats on the X chromosome *(fragile X)* [14, 15].

Problems Within the Uterine Environment

Anatomic abnormalities including congenital uterine anomalies, uterine synechiae, and fibroids can be diagnosed by *hysterosalpingography*. Available laboratory tests that can recognize immunologic risk factors are listed in alphabetical order below [16]:

- *Antinuclear antibodies* – The presence of ANA indicates there may be an underlying autoimmune process that affects the clotting off of the placenta and can lead to early pregnancy loss.
- *Antiphospholipid antibodies* – Antiphospholipid antibodies have a direct action on the blood vessel to cause clotting.
- *Antithyroid antibodies* – Women with thyroid antibodies face double the risk of miscarriage as women without them. Increased levels of thyroglobulin and thyroid microsomal (thyroid peroxidase) autoantibodies show a relationship in an increased miscarriage rate, and as many as 31% of women experiencing RSA are positive for one or both antibodies. Chances of a loss in the first trimester of pregnancy increase to 20%, and there is also an increased risk of postpartum thyroid dysfunction.

- *Embryotoxicity assay* – The embryotoxicity assay (ETA) is looking measured substances in the blood that kill embryos. Embryotoxic factors have been identified in as many as 60% of women with recurrent, unexplained miscarriage and also reported among women with endometriosis-associated infertility.
- *Immunoglobulin panel* – Hypogammaglobulinemia of lgA needs to be further evaluated to rule out IgA antibodies before treatment.
- *Lupus-like anticoagulant* – About 4% of women with recurrent miscarriage test positive for lupus-like anticoagulant and 9% of individuals diagnosed with SLE have a positive lupus anticoagulant test, or activated partial thromboplastin time (APTT). APTT is an adequate screening test for lupus-like anticoagulant antibodies, but there is a high incidence of false positives. Women who have a positive APTT should also have more specific tests, such as kaolin clotting time, Russel viper venom assay, and the platelet neutralization assay to confirm the presence of lupus anticoagulant antibody activity. And, since some women do not test positive until they are pregnant or have suffered a pregnancy loss, repeat testing during early pregnancy is highly recommended when there is a history of recurrent post-implantation pregnancy loss.
- *Natural killer activity* – Natural killer cell activity or activation assay (NKa) measures the killing activity (cytotoxicity) within each cell. Increased killing activity is associated with implantation failure and pregnancy loss. A value of greater than 105 killing with a target to effector ratio of 1:50 is considered abnormal. The NKa also measures the ability of IVIg to suppress the killing activity. Patients with high NK cell activity that suppress with IVIg in the NKa will respond very well to intravenous immunoglobulin (IVIg) therapy. In fact, the live birth rate with preconception IVIg is more than 80%, compared to 20% without treatment.
- *Reproductive immunophenotype* – White blood cells that belong to the innate or primitive immune system kill anything perceived as foreign. Some types of NK cells

produce a substance called tumor necrosis factor (TNF), which might be described as your body's version of chemotherapy and is toxic to a developing fetus. Patients who have high levels of these cells are at risk for implantation failure and miscarriage. The proportion of NK cells is determined by a reproductive immunophenotype (RIP) test, which looks for cells that have the CD56+ marker. An NK (CD56+) cell range above 12% is abnormal.

Inherited thrombophilic risk factors can be identified by performing a *Thrombophilia Panel.* Because hemostasis involves not only blood clotting but also dissolution of the clot once formed and damage to the blood vessel wall, increased thrombosis leading to recurrent pregnancy loss can result from defects in coagulation, fibrinolysis, platelet aggregation, and endothelial damage. Thrombophilia Panel contains gene mutations for ten genes involved in all aspects of normal hemostasis, including factor V G 1691A, factor V Hl299R (R2), factor II prothrombin G20210A, factor XIII V34L, fibrinogen -455G > A, PAI-1 4G/5G, HPAl alb (L33P), MTHFR C677T, and MTHFR A 1 298C [11, 12].

Treatment for Recurrent Pregnancy Loss

Effective treatment depends on the cause of the pregnancy loss. If the cause of the pregnancy loss is a problem within the embryo itself, elimination of the problem involves treatments including donor egg, donor sperm, or IVF with preimplantation genetic diagnosis (PGD). If, however, the cause is related to activated immune cells and their cytokines, treatments include intravenous immunoglobulin (IVIg), Intralipid, and/or steroids. If either acquired or inherited thrombophilia is causing clotting of the placental vessel and subsequent pregnancy loss, then heparin and aspirin are the treatment of choice.

IVIg and Intralipids have been used to successfully treat women with elevated circulating levels of NK cells, NK cell killing activity, and embryotoxins with live birth rates between 70% and 80% [8, 16]. In two studies women receiving aspirin alone or heparin plus aspirin for treatment of repeat pregnancy loss associated with antiphospholipid antibodies, heparin plus aspirin provided a significantly better outcome that aspirin alone (live birth rate of 80% vs 44%) [17, 18]. A study comparing live birth rates in women treated with heparin and aspirin with prednisone and aspirin showed 75% live births in both groups. However, both maternal complications and preterm delivery with premature rupture of membranes and toxemia of pregnancy were significantly higher in pregnant women treated with prednisone and aspirin compared with heparin and aspirin [19]. Therefore, the current recommendation for "first-attempt" treatment for repeat pregnancy loss associated with antiphospholipid antibodies is heparin and aspirin.

If the cause of the recurrent pregnancy loss resides within the uterine environment and if that cause cannot be corrected, then a host uterus may be a final solution for treatment.

References

1. Practice Committee of the American Society for Reproductive Medicine. Definitions of infertility and recurrent pregnancy loss. Fertil Steril. 2008;90:60S.
2. Clark DA, Daya S, Coulam CB, Gunby J, Recurrent Miscarriage Immunotherapy Trialists Group. Implication of abnormal human trophoblast karyotype for the evidence-based approach to the understanding, investigation, and treatment of recurrent spontaneous abortion. Am J Reprod Immunol. 1996;35:495–8.
3. Kirk EP, Chuong CJ, Coulam CB, Williams TJ. Pregnancy after metroplasty for uterine anomalies. Fertil Steril. 1993;59(6):1164–8.
4. Peters AJ, Lloyd RP, Coulam CB. Prevalence of out-of-phase endometrial biopsy specimens. Am J Obstet Gynecol. 1992;166:1738–45.
5. Pratt D, Novonty M, Kaberlein G, et al. Antithyroid antibodies and the association with nonorgan specific antibodies in recurrent pregnancy loss. Am J Obstet Gynecol. 1993;168:837–41.
6. Temple R, Aldridge V, Greenwood R, Heyburn P, Sampson M, Stanley K. Association between outcome of pregnancy and glycaemic control in early pregnancy in type I diabetes: population based study. BMJ. 2002;325:1275–6.

7. Glueck CJ, Wang P, Fontaine R, Tracy T, Sieve-Smith L. Metformin-induced resumption of normal menses in 39 of 43 (91%)previously amenorrheic women with polycystic ovary syndrome. Metabolism. 1999;48:1–10.
8. Coulam CB, Stephenson M, Stem JJ, Clark DA. Immunotherapy for recurrent pregnancy loss: analysis of results from clinical trials. Am J Reprod lmmunol. 1996;35:352–9.
9. Regan L, Rai R. Thrombophilia and pregnancy loss. J Reprod Immunol. 2002;55:163–80.
10. Hiller E, Pihusch R. Thrombophilia caused by congenital disorders of blood coagulation. Semin Thromb Hemost. 1998;116:26–32.
11. Goodman CS, Coulam CB, Jeyendran RS, Acosta VA, Roussev R. 2006Which thrombophilic gene mutations are risk factors for recurrent pregnancy loss? Am J Reprod lmmunol. 2006;56:230–6.
12. Coulam CB, Jeyendran RS, Fishel LA, Roussev RG. Multiple thrombophilic gene mutations rather than specific gene mutations are risk factors for recurrent miscarriage. Am J Reprod Immunol. 2006;55:60–368.
13. Visser JA, de Jong FH, Laven JSE, Themmen APN. Anti-Mullerian hormone: a new marker for ovarian function. Reproduction. 2006;131:1–9.
14. Gleicher N, Weghofer A, Barad DH. A pilot study of premature ovarian senescence: I. Correlation of triple CGG repeats on the FMRI gene to ovarian reserve parameters FSH and anti-Mullerian hormone. Fertil Steril. 2009;91:1700–6.
15. Gleicher N, Weghofer A, Barad DH. A pilot study of premature ovarian senescence. IL different genotype and phenotype for genetic and autoimmune etiologies. Fertil Steril. 2009;91:1707–11.
16. Coulam CB. Immunotherapy for recurrent spontaneous abortion. Early Pregnancy. 1995;1:1–13.
17. Kutteh WH. Antiphospholipid-associated recurrent pregnancy loss: treatment with heparin and low-dose aspirin is superior to low dose aspirin alone. Am J Obstet Gynecol. 1996;174:1584–9.
18. Rai R, Cohen H, Dave M, Regan L. Randomised controlled trial of aspirin and aspirin plus heparin in pregnant women with recurrent miscarriage associated with phospholipid antibodies (or antiphospholipid antibodies). Br Med J. 1997;314:253–7.
19. Cowchock FS, Reece EA, Balaban D, Branch OW, Plouffe L. Repeated fetal losses associated with antiphospholipid antibodies: a collaborative randomized trial comparing prednisone with low-dose heparin treatment. Am J Obstet Gynecol. 1992;166:1318–23.

Chapter 18
Elective Pregnancy Termination

Cassing Hammond and Sheila Mody

The Patient Requiring Abortion

Introductory Comments

An important part of helping a woman safely through any pregnancy involves knowing how to safely end that pregnancy. Although inducing delivery of a term or preterm infant prompts limited conceptual dissent, inducing abortion to end a medically troubled or undesired pregnancy troubles some physicians and preoccupies many politicians. Meanwhile, half of all pregnancies in the United States are unintended [1]. Twenty-two percent of all pregnancies and 40% of unintended pregnancies undergo pregnancy termination [2]. Each year in the United States, 2% of reproductive age women undergo abortion, and one half of those women will have had at least one prior abortion [3]. Nearly one third of all US women will undergo an abortion by age 45 [4].

The sheer volume of pregnancies that women choose to abort, that spontaneously abort, or that require abortion in order to preserve the health of the woman highlights the

C. Hammond (✉) · S. Mody
Department of Obstetrics and Gynecology, Northwestern Memorial Hospital, Northwestern University Feinberg School of Medicine, Chicago, IL, USA
e-mail: chammond@nm.org

J. V. Knaus et al. (eds.), *Ambulatory Gynecology*,
https://doi.org/10.1007/978-1-4939-7641-6_18

importance of creating practice algorithms reflecting patient's needs as well as the individual physician's skill-set. Patients confronting troubled or undesired pregnancies can choose from a variety of safe options throughout the first and second trimesters that skilled providers routinely accomplish in ambulatory settings.

Referral or Provision

Primary care providers decide whether to provide uterine evacuation based on local laws, their training, and the ability to maintain requisite skills. Most obstetrician-gynecologists (OBGYN) receive training in first-trimester surgical evacuation of the uterus and second-trimester induction during residency, but training in first-trimester medical abortion and second-trimester surgical abortion remains uneven.

Although 51% of US OBGYN residency programs in one survey offered routine abortion training, 64% trained fewer than half of their residents in second-trimester dilation and evacuation (D&E), the most common method of second-trimester abortion. Most residents who received D&E training performed fewer than five procedures during their residencies [5].

Roughly one third of all first-trimester abortion providers in the United States are not OBGYN trained [6]. Family medicine physicians account for the majority of abortion providers in Canada. Physician assistants and advanced practice nurses safely provide abortions, particularly first-trimester procedures, in states such as New Hampshire and Vermont. Unfortunately, most states permit only physicians to provide abortions, and some states have imposed training stipulations that effectively restrict the provision of abortion services to OBGYN specialists. These provisions increase the responsibility of those possessing such credentials to provide services.

Given the safety and ease of performing most first-trimester medical and surgical abortions, OBGYN physicians should have no trouble offering these services. Complex first-trimester or second-trimester procedures might warrant referral to a family planning specialist. Patients and providers requiring expert assistance in these circumstances can contact the National Abortion Federation, North America's largest professional abortion organization, or one of the numerous sections of family planning at academic medical centers throughout the United States.

Counseling

Patients undergoing any medical procedure deserve proper informed consent and pre-procedure counseling to assure they understand the nature and extent of the medical intervention proposed. Very little published data assess the differential impact of specific models of pre-abortion counseling. Certainly, counseling needs vary for the patient undergoing abortion due to pregnancy loss, fetal anomalies, or in later gestation. Most counseling strategies emphasize "meeting the patient where she is at" in a non-judgmental manner that promotes effective communication and addresses common fears, sadness, guilt, or a sense of loss. Physicians may perform this counseling themselves or delegate to other qualified personnel.

Recent reviews, including a review by the American Psychological Association, show no association between abortion and long-term psychiatric illness [7–9]. Postpartum women are much more likely to require psychiatric hospitalization than women undergoing induced abortion [10].

The most important predictor of psychological state after abortion is psychological state before abortion [11]. Factors suggesting a higher risk of difficulties coping post-abortion include preexisting mental disorder, lack of emotional support, fetal abnormality, advanced gestational age, and a history of present sexual, physical, or emotional abuse [12].

Although most abortion services offer coordinated counseling services, patients can also obtain assistance from online resources such as the group Exhale at www.4exhale.org.

First-Trimester Abortion

Medication Abortion in the First Trimester

Prevalence

The Food and Drug Administration approved mifepristone in September 2000 for first-trimester medication abortion. This approval greatly improved access to first-trimester abortion. By 2005, facilities offering medication abortion increased by 70%. Among 40 areas reporting surveillance data to CDC in 2012, 20% of first-trimester abortions were accomplished by medication abortion.[1]

Patient Selection

Patients considering medical abortion commonly have an ultrasound confirming an intrauterine pregnancy and gestational age. Most facilities perform medication abortion through 70 days of gestation for the mifepristone/misoprostol. Preliminary laboratory tests include hemoglobin or hematocrit and a blood type to determine need for anti-D immune globulin (Rhogam®). Medical contraindications to a medication abortion include but are not limited to ectopic pregnancy, severe anemia, and known coagulopathy [13]. In addition, patients unlikely to comply with appropriate follow-up after medication abortion should consider surgical abortion.

Technical Issues

Medications

Mifepristone and misoprostol are used for most medication abortions. Mifepristone competitively binds to the progesterone

[1] http://www.cdc.gov/mmwr/preview/mmwrhtml/ss6410al.htm?s_cid=ss6410a1_e.

receptor and competitively inhibits progestin. Misoprostol, discussed further below, is a prostaglandin El analogue.

Dosage

In 2016, the Food and Drug Administration updated its approved medication abortion regimen so that it complied with evidence-based regimens already used by most abortion providers in the United States. The new regimen uses a regimen of mifepristone 200 mg followed by misoprostol 800 μg buccally 24–48 h following mifepristone.[2] With this regimen fewer than 5% of patients require surgical intervention, and providers can offer medication abortion through 70 days LMP. Although medication abortion can be accomplished with misoprostol alone, the completion rate is lower compared to regimens that include mifepristone and misoprostol [14, 15].

Analgesia and Anesthesia

Nonsteroidal anti-inflammatory drugs (NSAIDS) do not inhibit the action of agents used in medication abortion [16]. Physicians can prescribe NSAIDS or narcotics undergoing medication abortion.

Post-procedure Follow-Up

Follow-up for medication abortion often involves an ultrasound 10–14 days after misoprostol to document completion. The most important sonographic criteria for completion of a medication abortion are the absence of a gestational sac. If an ultrasound report fails to demonstrate a sac but thickening of the endometrium, clinical symptoms should guide management. Promising alternatives for follow-up of medication abortion include combinations of patient observation, urine pregnancy testing, and clinical examination [17, 18]. Fjerstad et al. decreased the rate of

---

[2] Greene MG, Druzen JM. A new label for mifepristone. N Engl J Med 2016;374:2281.

serious infection by changing the administration of misoprostol from vaginal to buccal and prescribing 7 days of doxycycline [19]. The overall rate serious of infection remains very low regardless of whether the patient receives antibiotic prophylaxis.

Safety

Overall mortality from medication abortion is one death per 100,000 procedures or roughly the same mortality as for spontaneous abortion. Even the emergence of an obscure cluster of infectious deaths from *Clostridium sordellii* has failed to change overall maternal mortality rates [20]. As for all procedures, however, complications can arise. The most common complication is bleeding from incomplete abortion that requires D&C.

Surgical Abortion in the First Trimester

Prevalence

Surgical abortion is the most common method of abortion in the United States. According to the Centers for Disease Control and Prevention, 69.4% of first-trimester abortions were performed through suction curettage.[3]

Patient Selection

There are few contraindications to surgical abortion. Certain medically complex patients may be better candidates for surgical abortion compared to a medical abortion. Surgical abortion provides a controlled, scheduled procedure. Patients unlikely to comply with follow-up following medication abortions should undergo surgical abortion.

---

[3] http://www.cdc.gov/mmwr/preview/mmwrhtml/ss6410a1.htm?s_cid =ss6410a1_e.

Technical Issues

Procedure

Some providers incorporate cervical preparation for first-trimester surgical abortions. Cervical preparation may decrease operating time. However, since complications such as cervical lacerations are so rare, it is difficult to study whether cervical preparation decreases complication rates. Agents studied for preoperative cervical preparation before first-trimester surgical abortion include mifepristone, misoprostol, and osmotic dilators (see below) [21].

Providers mechanically dilate the cervix using graduated dilators. A plastic cannula is then passed into the uterine cavity. Cannula size corresponds in millimeters to the number of weeks gestational age plus/minus one. For example, a pregnancy 10 weeks gestation age can be evacuated using a 9, 10, or 11 flexible or rigid cannula.

Following cannula insertion the vacuum device is connected. Most providers in the United States utilize electric vacuum aspiration (EVA), though manual vacuum aspiration (MVA) is equally effective. The MVA, a self-locking syringe, creates 60 mmHg suction, the same vacuum pressure used with EVA. Procedure completion is confirmed by utilizing the cannula to sense whether the uterine sidewalls feel "gritty" and contracted. Providers also inspect the products of conception to confirm that the tissue is appropriate for gestational age. Clinically it is usually not necessary to send the products of conception to pathology for further evaluation; however many states require pathologic evaluation of specimens.

Analgesia and Anesthesia

Anesthesia for surgical first-trimester abortions ranges from paracervical block to general anesthesia. The following specific types of paracervical block might decrease pain scores: carbonated lidocaine, deep injection, and 4% intrauterine lidocaine infusion.

Conscious sedation with paracervical block is often utilized for first-trimester surgical abortions and decreases post-procedural pain [22]. Regimens usually combine a short-acting narcotic and anxiolytic, most commonly fentanyl and midazolam [23]. General anesthesia is rarely used for first-trimester surgical abortion; however it may be appropriate in specific circumstances such as extreme anxiety or medically complicated patients.

Post-procedure Follow-Up

Patients often receive prophylactic antibiotics following surgical abortion. If the patient is Rh negative, she should receive anti-D immune globulin (Rhogam®). Many providers offer a 2-week post-procedure visit, though little data documents its necessity.

Safety

First-trimester surgical abortion is one of the safest surgical procedures. Most surgical risks – including bleeding, infection, retained products of conception, and uterine perforation – complicate fewer than 1% of procedures.

Second-Trimester Abortion

Prevalence

Between 10% and 15% of abortions worldwide occur in the second trimester. In the United States, 12% of abortions occur after 13 weeks gestation, 3.7% at 16–20 weeks gestation, and 1.3% beyond 20 weeks [24]. Although this represents a small percentage of total abortions, it represents a large number of procedures.

Internationally, the small fraction of abortions occurring in the second trimester accounts for disproportionate morbidity and mortality. Two thirds of major abortion complications and half of abortion-related mortality occur in second-trimester abortions. Fortunately, countries with legal abortion services offer methods of second-trimester surgical and medical abortion with less morbidity and mortality than other major gynecologic and non-gynecologic procedures.

Medication Abortion in the Second Trimester

Background

The traditional safety advantage ascribed to surgical versus medical abortion in the second trimester has waned, thanks to mifepristone-based induction regimens that lessen induction-abortion intervals [25]. This means that patients can often choose whether to undergo medical or surgical abortion based on other, perceived advantages. Medical abortion, for example, usually results in delivery of an intact fetus. This might facilitate some patient's emotional recovery and also might permit more complete morphologic evaluation of the fetus.

Technical Issues

Throughout most of the twentieth century, physicians induced abortion in the second trimester by instillation of hypertonic saline or hyperosmolar urea into the amniotic sac to "salt out" the fetus. Oxytocin, the most commonly used induction agent at later gestational ages, fails to induce labor as effectively at midtrimester because the uterus has fewer oxytocin receptors. This results in prolonged induction-abortion intervals and greater risks, including hemorrhage and even water intoxication.

By the latter part of the twentieth century, prostaglandin agents replaced other methods used to induce second-trimester abortion. Gemeprost and misoprostol, both El agonists, induce labor more effectively and with fewer side effects than other prostaglandins or than oxytocin alone or oxytocin in combination [26, 27] with other types of classes of PG [28, 29].

Misoprostol induces abortion throughout pregnancy, though at different doses. It is thermostable, widely available, well tolerated, and inexpensive [30]. Many studies [31–33] document its safety and efficacy throughout the second trimester [34–36].

The Royal College of Obstetricians and Gynecologists (RCOG) and the American Congress of Obstetricians and Gynecologists recommend a regimen utilizing 400 μg of vaginal misoprostol every 3 h, up to five doses [37].[4] This results in median induction-abortion intervals of approximately 12–16 h [38]. Dosing intervals of every 3 h significantly shorten induction-abortion interval compared with six-hourly administration, without increasing side effects [33, 39]. Mifepristone, an antiprogestin that competitively blocks both progesterone and glucocorticoid receptors, quintuples sensitivity to PG 24–48 h after its administration [40]. The synergy between mifepristone and PG permits greater efficacy of PG at lower doses, minimizing side effects. The World Health Organization, RCOG, and ACOG recommend regimens in which mifepristone precedes use of either misoprostol or gemeprost [41, 42]. The most commonly used regimens administer mifepristone 200 mg followed by a loading dose of misoprostol 800 μg vaginally. Operators continue administering misoprostol 400 μg every 3 h up to a total of five doses of misoprostol. Inductions using mifepristone followed by PG require roughly half the time as inductions using PG alone, and roughly 95% of patients deliver within 24 h [43]. Studies of second trimester medical terminations using mifepristone and misoprostol report no maternal deaths and [44] complication rates similar to other induction regimens [38].

The decrease in induction-to-abortion time and side effects removes the most serious psychological and clinical hurdles obstetricians have previously confronted when considering induction.

[4] ACOG Practice Bulletin No 135: second-trimester abortion. Obstet Gynecol 2013;121:1394.

Analgesia and Anesthesia

Pain is the most common side effect of inducing abortion in the second trimester. Young women, patients with longer induction-abortion intervals, and patients at later gestational age report more pain with second-trimester induction [45]. Patients may choose from regimens similar to those offered to other laboring patients including intermittent intravenous narcotics or epidural anesthesia.

Post-procedure Follow-Up

Despite conventional instruction to follow-up at 2 weeks, no data substantiate utility of this visit.

Safety

Physicians have now largely abandoned the use of hyperosmolar instillations due to risks such as hypernatremia, coagulopathy, and massive hemorrhage [46]. Recent trials comparing hypertonic saline with more common induction with misoprostol and other El agonists reveal longer induction times and higher rates of both blood transfusion and retained placenta when instillation is used [47].

Misoprostol inductions less commonly require surgical intervention for delivery of the placenta than induction with other agents. In the largest trial evaluating this issue, 59% of placentas are delivered within 1 h of fetal expulsion, and the overall rate of surgical intervention for retained placenta was 6.14% (95% confidence interval: 3.00–9.26). The authors recommended that physicians observe non-bleeding patients for at least 4 h for spontaneous placental expulsion after fetal delivery [48].

Many physicians fear uterine rupture during medical abortion, particularly among patients with prior uterine scars. Uterine rupture occurs with all agents used to induce abortion and at all gestational ages. This is true of newer prostaglandin regimens, including PGE1 used both alone and in conjunction with mifepristone [49–51]. Because prior studies have excluded women with uterine scars, there is little evidence regarding the true risk of uterine rupture though most reports suggest a frequency of less than 1% in patients with prior cesarean. The impact of dosing regimen and dosing interval remains unclear [52, 53].

Surgical Abortion in Second Trimester

Background

Even if dilation and evacuation lacked its well-documented safety profile, many patients would prefer it to medical induction. Unlike medical abortion, an experienced provider can perform D&E in less than 30 min. This predictability and sense of control decrease the emotional burden posed by prolonged induction [54–56]. It also permits clinical staff the flexibility to schedule a procedure when support from other medical specialists, blood products, and other ancillary services might be more readily available than at the time of less predictable delivery – particularly important for conditions such as bleeding diathesis and cardiac conditions that pose the greatest risk immediately peripartum. The ability to perform D&E in outpatient facilities avoids the high cost associated with inpatient admission to a labor and delivery suite and assures that patients receive the attention of supportive staff [57].

When Grimes offered patients an informed choice between D&E and medical induction, 62% of women refused randomization [58]. Unfortunately, a woman's decision in most parts of the United States reflects more the availability of a skilled D&E provider rather than a true choice between methods.

Technical Issues

Methods

D&E consists two parts: mechanical or chemical dilation of the cervix followed by surgical evacuation of the uterus.

D&E-related morbidity, particularly the risk of cervical injury and uterine perforation, correlates with adequacy of cervical dilation. Most surgeons rely on osmotic dilators to soften and dilate the internal os.

There are three types of osmotic dilators, each useful in their ability to exert radial pressure for dilation and to soften the cervix by modifying cervical ground substance.

Laminaria: Laminaria tents (MedGyn: Lombard, IL, USA, and Norscan: Westlake Village, CA, USA), the most commonly used osmotic dilator, are cylindrical pieces of dried seaweed. Laminaria swell in response to cervical fluid and prompt the elaboration of F-series prostaglandins from cervical stroma. This ripens and dilates the cervix. Laminaria may be used alone or in combination with other osmotic dilators.

Dilipan-S™: Dilapan™ (J.C.E.C. Co., Inc., Kendall Park, NJ) devices are polyacrylonitrile rods that swell in response to fluid. Dilapan cause little change in cervical ground substance, achieving cervical dilation primarily by exerting radial force against the cervical os. Many providers use Dilapan in conjunction with laminaria, particularly for abortions of advanced gestational age that require greater cervical dilation.

Lamicel®: Lamicel®, dry polyvinyl alcohol sponges containing 450 mg of magnesium sulfate, are no longer available in the United States. They absorb fluid from the surrounding cervix, decoupling collagen cross linkages and increasing sensitivity to E series prostaglandins within the cervical stroma. Lamicel® often help ripen the cervix prior to placement of other osmotic dilators, such as Dilipan-S™, that exert greater radial force.

Operators place osmotic dilators according to a variety of protocols that vary the number of dilators, the number of sets of dilators, and the timing of sets of dilators. More advanced gestations require more dilators and more cervical preparation time, usually between 12 and 48 h. With the cervix sufficiently dilated, surgeons remove the fetus and placenta through a combination of vacuum and extraction.

Suction cannula up to 16 mm permit evacuation of gestations through the early second trimester. Later abortions usually require a surgeon experienced using one of a variety of fetal extractors – such as the Hern, Van Lith, Sopher, or Bierer forceps – to remove fetal parts. Intraoperative ultrasound might facilitate technically challenging extractions and might decrease the risk of uterine perforation among less experienced providers [59]. Many providers use perioperative uterotonic agents to decrease hemorrhage, particularly with more advanced gestational ages. Dilute oxytocin and dilute vasopressin injected during deep paracervical injection might help control blood loss [60]. Some providers administer oxytocin or vasopressin intravenously throughout the D&E procedure. No randomized controlled trials offer clear evidence of a superior agent or regimen during the second trimester.

Following D&E the surgeon should inspect evacuated products for major fetal parts such as the calvarium, thorax, four extremities, and pelvis to confirm the uterus is evacuated. Ultrasound offers a useful adjunct to confirm uterine evacuation, particularly when physicians evacuate anomalous pregnancies or pregnancies in which fetal demise results in substantial maceration of fetal anatomy. Unfortunately, small blood clots rapidly accumulate immediately post D&E, obscuring some fetal parts and mimicking placenta.

The most important measure of complete evacuation is the clinical assessment of an experienced surgeon who has inspected evacuated products.

Chemical Ripening

During the past decade, abortion providers have increasingly relied upon misoprostol, a synthetic PG E1 analogue, either as a sole ripening agent or as an adjunct to traditional mechanical and osmotic dilation. Same-day chemical agents obviate the need for multiple-day osmotic dilator protocols. This decreases the expense of second-trimester abortion and increases access for many patients. Despite its prevalent use, few studies compare the safety and efficacy of misoprostol vs osmotic dilation preceding second-trimester abortion [61–63]. Retrospective, observational studies document the safety of misoprostol and adequacy of misoprostol-induced cervical dilation when preceding second-trimester abortion [64, 65].

To date, only one randomized, double-blinded, controlled trial has compared misoprostol with the traditional practice of overnight laminaria before second-trimester surgical abortion. Patients at 13.0–16.0 weeks' gestation (n_84) received either 400 μg of vaginal misoprostol 3–4 h preoperatively or overnight laminaria. Although patients preferred same-day misoprostol, second-trimester abortions after same-day misoprostol took longer and were technically more challenging than those after overnight laminaria [66].

Misoprostol often serves as a useful adjunct to osmotic dilation when the cervix resists placement of adequate numbers of osmotic dilators. When to use misoprostol as an adjunct, in what dose, and via what route of delivery remain unclear. Only one randomized, double-blind, placebo-controlled trial has evaluated this issue. The trial compared preoperative cervical preparation with overnight laminaria and either buccal placebo or 400 μg of buccal misoprostol 90 min before second-trimester D&E at 16–21 weeks' gestation. Although some surgeons subjectively reported easier dilation after pretreatment with misoprostol, the study found no objective differences in cervical dilation measured by passage of rigid dilators, need for additional dilation, or duration of procedures at 19 weeks' gestation. Women receiving buccal misoprostol reported more side effects [67].

Investigators have evaluated several other pharmacologic agents as primary or adjunctive ripening agents including gemeprost, meteneprost, PG F2 alpha, and PG E2 suppositories [68–70]. Several studies suggest that mifepristone holds particular promise as a sole ripening agent and adjunct modality [71].

A recent randomized trial by Shaw and colleagues demonstrated that use of mifepristone in conjunction with Dilapan 24 h before second-trimester D&E was not inferior to 2 days of preparation with Dilapan.[5] A large, multicenter trial led by

[5] Shaw KA, Shaw JG, Hugin M et al. Adjunct mifepristone for cervical preparation prior to dilation and evacuation: a randomized controlled trial. Contraception. 2015;91:313.

Goldberg compared overnight osmotic dilation with adjuvant mifepristone given at the time of dilator insertion and adjuvant misoprostol given 3 h before the procedure. Although procedure times did not vary between groups, adjuvant mifepristone facilitated D&E later in gestation and did so without gastrointestinal and other side effects common with misoprostol preparation.[6]

Injections to Cause Fetal Demise

Injections to cause fetal demise preclude the possibility of live birth, might facilitate the performance of D&E, and help providers comply with legislation that often penalizes the safest methods of uterine evacuation. Many providers use them routinely before all second-trimester abortions, while others use them only in those cases where they perceive a direct advantage to the patient.

Physicians use either digoxin or potassium chloride (KCl) to induce demise. Digoxin is administered into the amniotic sac or directly into the fetus. KCl requires direct fetal intracardiac or intraumbilical injection. Ultrasound, though not mandatory, helps providers assess fetal position, amniotic fluid volume, and placenta location before the procedure. It can also confirm needle placement and direct injection of either agent.

Intracardiac KCl uniformly effects demise. Reported rates of demise with intrafetal and intra-amniotic digoxin vary. One of the few series evaluating timing and efficacy of intrafetal digoxin confirmed fetal demise in 43% of patients at 2 h, 75% of patients at 3 h, and 98% of patients at 5 h [72]. Another series evaluating intra-amniotic digoxin confirmed demise in 92% of cases at 24-h postinjection [73]. Both methods are safe, though most published data consists of retrospective case series with small sample size that make it

---

[6] Goldber AB, Fortin JA, Drey EA et al. Cervical preparation before dilation and evacuation using adjunctive misoprostol or mifepristone compared with overnight osmotic dilators alone: a randomized controlled trial. Obstet Gynecol. 2015;126:599.

difficult to evaluate rare outcomes. Several series have reported increased rates of either spontaneous abortion or preoperative contractions prompting hospital evaluation after feticidal injection [74].

Although many experienced providers believe that induced demise softens cortical bone thereby facilitating fetal extraction, only one published study has evaluated this assertion. This study randomly compared 126 women undergoing second-trimester D&E in which the study group received 1 mg intra-amniotic digoxin, while the control group received placebo. Investigators demonstrated no difference in procedure time, estimated blood loss, operator perceived difficulty, or frequency of complications [73].

Analgesia and Anesthesia

Providers offer a range of analgesic and anesthetic options during second-trimester surgical abortion. Most providers perform a paracervical block, though opinions vary regarding the number and location of injection sites, type of local anesthetic, and period of postinjection waiting time required for maximal efficacy. Many providers add uterotonic agents such as oxytocin or vasopressin into the paracervical block solution. A survey of providers from the National Abortion Federation indicated that most also offer conscious sedation during second-trimester procedures, particularly at later gestational ages. While data from the Joint Program on the Study of Abortion (JPSA) suggested a higher rate of major complications among patients receiving general anesthesia, more recent data fails to confirm higher rates of complications among patients receiving general anesthesia. Physicians offering sedation must have personnel and equipment to monitor level of sedation and postanesthesia care.

Post-procedure Follow-Up

Most complications from surgical abortion occur within 72 h of the procedure. All patients should be monitored immediately post procedure, the time dependent on the level of sedation, to assure limited bleeding and appropriate pain control. Perforations, particularly those associated with bowel injury, often present after patients would have returned home. Thus, patients should receive the name and number of the provider with access to someone on call 24 h daily. As with first-trimester surgical abortion, many providers administer prophylactic antibiotics around the time of second-trimester abortion.

Safety

Mortality with D&E abortion has remained constant since the 1980s. Lawson et al. from the CDC noted a reduction from 10.4 deaths per 100,000 cases between 1972 and 1976 to 3.3 deaths per 100,000 cases between 1977 and 1982 [75]. Only ten US women died as a result of complications among the roughly 850,000 induced abortions reported to CDC in 2004, the majority of those procedures accomplished by D&E [24]. This favorably compares with overall maternal mortality of roughly 12.1 maternal deaths per 100,000 live births [76]. D&E exerts little impact on subsequent pregnancy outcome. In a retrospective review by Kalish et al. of 600 patients undergoing D&E between 14 and 24 weeks, the overall rate of preterm birth in subsequent pregnancies was less than the overall rate of preterm birth for the general US population (6.5% versus 12.5%) [77]. Similarly, Jackson et al. compared subsequent pregnancy outcomes among 317 women undergoing second-trimester D&E with 170 matched control subjects who had experienced viable pregnancies without midtrimester D&E. Although patients with a history of prior D&E delivered slightly earlier in gestation than control subjects (38.9 versus 39.5 weeks gestation; $P = 0.001$), there was no statistically significant difference in birth weight, spontaneous preterm delivery, abnormal placentation, or overall rates of perinatal complications [78].

Other Resources

A large portion of American women require abortion care. Unfortunately, much of the information is tainted by political ideology rather than reflecting best evidence and best practice.

Patients and providers seeking quality information online should consider some of the following resources:

The National Abortion Federation – http://www.prochoice.org
The Association of Reproductive Health Professionals – http://www.arhp.org
The Society of Family Planning – http://www.societyfp.org
The American College of Obstetricians and Gynecologists – http://www.acog.org
Physicians for Reproductive Health – http://www.prh.org

References

1. Finer LB, Henshaw SK. Disparities in rates of unintended pregnancy in the United States, 1994 and 2001. Perspect Sex Reprod Health. 2006;38(2):90–6.
2. Jones RK, Zolna MR, Henshaw SK, Finer LB. Abortion in the United States: incidence and access to services, 2005. Perspect Sex Reprod Health. 2008;40(1):6–16.
3. Jones RK, Finer LB, Singh S. Characteristics of U.S. abortion patients, 2008. New York: Guttmacher Institute; 2010.
4. Guttmacher Institute. State facts about abortion. New York, http://www.quttmacher.org!pubslsfaalnewyork.html. 2006. Accessed 12 Apr 2010.
5. Eastwood KL, Kacmar JE, Steinauer J, Weitzen S, Boardman LA. Abortion training in the United States obstetrics and gynecology residency programs. Obstet Gynecol. 2006;108:303–8.
6. O'Connell K, Jones H, Simon M, Saporta V, Paul M, Lichtenberg ES. First trimester surgical abortion practices: a survey of National Abortion Federation members. Contraception. 2009;79(5):385–92.
7. Boonstra H, Gold R, Richards C, Finer L. Abortion in women's lives. New York: Guttmacher Institute; 2006.
8. Charles VE, Polis CB, Sridhara SK, Blum RW. Abortion and long-tern mental health outcomes: a systematic review of the evidence. Contraception. 2008;78:436–50.
9. American Psychological Association. Report of the APA Task Force on Mental Health and Abortion. (Online). Cited June 2010. URL http://www.apa.org/pi/women/programs/aborti on/index.aspx (n.d.)

10. Hogue C, Boardman L, Stotland N. Answering questions about long-term outcomes. In: Paul M, et al., editors. Management of unintended and abnormal pregnancy: comprehensive abortion care. Oxford: Wiley Blackwell; 2009. p. 259.
11. Breen AN, Mourn T, Bodtker AS, Ekeberg O. Predictors of anxiety and depression following pregnancy termination: a longitudinal five-year follow-up study. Acta Obstet Gynecol Xcand. 2006;85:317–23.
12. Baker A, Beresford T. Informed consent, patient education, and counseling. In: Paul M, et al., editors. Management of unintended and abnormal pregnancy: comprehensive abortion care. Oxford: Wiley Blackwell; 2009. p. 57.
13. American College of Obstetrics and Gynecology. Medical management of abortion. ACOG Pract Bull. 2005;677:1–12.
14. Jain JK, Dutton C, Harwood B, Meckstroth KR, Mishell DR Jr. A prospective randomized, double blinded, placebo-controlled trial comparing mifepristone and vaginal misoprostol to vaginal misoprostol alone for elective terminations of early pregnancy. Hum Reprod. 2002;17:1477–821.
15. Carbonell JL, Rodriguez J, Velazco A, Tanda R, Sanchex C, Barambio S, Chami S, Valero F, Mari J, de Vargas F, Salvador I. Oral and vaginal misoprostol 800 micrograms every 8 h for early abortion. Contraception. 2003;67(6):457–62.
16. Crenin MD, Shulman. Effect of non-steroidal anti-inflammatory drugs on the action of misoprostol in regimen for early abortion. Contraception. 1997;56:165–8.
17. Clark W, Bracken H, Tanenhaus J, Schweikert S, Lichtenberg ES, Winikoff B. Alternatives to routine follow-up visit for early medical abortion. Obset Gynecol. 2010;115(2 pt 1):264–72.
18. Perriera LK, Reeves MF, Chen BA, Hohmann HL, Hayes J, Crenin MD. Feasibility of telephone follow up after medication abortion. Contraception. 2010;81(2):143–9.
19. Fjerstad M, Trussell J, Sivin I, Lichtenberg ES, Cullins V. Rates of serious infection after changes in regimens for medical abortion. N Engl J Med. 2009;361(2):145–51.
20. Fischer M, et al. Fatal toxic shock syndrome associated with Clostridium sordellii after medical abortion. N Engl J Med. 2005;353:2352–60.
21. Kapp N, Lohr PA, Ngo TD, Hayes JL. Cervical preparation for first trimester surgical abortion. Cochrane Database Syst Rev. 2010;17:2.

22. Renner RM, Jensen JT, Nichols MD, Edelman AB. Pain control in first-trimester surgical abortion: a systematic review of randomized controlled trials. Contraception. 2010;81(5):372–88.
23. O'Connell K, Jones HE, Simon M, Saporta V, Paul M, Lichtenberg ES, National Abortion Federation Members. First-trimester surgical abortion practices: a survey of National Abortion Federation members. Contraception. 2009;79(5):385–92.
24. Strauss L, Gamble S, Parker W, et al. Abortion surveillance-United States. MMWR Morb Mortal Wkly Rep. 2007;56(55–91):1–33.
25. Hammond C. Recent advances in second-trimester abortion: an evidence-based review. Am J Obstet Gynecol. 2009;200:347–56.
26. Su LL, Biswas A, Choolani M, Kalaichelvan V, Singh K. A prospective, randomized comparison of vaginal misoprostol versus intra-amniotic prostaglandins for midtrimester termination of pregnancy. Am J Obstet Gynecol. 2005;193:1410–4.
27. Owen J, Hauth JC. Vaginal misoprostol vs concentrated oxytocin plus low-dose prostaglandin E2 for second trimester pregnancy termination. J Matern Fetal Med. 1999;8:48–50.
28. Andersen LF, Poulsen HK, Sorensen SS, Christensen BM, Sponland G, Skjeldestad FE. Termination of 2nd trimester pregnancy with gemeprost vaginal pessaries and intra-amniotic Pgf2-alpha: a comparative study. Eur J Obstet Gynecol Reprod Biol. 1989;31:1–7.
29. Cameron IT, Baird DT. The use of 16, 16-dimethyl-trans-delta-2 prostaglandin-El methyl-ester (gemeprost) vaginal pessaries for the termination of pregnancy in the early 2nd trimester: a comparison with extra-amniotic prostaglandin-E2. Br J Obstet Gynaecol. 1984;91:1136–40.
30. Blanchard K, Clark S, Winikoff B, Gaines G, Kabani G, Shannon C. Misoprostol for women's health: a review. Obstet Gynecol. 2002;99:316–32.
31. Ramin KD, Ogburn PL, Daninlenko DR, Ramsey PS. High-dose oral misoprostol for mid-trimester pregnancy interruption. Gynecol Obstet Investig. 2002;54:176–9.
32. Bebbington MW, Kent N, Lim K, et al. A randomized controlled trial comparing two protocols for the use of misoprostol in midtrimester pregnancy termination. Am J Obstet Gynecol. 2002;187:853–7.
33. Wong KS, Ngai CSW, Yeo ELK, Tang LCH, Ho PC. A comparison of two regimens of intravaginal misoprostol for termination of second trimester pregnancy: a randomized comparative trial. Hum Reprod. 2000;15:709–12.

34. Jain JK, Mishell DR. A comparison of intravaginal misoprostol with prostaglandin E2 for termination of second-trimester pregnancy. N Engl J Med. 1994;331:290–3.
35. Herabutya Y, Prasertsawat PO. Second trimester abortion using intravaginal misoprostol. nt J Gynaecol Obstet. 1998;60:161–5.
36. Dickinson JE, Evans SF. The optimization of intravaginal misoprostol dosing schedules in second trimester pregnancy termination. Am J Obstet Gynecol. 2002;186:470–4.
37. Hammond C. Recent advances in second trimester abortion. Am J Obstet Gynecol. 2009;200(4):347–56.
38. Ashok PW, Templeton A, Wagaarachchi PT, Flett GMM. Midtrimester medical termination of pregnancy: a review of 1002 consecutive cases. Contraception. 2004;69:51–8.
39. Pongsatha S, Tongsong T. Intravaginal misoprostol for pregnancy termination. Int J Gynaecol Obstet. 2004;87:176–7.
40. Bygdeman M, Swahn ML. Progesterone receptor blockage: effect on uterine contractility and early pregnancy. Contraception. 1985;32:45–51.
41. World Health Organization. Safe abortion: technical and policy guidance for health systems. Geneva: World Health Organization; 2003.
42. Royal College of Obstetricians and Gynecologists. The care of women requesting induced abortion. London: Royal College of Obstetricians and Gynecologists; 2004.
43. Tang OS, Chan CCW, Kan ASY, Ho PC. A prospective randomized comparison of sublingual and oral misoprostol when combined with mifepristone for medical abortion at 12–20 weeks gestation. Hum Reprod. 2005;20:3062–6.
44. Rose SB, Shand C, Simmons A. Mifepristone-and misoprostol-induced mid-trimester termination of pregnancy: a review of 272 cases. Aust N Z J Obstet Gynaecol. 2006;46:479–85.
45. Hamoda H, Ashok PW, Flett GM, Templeton A. Analgesia requirements and predictors of analgesia use for women undergoing medical abortion up to 22 weeks of gestation. BJOG. 2004;111:996–1000.
46. Kafrissen ME, Barke MW, Workman P, et al. Coagulopathy and induced abortion methods: rates and relative risks. Am J Obstet Gynecol. 1983;147:344–5.
47. Kapp N, Todd CS, Yadgarova KT, et al. A randomized comparison of misoprostol to intrauterine instillation of hypertonic saline plus a prostaglandin F2 analogue for second trimester induction termination in Uzbekistan. Contraception. 2007;76:461–6.

48. Green J, Borgatta L, Sia M, et al. Intervention rates for placental removal following induction abortion with misoprostol. Contraception. 2007;76:310–3.
49. Marinoni E, Santoro M, Vitagliano MP, Patella A, Cosmi EV, Ci Lorio R. Intravaginal gemeprost and second-trimester pregnancy termination in the scarred uterus. Int J Gynaecol Obstet. 2007;97:35–9.
50. Daponte A, Nzewenga G, Dimopoulos KD, Guidozzi F. The use of vaginal misoprostol for second trimester pregnancy termination in women with previous single cesarean section. Contraception. 2006;74:324–7.
51. Shammas AG, Momani MD. Misoprostol for termination of second trimester pregnancy in a scarred uterus. Saudi Med J. 2006;27:1173–6.
52. Mazouni C, Provensal M, Porcu G, et al. Termination of pregnancy in patients with prior cesarean section. Contraception. 2006;73:244–8.
53. Daskalakis GJ, Mesogitis SA, Papantoniou NE, Moulopoulos GG, Papapanagiotou AA, Antsaklis AJ. Misoprostol for second trimester pregnancy termination in women with prior cesarean section. BJOG. 2005;112:97–9.
54. Freeman EW. Abortion: subjective attitudes and feelings. Fam Plan Perspect. 1978;10:150–5.
55. Rooks JB, Cates W. Emotional impact of D and E vs instillation. Fam Plan Perspect. 1977;9:276–7.
56. Kaltreider NB, Goldsmith S, Margolis AJ. The impact of midtrimester abortion techniques on patients and staff. Am J Obstet Gynecol. 1979;135:235–8.
57. Cowett A, Golub R, Grobman W. Cost-effectiveness of dilation and evacuation versus the induction of labor for second-trimester pregnancy termination. Am J Obstet Gynecol. 2006;194:768–73.
58. Grimes DA, Smith MS, Witham AD. Mifepristone and misoprostol versus dilation and evacuation for midtrimester abortion: a pilot randomized controlled trial. BJOG. 2004;111:148–53.
59. Darney PD, Sweet RL. Routine intraoperative ultrasonography for second trimester abortion reduces incidence of uterine perforation. J Ultrasound Med. 1989;8:71–5.
60. Schulz KF, Grimes DA, Christensen DD. Vasopressin reduces blood loss from second-trimester dilatation and evacuation abortion. Lancet. 1985;2:353–6.

61. Maclsaac L, Grossman D, Balistreri E, Darney P. A randomized controlled trial of laminaria, oral misoprostol, and vaginal misoprostol before abortion. Obstet Gynecol. 1999;93:766–70.
62. Ngai SW, Chan YM, Tang OS, Ho PC. The use of misoprostol for pre-operative cervical dilatation prior to vacuum aspiration: a randomized trial. Hum Reprod. 1999;14:2139–42.
63. El-Refaey H, Calder L, Wheatley DN, Templeton A. Cervical priming with prostaglandin El analogues, misoprostol and gemeprost. Lancet. 1994;343:1207–9.
64. Todd CS, Soler M, castleman L, Rogers MK, Blumenthal PD. Buccal misoprostol for second trimester pregnancy termination. Contraception. 2002;65:415–8.
65. Patel A, Talmont E, Morfesis J, et al. Adequacy and safety of buccal misoprostol for cervical preparation prior to termination of second trimester pregnancy. Contraception. 2006;73:420–30.
66. Goldberg A, Drey E, Whitaker A, Kang M, Meckstroth K, Darney P. Misoprostol compared with laminaria before early second trimester surgical abortion: a randomized trial. Obstet Gynecol. 2005;106:234–41.
67. Edelman A, Buckmaster J, Goetsch M, Nichols M, Jensen J. Cervical preparation using laminaria with adjunctive buccal misoprostol before second-trimester dilation and evacuation procedures: a randomized clinical trial. Am J Obstet Gynecol. 2006;194:425–30.
68. Darney PD, Dorward K. Cervical dilation before first-trimester elective abortion: a controlled comparison of meteneprost, laminaria and hypan. Obstet Gynecol. 1987;70:397–400.
69. Chen JK, Elder MG. Preoperative cervical dilatation by vaginal pessaries containing prostaglandin El analogue. Obstet Gynecol. 1983;62:339–42.
70. Lauersen HN, Den T, Iliescu C, et al. Cervical priming prior to dilatation and evacuation: a comparison of methods. Am J Obstet Gynecol. 1982;14:890–4.
71. Carbonell J, Gallego F, Llorente M, et al. Vaginal vs sublingual misoprostol with mifepristone for cervical priming in second-trimester abortion by dilation and evacuation: a randomized clinical trial. Contraception. 2007;75:230–7.
72. Hammond C, Chasen S. Dilation and evacuation. In: Paul M, Lichtenberg S, Borgatta L, et al., editors. Management of unintended and abnormal pregnancy: comprehensive abortion care. Oxford: Wiley Blackwell; 2003. p. 167.

73. Jackson RA, Teplin VL, Drey EA, et al. Digoxin to facilitate late second-trimester abortion: a randomized, masked, placebo-controlled trial. Obstet Gynecol. 2001;97:471–6.
74. Molaei M, Jones HE, Weiselberg T, et al. Effectiveness and safety of digoxin to induce fetal demise prior to second-trimester abortion. Contraception. 2008;77:223–5.
75. Lawson HW, Frye A, Atrash HK, et al. Abortion mortality, United States, 1972–1987. Am J Obstet Gynecol. 1994;171:1365–72.
76. Hoyert DL. Maternal mortality and related concepts: National Center for Health Statistics. Vital Health Stat. 2007;3:33.
77. Kalish RB, Chasen ST, Rosenzweig LB, Rashbaum WK, Chervenak FA. Impact of midtrimester dilation and evacuation on subsequent pregnancy outcome. Am J Obstet Gynecol. 2002;187:882–5.
78. Jackson JE, Grobman WA, Haney E, Casele H. Mid-trimester dilation and evacuation with laminaria does not increase the risk for severe subsequent pregnancy complications. Int J Gynaecol Obstet. 2007;96:12–5.

Chapter 19
Clinical Genetics for the Gynecologist

Valerie P. Grignol and Doreen M. Agnese

Family history has long been recognized as a significant risk factor for cancer development, and in some families (approximately 10%), a genetic mutation predisposing to increased risk may be responsible. Several highly penetrant genes, those associated with a very high risk of cancer, have been described in breast and gynecologic cancers (Table 19.1). Clustering of cancers in families in whom no high penetrance gene mutation is found suggests there may be other causes, and currently it is thought that a number of lower-penetrance genes may explain these cases. Recent advances in technology have made more extensive genetic testing possible, and this has increased the complexity of decision-making. Hereditary syndromes associated with breast and gynecologic cancer risks are described below, including management recommendations when available.

V. P. Grignol
Ohio State University, Department of Surgery, Columbus, OH, USA

D. M. Agnese (✉)
The Ohio State University, Surgical Oncology and Human Genetics, Columbus, OH, USA
e-mail: Doreen.Agnese@osumc.edu

J. V. Knaus et al. (eds.), *Ambulatory Gynecology*, https://doi.org/10.1007/978-1-4939-7641-6_19

Table 19.1 Hereditary breast and gynecologic cancer syndromes, associated genetic mutations, and risks

Syndrome	Mutation	Lifetime cancer risk		
		Breast	Ovarian	Endometrial
Hereditary breast and ovarian cancer syndrome	*BRCA 1*, *BRCA 2*	45–80%	20–40%	N/A
Lynch syndrome	*MLH1*, *MSH2*, *MSH6*, *PMS2*	14%	12%	42%
Cowden	*PTEN*	25–50%	N/A	30%
Hereditary diffuse gastric cancer syndrome	*CDH1*	30–50%	N/A	N/A
Peutz-Jeghers	*STK11*	32–54%	18–20%	9%
Li-Fraumeni	*TP53*	~22%	Unknown	Unknown
Fanconi anemia	*PALB2*[a]	33–58%	Unknown	N/A

[a]Syndrome has other associated mutations of unclear significance at this time

Hereditary Breast and Ovarian Cancer Syndrome (HBOC)

An autosomal dominant pattern of breast cancer was first described in 1988 and subsequent linkage to the *BRCA1* and *BRCA2* genes demonstrated [1–4]. In the general population, mutations are found in about 1 in 400 individuals (about 0.25%), but are much more common in Ashkenazi Jewish individuals (1 in 40, or 2.5%) due to the founder effect [5–7]. Clinical criteria that predict a likelihood of carrying a mutation include individuals with early onset breast cancer (diagnosed under age 45–50), ovarian cancer at any age, bilateral breast cancer, a history of both breast and ovarian cancer, male breast cancer, and triple negative breast cancer under the age of 60.

The lifetime risk of developing breast cancer in women who carry a mutation in *BRCA1* or *BRCA2* is approximately 45–80%; the risk of development of a cancer in the contralateral breast is approximately 20% and increases up to 60% as age of first diagnosis decreases [8]. The lifetime risk of developing ovarian cancer (including Fallopian tube cancer and primary peritoneal carcinoma) is 18–54% in *BRCA1* carriers and 2.4–21% in *BRCA2* carriers [9, 10]. An increased risk of cancers of the male breast, pancreas, and prostate and melanoma has also been described, particularly for *BRCA2* mutation carriers [11, 12].

Management options include increased surveillance, chemoprevention, and risk-reducing surgery. Screening for breast cancer includes annual mammography and MRI as well as clinical examination. Screening for ovarian cancer is not recommended, as it has not been associated with earlier detection or survival advantage. Tamoxifen and other similar drugs can be used for chemoprevention of breast cancer. Oral contraceptives have been shown to lower risk of ovarian cancer with longer durations of use associated with greater protection. The current formulations have not been associated with increased risk for breast cancer [13]. Risk-reducing mastectomy has been shown to reduce breast cancer risk by 90–95%. Risk-reducing salpingo-oophorectomy significantly lowers ovarian cancer risk and when performed at early age may also reduce breast cancer risk [14].

Lynch Syndrome

Lynch syndrome is an autosomal dominant hereditary syndrome caused by germline mutations in the mismatch repair genes (*MLH1*, *MSH2*, *MSH6*, *PMS2*). It is characterized by predominantly right-sided colon cancer, endometrial cancer, ovarian cancer, and other extracolonic cancers (renal pelvis, ureter, small bowel, and pancreas). Endometrial cancer is the second most common cancer in this syndrome with lifetime risk estimates of 42% [15, 16]. Lifetime risk estimates for ovarian cancer are 12%. Ovarian cancers associated with mismatch repair genes are often low stage with improved prognosis [17]. Although the issue of breast cancer risk in Lynch syndrome has been controversial, recent studies have shown a twofold increased risk for breast cancer as well [18, 19]. Many centers test all colon and endometrial cancers with IHC for mismatch repair (MMR) genes or microsatellite instability (MSI) of the tumor, regardless of history, on routine pathologic analysis in an effort to identify hereditary cases [20, 21].

In addition to surveillance colonoscopy, every 1–2 years beginning at age 25, risk-reducing hysterectomy and bilateral salpingo-oophorectomy should be considered in women who have completed childbearing. Patients should be aware that dysfunctional uterine bleeding should be evaluated without delay. There is no evidence to support routine screening for endometrial or ovarian cancers [22].

Li-Fraumeni Syndrome

Li-Fraumeni syndrome is a rare syndrome caused by germline mutation in the *TP53* gene. Characteristic tumors include early onset breast cancer (often under age 35), sarcoma, brain tumors, leukemia, and adrenocortical carcinoma [23, 24]. Testing is generally recommended for women with breast cancer diagnosed under age 35 when *BRCA* testing is negative. Affected individuals should be made aware of symptoms associated with cancers seen in the syndrome. Screening for breast cancer with annual MRI and mammogram is recommended, and risk-reducing mastectomy may be considered. The screening for other associated cancers is limited, but annual whole body MRI is performed at some centers [25].

Cowden Syndrome

Cowden syndrome is an autosomal dominant condition caused by mutations in the *PTEN* gene. It is a syndrome of benign overgrowths (multiple hamartomas, trichilemmomas, papillomatous papules, uterine fibroids) and increased risk for several types of cancers, including breast, thyroid, and endometrial cancer. The lifetime risk of breast cancer is estimated to be between 25% and 50% [26, 27]. The lifetime risk of endometrial cancer is 30% beginning at age 25 [28]. Screening recommendations include clinical breast examinations every 6–12 months beginning at age 25, annual mammography and breast MRI beginning at age 30–35 (individualized based on family history), and patient education about dysfunctional uterine bleeding. Annual random endometrial biopsies and/or ultrasound and risk-reducing hysterectomy may be considered [25].

PALB2-Associated Breast Cancer

PALB2 (partner and localizer of *BRCA2*) has recently been recognized as an important cause of hereditary breast cancer. Homozygous mutations in *PALB2* cause Fanconi anemia. Heterozygous mutations are associated with increased cancer risks. The phenotype is similar to that seen in *BRCA2* mutation carriers. The lifetime breast cancer risk ranges from 33%, for those with no family history of breast cancer, to 58%, for those with family history [29]. There is an increased risk of male breast cancer [30] and pancreatic cancer as well [31, 32]. The risk of ovarian is unclear. Breast cancer risk management is similar to that for BRCA mutation carriers. The role of pancreatic cancer screening is not well described.

Diffuse Gastric and Lobular Breast Cancer Syndrome

Hereditary diffuse gastric cancer syndrome is an autosomal dominant condition caused by mutations in the *CDH1* gene. It is characterized by diffuse, poorly differentiated invasive adenocarcinoma of the stomach (linitis plastica). The risk of diffuse gastric cancer is as high as 83% [33], and early risk-reducing gastrectomy is recommended due to the ineffectiveness of screening. The lifetime risk for invasive lobular cancer in affected females is 30–50% [34], and management guidelines are similar to those previously described. Rarely *CDH1* mutations have been found in families with lobular breast cancers and no gastric cancers [35].

Peutz-Jeghers Syndrome

Peutz-Jeghers syndrome is an autosomal dominant condition caused by germline mutations in the *STK11* gene. This syndrome is characterized by melanocytic macules on the lips and perioral region and hamartomatous GI polyps. Although the most common associated malignancies are those of the GI tract, malignancies of the breast and ovary have also been observed, with cumulative risk estimates of 32–54% and 21%, respectively [36–38].

Moderate- and Low-Penetrance Breast and Gynecologic Cancer Susceptibility Genes

A number of lower-penetrance genes are associated with more moderate cancer risks have been seen more frequently in families who underwent genetic testing and were negative for mutations in highly penetrant genes. The value of identification of mutations in these genes is currently unclear, as the evidence regarding risk is limited and management guidelines may not exist. These genes may operate in a polygenic model where multiple genes contribute to an individual's increased risk [39]. Some of the low-penetrance genes associated with breast cancer risk (relative risk of 1.5–2) include *ATM*, *CHEK2*, *BARD1*, and *NF1*. Low- to moderate-penetrance genes associated with ovarian cancer include *RAD51C*, *RAD51D*, and *BRIP-1*, which interestingly are associated with the Fanconi anemia pathway. A moderate-penetrance gene associated with endometrial cancer, *EPCAM*, is part of the Lynch pathway. These lists continue to expand.

Genetic Testing

Knowledge of the features associated with the hereditary syndromes described above is essential to identifying individuals that would benefit from referral for genetic counseling and possible testing. Patients with ovarian cancer diagnosed at any age should be referred, regardless of family history. Referral is recommended for those with breast cancer and either a known familial mutation, two primary breast cancers, diagnosis under age 50, or a triple negative breast cancer under age 60. Patients with breast cancer at any age with at least one close relative diagnosed with breast cancer ≤50 and ovarian cancer at any age or two relatives with breast and/or pancreatic cancer should also be referred. Referral should also be considered in patients with breast cancer at any age and a family history of three or more cases of pancreatic cancer, prostate cancer, sarcoma, adrenal cortical carcinoma, brain tumors, endometrial cancer, thyroid cancer, diffuse gastric cancer, ovarian cancer, and/or male breast cancer [25].

Referral should be considered for anyone diagnosed with endometrial cancer under age 50, a tumor that is MSI-high or demonstrates loss of IHC for one or two of the MMR genes, a personal history of Lynch-related cancers, a first-degree relative with a Lynch-related cancer diagnosed under age 50, or two first- or second-degree relatives diagnosed with Lynch-related cancers [22].

Patients without cancer who have a family history meeting the above criteria may also be referred. A careful history and physical examination should be performed to identify other features suggestive of a particular hereditary cancer syndrome, for instance, dermatologic manifestations, hamartomatous polyps, and macrocephaly. These benign conditions in addition to a strong family history of specific types of cancer can help to direct genetic testing.

Once the possibility of a hereditary cancer syndrome is identified, the patient should be evaluated by a health professional with expertise in cancer genetics. An expanded pedigree including affected and unaffected individuals will be developed from a detailed history as it pertains to cancer risk, and medical records will be obtained to document reports of cancers. Documentation with medical records is important when possible, since many cancers are misreported by family history, and the specific pathology will determine the genetic risk. The medical professional ordering the test should be well versed in discussing the risks and benefits of each of the testing options and disclosing and interpreting results in the context of the family history. A discussion of risk as well as screening and prevention options should also be provided. Finally the decision to test other family members should be discussed.

Testing Options

Traditionally, single gene testing or sequential gene testing has been employed. Based on analysis of the family history, a specific gene or genes are tested. If testing is negative for the first syndrome, testing for other syndromes is considered. These methods are most appropriately applied to those in whom a single syndrome is being considered.

Multi-gene or panel testing has become possible in recent years due to advances in genetic sequencing technology combined with the exponential discovery of new mutations. Multi-gene testing is useful in patients who meet the specific criteria for more than one cancer syndrome. The number of genes tested ranges from 7 to 60 genes. Some panels include only high-risk genes, for which data is available that describes relative risks for associated cancers and testing results can aid in medical decision-making. Other panels also include more moderate-risk genes and limited evidence genes of unclear actionability.

More extensive gene testing leads to a greater likelihood of identifying variants of uncertain significance (VUS). These variants are commonly single-nucleotide polymorphisms in the sequence of the gene which may or may not affect the function of the protein. Associated risk of cancer is unknown.

With panel testing, the risk of finding VUS is about 30% [40]. These results may lead to significant anxiety for the affected individual and, if misinterpreted by a health-care provider not well versed in genetics, could lead to unnecessary testing and treatments.

In the future, more extensive testing will almost certainly aid in refining risk prediction, widening the applicability to the general population. As more data is collected on these more recently described mutations and variants, the related cancer risks and appropriate screening and preventive measures will become clearer. The risks and benefits of each testing method need to be discussed in detail with the patient so that the most appropriate method for that individual is selected.

References

1. Newman B, Austin MA, Lee M, King MC. Inheritance of human breast cancer: evidence for autosomal dominant transmission in high-risk families. Proc Natl Acad Sci U S A. 1988;85(9):3044–8.
2. Hall JM, Lee MK, Newman B, Morrow JE, Anderson LA, Huey B, et al. Linkage of early-onset familial breast cancer to chromosome 17q21. Science. 1990;250(4988):1684–9.
3. Narod SA, Feunteun J, Lynch HT, Watson P, Conway T, Lynch J, et al. Familial breast-ovarian cancer locus on chromosome 17q12-q23. Lancet. 1991;338(8759):82–3.
4. Wooster R, Neuhausen SL, Mangion J, Quirk Y, Ford D, Collins N, et al. Localization of a breast cancer susceptibility gene, BRCA2, to chromosome 13q12-13. Science. 1994;265(5181):2088–90.
5. Whittemore AS, Gong G, John EM, McGuire V, Li FP, Ostrow KL, et al. Prevalence of BRCA1 mutation carriers among U.S. non-Hispanic whites. Cancer Epidemiol Biomark Prev. 2004;13(12):2078–83.
6. Prevalence and penetrance of BRCA1 and BRCA2 mutations in a population-based series of breast cancer cases. Anglian Breast Cancer Study Group. Br J Cancer 2000 Nov;83(10):1301–8.
7. Struewing JP, Hartge P, Wacholder S, Baker SM, Berlin M, McAdams M, et al. The risk of cancer associated with specific mutations of BRCA1 and BRCA2 among Ashkenazi Jews. N Engl J Med. 1997;336(20):1401–8.

8. Malone KE, Begg CB, Haile RW, Borg A, Concannon P, Tellhed L, et al. Population-based study of the risk of second primary contralateral breast cancer associated with carrying a mutation in BRCA1 or BRCA2. J Clin Oncol. 2010;28(14):2404–10.
9. Antoniou A, Pharoah PD, Narod S, Risch HA, Eyfjord JE, Hopper JL, et al. Average risks of breast and ovarian cancer associated with BRCA1 or BRCA2 mutations detected in case series unselected for family history: a combined analysis of 22 studies. Am J Hum Genet. 2003;72(5):1117–30.
10. Chen S, Parmigiani G. Meta-analysis of BRCA1 and BRCA2 penetrance. J Clin Oncol. 2007;25(11):1329–33.
11. Brose MS, Rebbeck TR, Calzone KA, Stopfer JE, Nathanson KL, Weber BL. Cancer risk estimates for BRCA1 mutation carriers identified in a risk evaluation program. J Natl Cancer Inst. 2002;94(18):1365–72.
12. Tai YC, Domchek S, Parmigiani G, Chen S. Breast cancer risk among male BRCA1 and BRCA2 mutation carriers. J Natl Cancer Inst. 2007;99(23):1811–4.
13. Iodice S, Barile M, Rotmensz N, Feroce I, Bonanni B, Radice P, et al. Oral contraceptive use and breast or ovarian cancer risk in BRCA1/2 carriers: a meta-analysis. Eur J Cancer. 2010;46(12):2275–84.
14. Rebbeck TR, Friebel T, Lynch HT, Neuhausen SL, van 't Veer L, Garber JE, et al. Bilateral prophylactic mastectomy reduces breast cancer risk in BRCA1 and BRCA2 mutation carriers: the PROSE study group. J Clin Oncol. 2004;22(6):1055–62.
15. Watson P, Lynch HT. Cancer risk in mismatch repair gene mutation carriers. Familial Cancer. 2001;1(1):57–60.
16. Brown GJ, St John DJ, Macrae FA, Aittomaki K. Cancer risk in young women at risk of hereditary nonpolyposis colorectal cancer: implications for gynecologic surveillance. Gynecol Oncol. 2001;80(3):346–9.
17. Grindedal EM, Renkonen-Sinisalo L, Vasen H, Evans G, Sala P, Blanco I, et al. Survival in women with MMR mutations and ovarian cancer: a multicentre study in lynch syndrome kindreds. J Med Genet. 2010;47(2):99–102.
18. Win AK, Lindor NM, Young JP, Macrae FA, Young GP, Williamson E, et al. Risks of primary extracolonic cancers following colorectal cancer in lynch syndrome. J Natl Cancer Inst. 2012;104(18):1363–72.
19. Engel C, Loeffler M, Steinke V, Rahner N, Holinski-Feder E, Dietmaier W, et al. Risks of less common cancers in

proven mutation carriers with lynch syndrome. J Clin Oncol. 2012;30(35):4409–15.
20. Vilar E, Gruber SB. Microsatellite instability in colorectal cancer-the stable evidence. Nat Rev Clin Oncol. 2010;7(3): 153–62.
21. Gwin K, Wilcox R, Montag A. Insights into selected genetic diseases affecting the female reproductive tract and their implication for pathologic evaluation of gynecologic specimens. Arch Pathol Lab Med. 2009;133(7):1041–52.
22. Provenzale D, Gupta S, Ahnen DJ, Bray T, Cannon JA, Cooper G, et al. Genetic/familial high-risk assessment: colorectal version 1.2016, NCCN clinical practice guidelines in oncology. J Natl Compr Cancer Netw. 2016;14(8):1010–30.
23. Li FP, Fraumeni JF Jr. Soft-tissue sarcomas, breast cancer, and other neoplasms. A familial syndrome? Ann Intern Med. 1969;71(4):747–52.
24. Garber JE, Goldstein AM, Kantor AF, Dreyfus MG, Fraumeni JF Jr, Li FP. Follow-up study of twenty-four families with Li-Fraumeni syndrome. Cancer Res. 1991;51(22):6094–7.
25. National Comprehensive Cancer Network. NCCN Clinical Practice Guidelines in Oncology: Genetic/Familial High-Risk Assessment: Breast and Ovarian. Version 2 2016;. Accessed 31 July 2016.
26. Tsou HC, Teng DH, Ping XL, Brancolini V, Davis T, Hu R, et al. The role of MMAC1 mutations in early-onset breast cancer: causative in association with Cowden syndrome and excluded in BRCA1-negative cases. Am J Hum Genet. 1997;61(5):1036–43.
27. Hobert JA, Eng C. PTEN hamartoma tumor syndrome: an overview. Genet Med. 2009;11(10):687–94.
28. Tan MH, Mester JL, Ngeow J, Rybicki LA, Orloff MS, Eng C. Lifetime cancer risks in individuals with germline PTEN mutations. Clin Cancer Res. 2012;18(2):400–7.
29. Antoniou AC, Casadei S, Heikkinen T, Barrowdale D, Pylkas K, Roberts J, et al. Breast-cancer risk in families with mutations in PALB2. N Engl J Med. 2014;371(6):497–506.
30. Ding YC, Steele L, Kuan CJ, Greilac S, Neuhausen SL. Mutations in BRCA2 and PALB2 in male breast cancer cases from the United States. Breast Cancer Res Treat. 2011;126(3):771–8.
31. Jones S, Hruban RH, Kamiyama M, Borges M, Zhang X, Parsons DW, et al. Exomic sequencing identifies PALB2 as a pancreatic cancer susceptibility gene. Science. 2009;324(5924):217.

32. Slater EP, Langer P, Niemczyk E, Strauch K, Butler J, Habbe N, et al. PALB2 mutations in European familial pancreatic cancer families. Clin Genet. 2010;78(5):490–4.
33. Benusiglio PR, Malka D, Rouleau E, De Pauw A, Buecher B, Nogues C, et al. CDH1 germline mutations and the hereditary diffuse gastric and lobular breast cancer syndrome: a multicentre study. J Med Genet. 2013;50(7):486–9.
34. McVeigh TP, Choi JK, Miller NM, Green AJ, Kerin MJ. Lobular breast cancer in a CDH1 splice site mutation carrier: case report and review of the literature. Clin Breast Cancer. 2014;14(2):e47–51.
35. Xie ZM, Li LS, Laquet C, Penault-Llorca F, Uhrhammer N, Xie XM, et al. Germline mutations of the E-cadherin gene in families with inherited invasive lobular breast carcinoma but no diffuse gastric cancer. Cancer. 2011;117(14):3112–7.
36. Giardiello FM, Brensinger JD, Tersmette AC, Goodman SN, Petersen GM, Booker SV, et al. Very high risk of cancer in familial Peutz-Jeghers syndrome. Gastroenterology. 2000;119(6):1447–53.
37. Hearle N, Schumacher V, Menko FH, Olschwang S, Boardman LA, Gille JJ, et al. Frequency and spectrum of cancers in the Peutz-Jeghers syndrome. Clin Cancer Res. 2006;12(10):3209–15.
38. Lim W, Olschwang S, Keller JJ, Westerman AM, Menko FH, Boardman LA, et al. Relative frequency and morphology of cancers in STK11 mutation carriers. Gastroenterology. 2004;126(7):1788–94.
39. Hollestelle A, Wasielewski M, Martens JW, Schutte M. Discovering moderate-risk breast cancer susceptibility genes. Curr Opin Genet Dev. 2010;20(3):268–76.
40. LaDuca H, Stuenkel AJ, Dolinsky JS, Keiles S, Tandy S, Pesaran T, et al. Utilization of multigene panels in hereditary cancer predisposition testing: analysis of more than 2,000 patients. Genet Med. 2014;16(11):830–7.

Chapter 20
Female Sexual Dysfunction

Barbara Levy

Wide publicity prior to FDA panel meetings and the subsequent approval of flibanserin as the first specific medication for the treatment of female sexual desire disorder has created a heightened awareness of women's sexual concerns. Low libido and complaints about sexual dysfunction are common. They are often non-specific. Patients and providers may be uncomfortable talking about sexuality which makes addressing this important health issue problematic. First, it is useful to understand research models of female sexual function. The classical linear model with progression from stimulation to arousal, plateau, and orgasm is not all that helpful clinically in determining etiology and treatment for our patients. The biopsychosocial model considers physical, psychological, relational, and situational determinants. Focusing on the history (or understanding "her" story) as it relates to these four components will generally uncover the source and inform the treatment for the patient's complaints. Secondly, considering the patient's age and physiological status will direct further investigation. DSM V has reclassified female sexual dysfunction into three domains: female sexual interest/arousal disorder, genito-pelvic pain/penetration disorder, and female orgasmic disorder. Superimposing this framework on the

---

B. Levy (✉)
The American College of Obstetricians and Gynecologists,
Washington, DC, USA
e-mail: blevy@acog.org

J. V. Knaus et al. (eds.), *Ambulatory Gynecology*,
https://doi.org/10.1007/978-1-4939-7641-6_20

biopsychosocial model makes identification of the etiology and formulation of a treatment plan for specific complaints considerably easier than most of us fear. Finally, it is important to be sensitive to the patient's social and medical history. We should not assume that she has a male partner – or any partner at all.

Sexual Interest/Arousal Disorder

DSM-IV divided this into two categories – hypoactive sexual desire disorder (HSDD) and sexual aversion disorder (SAD). Lack of interest in pleasurable experiences is a hallmark symptom of depression, but HSDD and SAD may result from experiences and attitudes occurring during childhood. Strictly religious upbringing or parental attitudes that demonize women who enjoy sexual encounters can have lifelong psychological effects. Not uncommonly, the powerful hormonal determinants of attraction in a new relationship will mask these underlying psychological barriers. Once the relationship matures, however, the "lust" driven by phenylethylamine (PEA) drifts into the more comfortable, stable relationship, and barriers to receiving pleasure and enjoying sexuality can emerge. Childhood physical, sexual, and/or emotional abuse are also powerful and deep-seated sources of desire disorder. Sexual aversion is a psychiatric illness and requires referral to a qualified sexual therapist (www.aasect.org). HSDD may be successfully treated by an experienced and interested psychotherapist without additional training in sexual therapy. Attempts to treat female desire disorder pharmacologically have largely been unsuccessful. However, flibanserin, a serotonin 5HT 1a agonist, was FDA approved in August of 2015 for the treatment of premenopausal women with bothersome desire disorder. Flibanserin requires daily dosing, and its acceptance has been hindered to some degree by the prohibition of alcohol intake during use as well as the side effect profile. In addition, several trials have demonstrated a modest improvement in desire for estrogen-repleted surgically menopausal women when treated with supraphysiological doses of testosterone. Off-label use of compounded testosterone or reduced doses of products available for testosterone deficiency in men may be useful. Although generally available laboratory assays for serum or salivary testosterone levels are not particularly useful for the diagnosis of HSDD, if commercial testosterone products are prescribed, testing to identify excessively high levels of testosterone before irreversible physiological changes occur (voice lowering, male-pattern hair loss) is advisable.

Arousal Disorder

Arousal disorder in women is analogous to erectile dysfunction in men. For women, it is somewhat difficult to separate this condition from primary desire disorder, especially once a pattern of poor arousal, dryness, and resultant dyspareunia has been established. Difficulty in distinguishing desire from arousal in women likely contributed to the decision to combine these conditions into a single category in DSM V. Arousal occurs secondary to genital vasodilation and tissue engorgement. Any physiological disorder that diminishes blood flow may cause arousal disturbance. Smoking, diabetes, hypertension, and hypoestrogenism all reduce genital blood flow. Failure to lubricate in a woman who has a desire for sexual activity is the hallmark of arousal disorder. Treatment consists of efforts to increase blood flow and sensitivity. Lifestyle changes – increased exercise and discontinuation of smoking – are useful. Estrogen for menopausal women but also for new mothers who are nursing or young women on progestin-dominant combined oral contraceptives is quickly effective in providing lubrication and increased elasticity to the introitus and vagina. Intermittent suction applied directly to the clitoris either through oral sex or with a vacuum device may improve engorgement. This is especially helpful for women who are not candidates for estrogen therapy. Off-label use of the phosphodiesterase inhibitors (sildenafil and others) may be considered as well. Over-the-counter "warming gels" and topical irritants create engorgement but may cause burning discomfort for many. They may be helpful for some women; however the very act of applying them and rubbing them into the external genitalia, focusing attention on sensation, may be key to their efficacy.

Decreased Sensation

The perception that the vagina and external genitalia have diminished sensation may have physiological, neurological, or supratentorial etiologies. Unlike penile erection in men, for women, there is little direct feedback regarding her body's arousal. Not infrequently there is a disconnect between the sensory afferent input and higher level awareness and interpretation of the physiological state of arousal. A thorough physical and neurological examination is essential. Evaluate the sensory nerves, correct any inflammatory skin conditions, and work on methods to increase blood flow to the genitalia. If the problem persists, referral to a therapist who can assess barriers to intimacy and sexuality will be most successful.

Pain Disorders

Pain is a powerful suppressor of desire and should be considered in any patient presenting with "low libido." Understanding the cause will require a careful clinical history. Is the pain of recent onset or lifelong? Is it related to childbirth, traumatic delivery, nursing, or menopause? Pain with penetration may be due to vulvovaginitis – chemical, infectious, or atrophic. Ask about hygiene habits. Dryness and pain with penetration are not uncommonly due to contact dermatitis and irritation from soaps, scrubbing, daily use of pantyliners, or the so-called feminine hygiene products. Chemicals in swimming pools and hot tubs may also contribute to chronic vulvar irritation.

Consider vulvar dystrophies as well. Untreated lichen sclerosus or hypertrophic dystrophy will result in fibrosis, lack of elasticity, loss of normal architecture, and painful fissures. Since this frequently occurs in postmenopausal women, treatment should address both the fibrosis and the hypoestrogenic atrophy for optimal improvement.

Vulvar vestibulitis is a poorly understood condition that occurs more often in younger women, often subsequent to vulvar infections or postpartum. It is characterized by point tenderness (often a searing, burning sensation) surrounding the introitus and specifically arising from the vestibular glands. The gland necks may or may not be erythematous, but careful examination with a moistened Q-tip will disclose the classic distribution. Early conservative treatment with topical steroid ointment, avoidance of topical irritants, and hydroxyzine may avoid surgery for these women. In many cases, however, vestibulectomy is ultimately required for resolution of symptoms.

Vulvodynia, a more generalized pain syndrome involving the entire vulvar region, may be the source of painful penetration. This condition is associated with many other pain syndromes including endometriosis and interstitial cystitis (painful bladder syndrome). Central pain sensitization results in hyperesthesia and allodynia. Pudendal neuropathy should also be considered – especially in bicyclists. Treatment generally consists of off-label use of neuromodulators such as tricyclic antidepressants, gabapentin, or duloxetine.

Vaginismus may bc primary or secondary. Patients may be unable to tolerate any vaginal penetration including pelvic examinations or use of tampons. Evaluate these women for childhood sexual abuse. Ask about previous attempts at vaginal penetration – including medical examinations – that may have been painful or may have generated fear and anxiety. Women with strong aversion to or suppression of their sexuality may present with primary vaginismus. Secondary vaginismus can occur after many years of satisfying sexual function as a result of pelvic reconstructive surgery, vulvar dystrophy, or vulvovaginal atrophy causing pain with penetration. Pain, or fear of pain, can elicit powerful reflex spasm of the levator ani musculature. Secondary vaginismus may occur during sexual activity and may not be reproduced during pelvic examination in the office.

Treatment of vaginismus includes pelvic floor physical therapy using biofeedback techniques. It is essential that the partner attends at least one physical therapy session to become knowledgeable about techniques to prevent levator spasm and desensitize the reflex. It is important for the couple to engage in sexual activity with a pact to avoid any attempt at penetration. This serves to reawaken sexual desire and arousal by eliminating the fear of pain. Intimacy and good communication in the relationship are strong predictors of quick and successful treatment. Relationship difficulties, on the other hand, make successful treatment problematic. Counseling and psychological evaluation and treatment may be necessary for resolution of vaginismus – particularly in women with a history of abuse.

Deep Dyspareunia

Sometimes called "bump dyspareunia," this may occur as a result of poor arousal or fixation of the pelvic organs due to endometriosis, adhesions, or post-hysterectomy scarring. During normal arousal, the vagina increases in length by approximately 30%, while the uterus and cervix lift up and out of the cul-de-sac. This normal arousal process helps to explain why all women with retroverted uteri – even women with an obliterated cul-de-sac – do not experience deep dyspareunia. When taking her history, ask the patient about foreplay, adequate lubrication, and arousal prior to penetration. On the physical examination, look for point tenderness along the cuff or painful nodularity along the uterosacral ligaments. Treatment consists of addressing any pelvic pathology and addressing the arousal disorder if present. While there are surgical procedures to elevate and alter the position of uterine retroversion, they are very rarely necessary if adequate arousal can be achieved.

Pain with Orgasm

Strong contraction of the myometrium and levator ani musculature occurs with orgasm. Specific organic pathology – especially adenomyosis or degenerating uterine fibroids – may cause pain with or after orgasm. Women with pelvic floor tension myalgia may also experience aching and pain in the pelvis after orgasm. A directed careful physical examination should be able to distinguish uterine from pelvic floor pain. Begin with a single digit examination of each pelvic floor muscle before touching the cervix and uterus. Because compressing a tender uterus will often trigger pelvic floor muscle spasm, it is important to assess the muscles for tone and discomfort prior to the traditional bimanual examination. Pelvic floor tension myalgia is treated with physical therapy and biofeedback, while uterine pathology will require medical or surgical intervention.

Pain with sexual activity can lead to disorders of both desire and arousal. Evaluation of painful sex requires patience with careful attention to the medical history (her story) as well as a detailed physical examination. Treatment of painful sexual disorders is multidisciplinary and requires commitment by the patient and her partner as well as the medical team.

Anorgasmia

Once again, this may be primary or secondary. In previously orgasmic patients, failure to achieve orgasm is most often drug related. Selective serotonin reuptake inhibitors (SSRIs), tricyclic antidepressants, and various other drugs commonly disrupt orgasm. Treatment may be difficult in that discontinuation of the medication may result in worsening depression – often itself a source of desire disorder. Switching classes of antidepressants to some less likely to disrupt orgasm such as bupropion or atypical antidepressants like trazodone may be successful. There is some limited evidence that off-label use of sildenafil in low doses may reverse the effect of SSRIs on orgasmic function [1, 2].

Primary anorgasmia is more problematic. It may be related to sexual inexperience and ignorance. In this case education, use of a vibrator and specific permission to engage in self-exploration may be all that is required. In other situations, however, evaluation and management by a trained sexual therapist will likely be required. Educational materials and video assistance for patients can be found at www.bettersex.com.

Specific Patient Issues

Perimenopausal and menopausal women have many interrelated issues that may result in sexual dysfunction. Body image and self-esteem problems may result in feelings of unattractiveness which limits interest in sexual activity. Testosterone levels do decline very gradually throughout a woman's reproductive lifetime. Unlike the relatively abrupt drop in estrogen with menopause, testosterone levels naturally decrease quite slowly. Some common medications – specifically oral contraceptives and oral estrogen products – increase sex hormone-binding globulin which may result in a dramatic decrease in available (free) testosterone. Some women are particularly sensitive to this and will report rapid loss of sexual desire whenever they take these medications. Other delivery routes – transdermal or transvaginal – for menopausal women will avoid this concern. Other issues as women age also directly affect sexual function. Diminished blood flow, urogenital atrophy (genitourinary syndrome of menopause), as well as increasing numbers of physical impairments such as arthritis, diabetes, and cardiovascular disease may make it challenging to engage in comfortable and satisfying sexual activity. Fatigue, insomnia, and depression are all more common with age. Many medications may interfere with sexual function, and finally there may be issues with a partner's health or availability.

Relationship issues may interfere with sexual function at any time. For many women, a sense of intimacy and trust are essential for desire and arousal. The brain is the most critical sexual organ in the body. Negative thoughts and feelings, as well as anger, are powerful inhibitors of sexual desire, arousal, and sensation. Careful history taking may reveal deep-seated anger and insecurity in the relationship.

Many women describe profound reduction in sexual desire after childbearing. While some of this is likely hormonal, much of it may be situational as the demands of motherhood and fatigue force almost all emotional energy to be focused on the baby and household with little left for the relationship. This is a vulnerable time for many couples. Especially as families are geographically isolated with few support systems, mothers and fathers both suffer. Attention to the relationship – date nights and scheduled overnight times away from the children – may help to preserve and encourage healthy sexuality during many difficult years.

Conclusions

Female sexual function is complex. It is crucial to consider the "whole woman" and her context not just hormones and genitalia in assessing sexual complaints. The nonlinear biopsychosocial model works best in assessing and treating female sexual health concerns.

References

1. Nurnberg HG, Hensley PL, Gelenberg MD, et al. Treatment of antidepressant associated sexual dysfunction with sildenafil: a Randomized Trial. JAMA. 2003;289:56–64.
2. Nurnberg, et al. Sildenafil treatment of women with antidepressant associated sexual dysfunction: a randomized trial. JAMA. 2008;300:395–404.

Chapter 21
Sexual Minority Health

Megan Harrington and Katherine A. O'Hanlan

A number of studies [18–20, 78] have described lesbians in the United States as an underserved patient population. Among women in the United States, having a sexual orientation other than heterosexual is associated with increased rates of poor physical and mental health [19]. This chapter will provide background to the ways that lesbians in the United States have been shown to be underserved in terms of health care and describe what clinicians can do to improve the quality of care provided to lesbian women, including detailed recommendations for gynecologic care in the outpatient setting.

Barriers to Care

Access to health care for lesbians is often reported to be a considerable issue, which negatively affects health outcomes; there are a variety of reasons for this as lesbian women

M. Harrington
Stanford Hospital, Stanford, CA, USA

K. A. O'Hanlan (✉)
Laparoscopic Institute for Gynecology and Oncology, Department of Gynecologic Oncology, Portola Valley, CA, USA

J. V. Knaus et al. (eds.), *Ambulatory Gynecology*,
https://doi.org/10.1007/978-1-4939-7641-6_21

describe both financial and cultural barriers to attaining proper health-care services [45]. Fear of discrimination from practitioners, often based on past experience, is a large concern for lesbian women [18]. Additionally, the real or perceived experience of social stigma or discrimination, which many lesbians are familiar with, often results in negative psychologic and physiologic changes [58]. Lack of adequate insurance coverage is also problematic for a disproportionate number of lesbians as compared to heterosexual women (harrisinteractive.com, 2005). Lesbian women may often have trepidation about disclosing their sexual orientation to friends, family, coworkers, and acquaintances due to fear of stigma and/or discrimination. This apprehension certainly applies to their health-care providers as well. A majority of lesbian women report a preference for receiving care from a lesbian provider; however, they also report having limited success in finding one [45]. If lesbian patients do not feel comfortable disclosing their orientation to their providers, then they cannot be appropriately assessed and cared for based on their individual needs.

Many lesbian women and the providers who care for them are not even aware of the unique health risks of this patient population. Both providers and patients are often unaware of the proper preventative health screening exams called for in lesbian women [73]. The foremost example is the common misperception that lesbian women do not need regular cervical cytology smears because they do not have intercourse with men. On the contrary, lesbians need to be screened regularly as the human papilloma virus can be transmitted between women [2, 15, 38, 70, 87]. Additionally, a significant portion of lesbian-identified women have had sex with men [1]. Both of these justify the need for regular cervical screening.

Another contributing factor leading to this gap in clinical understanding of lesbian health requirements is the lack of curriculum dedicated to the needs of the lesbian population in nursing and medical education [42, 60, 61, 71]. Due to this lack of understanding of lesbian health needs among patients and providers, lesbian women seek and receive less necessary preventative care, a distinct factor resulting in poorer physical and mental health [18, 20, 46, 47, 56, 79].

An additional critical element for lesbians having access to health care is the ability to obtain adequate health insurance coverage; this lack of access has been tied to a lack of spousal insurance benefits prior to widespread recognition of same-sex marriage. Now that there is federal recognition of marriage equality for same-sex couples, and with the passing of the Affordable Health Care Act, further research is needed to assess how opportunity for improved insurance access has made an impact in lesbian health.

This population has unique health concerns; however there is a dearth of research and ongoing studies being done to provide the data necessary to understand and appropriately treat lesbian women [17, 29, 62].

Studying and understanding the varying needs of lesbian women is the foundation to improving care. Putting processes in place to best address these specific needs will enhance the physical and mental health of this population. Addressing the specific barriers to care – including poorly informed providers, historical lack of health insurance, and the effects of discrimination – is critical for enhanced access to care and improved health outcomes.

There are many things that clinicians can do to educate themselves, to make their practice more lesbian friendly, and to advocate for lesbian and bisexual women with regard to improving health-care outcomes.

Providing Culturally Competent Care

It has been argued that it is necessary to regard lesbians as a distinct cultural minority, which, as with other minorities, requires culturally competent care [21, 29, 60, 61]. Cultural competence is defined as:

Having a defined set of values and principles, and demonstrate behaviors, attitudes, policies and structures that enable them to work effectively cross-culturally.
Having the capacity to (1) value diversity, (2) conduct self assessment, (3) manage the dynamics of difference, (4) acquire and institutionalize cultural knowledge and (5) adapt to diversity and the cultural contexts of the communities they serve.
Incorporating the above in all aspects of policy-making, administration, practice, service delivery and involve systematically consumers, key stakeholders and communities [67].

Practicing with cultural competence is important to help alleviate rather than exacerbate the effects of health disparities [82].

A thoughtful yet succinct examination of the current literature is an essential step in understanding the unique concerns of this particular subset of women. Research focusing on the health and health behaviors of lesbian women began in earnest in the mid-1990s. It is worthwhile to remark on the considerable effort that has been taken to include questions about sexuality into women's health research. Throughout the 1980s and 1990s, most research dollars allocated to studying health and homosexuality were spent addressing male homosexuality as the primary or secondary focus, with the overwhelming majority of funding going to HIV/AIDS [28]. Lesbian health researchers keenly understood that lesbians would be more appropriately studied as a distinct subgroup of women, instead of in relation to gay men. They began this process of studying lesbian health under the umbrella of women's health advocacy, which was a burgeoning specialty at this time. Support for studying lesbian health in this manner increased in the 1990s, and the administration at the Department of Health and Human Services (DHHS) was responsive to this growing interest within women's health. After much political wrangling, demographic questions regarding sexual orientation were added to the Women's Health Initiative (WHI) and Nurses' Health Study (NHS).

This is significant as both are large National Institute of Health (NIH)-funded studies that have provided the greatest sources of information regarding how self-identified lesbians are compared with heterosexual women in regard to health behaviors and risks for certain diseases [28]. In 1999, under the direction of the Institute of Medicine (IOM), the National Academy Press published *Lesbian Health: Current Assessment and Directions for the Future* [83] which clarified that certain health risks, including nulliparity, minority stress, and barriers to health care, were overrepresented among lesbian women and discussed whether these health risks contribute to worse health outcomes for lesbians and require additional research [28].

With government requirements for electronic health records, there has been a focus on improving options for self-identification regarding sexual orientation and gender identity [24]. A recent study out of UC Davis Health Center showed that allowing patients to self-identify their sexual orientation and gender identity has led to significant improvements in the cultural climate for LGBT patients [8].

Health Disparities

In 2000, the Minority Health and Health Disparities Research and Education Act was passed. Within this document, health disparities are defined as "disparity in the overall rate of disease incidence, prevalence, morbidity, mortality, or survival rates in the population as compared to the health status of the general population" [64]. The Women's Health Initiative (WHI) and the Nurses' Health Study II (NHS) have supplied a large body of empirical evidence, which illustrates the health-care inequities facing the lesbian population.

The study "Sexual Orientation and Health: Comparisons in the Women's Health Initiative Sample" [85] compared heterosexual and nonheterosexual women aged 50–79 for psychosocial risk factors, screening practices and other healthrelated behaviors associated with increased risk for developing reproductive cancers, cardiovascular disease, and mental health disorders. The data revealed that sexual minorities had higher risks in relation to increased alcohol consumption, infrequent Pap smears, past or current smoking, obesity, and nulliparous status. These factors contribute to increased risk for breast, ovarian, and colon cancer and highlight the need for regular preventative health screenings, including clinical breast examination, mammography, Pap and pelvic exams, and colonoscopies. Additionally, this study notes higher rates of depression among lesbians, consistent with many other studies [3, 19, 47]. It was also noted in this data that many lesbian women are living with partners and are raising children, highlighting the impact of these health disparities on lesbian families [85].

Women aged 32–51 years old were analyzed in "Sexual Orientation, Health Risk Factors and Physical Functioning in the Nurses' Health Study II" [9]. The researchers examined the association between sexual orientation and breast cancer risk factors, cardiovascular disease risk factors, mental health status, and health-related functioning within this group. Similar to the older women examined in the Valanis study, the lesbians in the NHS II had a higher incidence of nulliparity and high daily alcohol intake, resulting in increased risk for breast cancer compared to heterosexual women.

Lesbians in this study also had a higher prevalence of several CVD risk factors including higher body mass index (BMI) and prevalence of current tobacco use. This study also recognizes that lesbian women are more likely to report depression and use antidepressant medication [9].

The lifetime sexual behavior in self-identified lesbian women often does not correlate neatly with the expected norm that they only have sex with women. Several studies have shown that lesbian women have had at least one male sexual partner in their lifetime [1, 38, 46]. This is important to take note of, as there are misconceptions among health-care providers that lesbian women do not need STI screenings, including regular Pap smears [38]. In fact, even among lesbians who have only had sex with women, transmission of HPV,

HIV, gonorrhea, chlamydia, and trichomoniasis has been documented, though these are far less likely to be transmitted between women [1, 38, 54]. Regular Pap screenings for lesbian patients should be conducted under the same guidelines as heterosexual women [55, 70].

Minority stress, or the discrimination and stigma accompanying minority sexual orientation, is widely thought to be directly related to a higher prevalence of mental disorders, specifically anxiety and depression, among lesbian women [58, 63]. In their study "Mental Health Correlates of Perceived Discrimination among Lesbian, Gay and Bisexual Adults in the United States" [58], Mays and Cochran found that:

> Homosexual and bisexual individuals more frequently than heterosexual persons reported both lifetime and day-to-day experiences with discrimination. Approximately 42% attributed this to their sexual orientation, in whole or part. Perceived discrimination was positively associated with both harmful effects on quality of life and indicators of psychiatric morbidity in the total sample. Controlling for differences in discrimination experiences attenuated observed associations between psychiatric morbidity and sexual orientation.

The authors conclude their discussion by calling for public health efforts to improve the mental health of this population, with "interventions to either prevent or treat stress sensitive disorders" for this population.

A summary of the research to date demonstrates that lesbian women exhibit higher rates of smoking [40], alcohol abuse [39, 77], obesity [89], and depression [47, 63] as compared to heterosexual women. Additionally, there are higher incidence and risk factors for certain types of cancer and cardiovascular disease among lesbian women [13, 22, 23, 56, 75], but there has been little research in understanding the phenomena behind those statistics.

Limitations to Research

Studies until this point have been limited in regard to generalizability due to a lack of standardized definitions [6]. When literature uses the term "lesbian," it isn't clear what population is being referenced. In the publication, *Lesbian Health: Current Assessment and Directions for the Future* [83], Solarz identified methodologic topics that require further understanding. One area of concern was the need for standardizing the definition and assessment of sexual orientation among women. In the article titled "Methodologic Concerns in Defining Lesbian for Health Research" [6], Brogan et al. discuss that some variation in the definitions of the term lesbian may be employed to most accurately measure the phenomenon a particular study is measuring. The authors agree with a building consensus that sexual orientation can be defined by self-identification, sexual behavior, and sexual attraction; however meeting all three definitions is not needed or may not be appropriate for most research purposes. Using familiar examples, if the outcome of the research is to determine health-seeking behavior, then self-identification is the important measurement factor as it can affect social factors such as stigmatization. However, if the study outcome is designed to measure incidence of STIs, then sexual behavior is the important operational definition.

In an article by Young and Meyer [90], the authors argue against the limitation of definitions based solely on a behavior. They declare that identity often, but not always, informs behavioral decisions, therefore making conclusions about outcomes that stem from behavioral definitions imprecise. For the purposes of this chapter, "lesbian" is defined primarily in terms of self-identification, as the social factors that accompany this identity are acutely enmeshed with the inequities lesbian women face in health care and to a large extent are equally a part of potential solutions.

Role of Clinicians

Clinicians providing gynecologic care should carefully consider how we could improve the well-being of our lesbian patients. Advocacy for clients' physical health needs within the confines of the exam room is only a part of the care clinicians could be providing. Understanding clients' daily stressors, their relative ability to cope with these pressures, and the extent to which their physical and mental health may be affected is a fundamental aspect of our profession.

Susan Roberts outlined several recommendations for lesbian health that clinicians can commit to in their practice [76]. These recommendations include office forms and educational materials that are inclusive or gender neutral.

When asking about sexual health, she recommends that practitioners use an open and unassuming phrase such as "do you have sex with men, women, or both?" which allows for an opportunity to disclosure. Performing a detailed sexual history is important, with the understanding that lesbian-identified women may currently or in the past have had male partners, and this can affect the type of screening and examination that should be conducted. Clinicians should be aware that depression, alcohol abuse, and minority stress are all significantly represented in this population, and one should have culturally sensitive resources available. It is important to be alert to the varying ways that lesbians form families and to the stressors caused by lack of legal recognition of this family unit.

Guidelines for the Clinical Management of Lesbian and Sexual Minority Patients

Dysmenorrhea/Pelvic Pain

Severe dysmenorrhea was reported by 38–54% of surveyed lesbians [5, 44, 57]. The reported rates of nulliparity, severe dysmenorrhea, and hysterectomy suggest a high rate of endometriosis or adenomyosis among lesbian respondents [44]. Minimally invasive surgical therapy for debilitating menstrual pain not responding to pharmacologic or noninvasive therapies should be offered to women who have elected not to bear children or who have completed childbearing.

Menstruation

There is no evidence for differences in menstrual irregularities or menstrual prodromata as serum hormone levels of testosterone, androstenedione, estradiol, and progesterone were measured at the same time in the menstrual cycle and were found to be the same among lifelong adult lesbians, lesbians who realized their orientation as adults, and heterosexual women [16].

Sexually Transmitted Diseases and Vaginitis

The incidence of vaginitis and sexually transmitted diseases is low in the lesbian population; however, every category of infection has been diagnosed and reported in lesbians. Exclusive lesbian sexual activity (sexual activity with women only) is associated with the lowest rates of infection although exclusive lesbians have been diagnosed with bacterial vaginosis [4, 54], trichomonas [43], human papilloma virus [70], and AIDS [53]. Women who identified as bisexual were more likely than women who identified as lesbian to contract trichomonas, yeast, herpes, and gonorrhea, with rates of infection correlating with extent of their sexual activity with men [44]. Chlamydia, syphilis, and gonorrhea screening is not productive among all lesbians [43, 81] but should be offered to lesbians with a history of these infections, symptoms, or signs of them or who have been recently sexual with men. The incidence of bacterial vaginosis is higher among women sexually active with women, with the thought that the infection is being repeatedly transferred between partners if both partners are not effectively treated [54].

Herpes affected 7.4% of screened lesbians [81] and may be transmitted by lesbian sexual activity [44]. Because herpes virus can be spread by orogenital sex, lesbians with either oral or genital lesions should refrain from sexual activity during times of clinical ulcers and be informed about the risk of occult transmission during subclinical disease.

The human immunodeficiency disease virus (HIV) has been identified in menstrual blood, the white blood cells of vaginal effluent, and saliva. It is thus reasonable to expect that the virus is transmissible during lesbian sexual activity, and possibly more so during menses, during vaginitis (more WBCs present), or after traumatic sexual behavior. Woman-to-woman sex is believed to confer a very low risk for contracting the AIDS virus because women in general rarely transmit the virus to their male partners and because saliva has active antibodies, which make the oral route a less likely route of viral entry. There are, however, many cases of suspected sexual transmission by lesbian sex [53, 65, 72] and a report of HIV transmission to an exclusive lesbian [84]. In addition, there are other risks for HIV within the lesbian population, such as needle sharing among injection drug users, sex with men, bisexual men, or injection drug-using men or women [10, 26]. Until more specific investigation of the lesbian population is undertaken, it is prudent to recommend safer sex precautions to lesbians, similar to those heterosexual women must use. Safer sex among lesbians has not been rigorously defined or studied, but most agree that hand-washing and the use of condoms covering any items inserted into the vagina are important.

Obesity

A study of college-aged women demonstrated that lesbians weighed slightly but significantly more, identified a significantly heavier ideal body weight, and expressed less concern for appearance and thinness than their heterosexual peers [36]. This is likely due to the notion that many lesbians do not adhere to popular standards of women's attractiveness, e.g., tiny waistlines, large breasts, and long hair [89]. It should be emphasized that weight issues should become a focus because of the associated increase in hypertensive disorders, diabetes, risk for surgical complications, as well as risk for breast, colon, and endometrial cancers, [37] heart disease, and gall stone formation [66, 85]. Clinicians should advise lesbian patients who are obese to modify their eating habits and exercise to reduce their disease risks. Further research regarding culturally competent interventions in the lesbian and bisexual population is necessary to combat obesity [74].

Neoplastic Diseases

Ovary

High parity, long duration of oral contraceptive use, tubal ligation, and rural living all reduce the risk of developing ovarian carcinoma [14, 37]. Lesbians seem to cluster in the cities, are unlikely to have used oral contraceptives extensively, are frequently nulliparous, and thus are at higher risk of ovarian cancer. Clinicians should counsel lesbians to consider taking oral contraceptives for 5 and preferably 10 years, if they have multiple risk factors for ovarian cancer and especially an extensive family history of it. Oophorectomy, and consider hysterectomy, for women with extensive family histories or documented familial ovarian carcinoma syndrome should be performed when fertility is complete.

Endometrium

The risk factors for endometrial cancer include obesity, a high fat diet, and low parity, all common features of the lesbian demographic profile, suggesting a higher risk for this gynecologic cancer as well [37]. Extended use of oral contraceptives exerts a protective effect, but many lesbians have never needed this.

Cervical Dysplasia

Sex with men and smoking are both risk factors for contracting the human papilloma virus, the initiating agent for cervical and vulvar dysplasias and cancers [37]. It has been demonstrated that lesbians smoke more than heterosexual women [40]. Because 77–91% of lesbians have had at least one prior sexual experience with men [5, 7, 12], continued surveillance by routine Pap smear is indicated. Most lesbians do not know the risk factors for cervical cancer and do not perceive themselves to be at risk [73]. It has been reported that lesbians can contract HPV through sexual contact exclusively with women [70].

The interval between Pap smears was reported for lesbians to be nearly three times that for heterosexual women [81]. As many as 5–10% of lesbian respondents in two large surveys had never had a Pap smear or had one over 10 years ago [5, 7]. It appears prudent to stratify patients based on their clinical histories, recommending yearly Pap tests to women with *any* of the known risk factors for cervical cancer and offering triennial Pap smears to those lesbians with none of the risk factors and a history of normal Pap smears over the 3 prior years.

Breast

Risk factors for breast cancer include nulliparity or delayed parity, alcohol use, obesity, and high fat intake [37, 50, 88]. One-fourth of lesbians over age 40 in the Michigan study had never had a mammogram [7]. The lack of appropriate use of screening modalities, combined with an apparent concentration of risk factors, may indicate a hidden epidemic of breast cancer among lesbians.

Colon

Obesity, a high fat diet, a history of colon polyps, smoking, and high alcohol intake have been shown to increase risk for colon carcinoma [11, 32, 33]. Stool guaiac screening has been shown to result in earlier diagnosis of colon cancer and subsequent higher survival rates [30]. Digital rectal exam revealing polyps or a lesion may be the earliest sign of a small cancer and is an important part of the annual exam.

Coronary and Cerebrovascular Diseases

Smoking and obesity are two major risk factors for coronary artery disease [49, 52]. Considering these factors, there are higher incidence and risk factors for certain types of cancer and cardiovascular disease among lesbian women [13, 22, 23, 56, 75], especially if they defer seeing a clinician until symptoms or signs become extreme or acute [35, 69, 80].

Clinical assessment of the serum cholesterol, blood pressure, weight, exercise, and dietary history is part of routine annual screening checkups which lesbians miss if they forego annual doctor visits.

Insemination

Lesbians seeking fertility should be encouraged to use formal fertility services licensed by the American Blood Bank Association. This will establish their parental roles; avoid propagation of sexually transmitted diseases, undiagnosed genetic disorders, and oversaturation of an area with offspring from one donor; and avoid paternity suits. In three surveys since 2000, 55–84% of gynecologists said that they would inseminate or offer advanced reproductive services to lesbians [48]. Recently the American College of Obstetricians and Gynecologists added sexual orientation and gender expression to its nondiscrimination policy.

Obstetric Care

There are no specific obstetric risk factors conferred by lesbian sexual orientation. However, clinicians should understand the legal rights of lesbians in their respective state with regard to legal contracts for durable powers of attorney for health care, as well as parental rights for non-gestational parent. Laws regarding recognition of rights for same-sex couples are rapidly changing, and it is critical that clinicians keep up to date and encourage all lesbian couples to understand the laws of their state and plan for all medical and legal scenarios, especially prior to planned gynecologic or obstetric procedures.

Transsexuals

Transsexual individuals have a strong belief, often from childhood onward, that they were born into a body with the wrong sex. The vast majority is heterosexual to their identified gender, but a few have a homosexual orientation. Gender identity is thought to develop as various sex hormones affect the developing fetal brain [31, 91]. Many studies of the multiple sexually dimorphic nuclei in the brain suggest that transsexuals possess the neuroanatomy appropriate to their self-perceived gender, not their phenotypic gender [27, 31, 91]. The obstetrician-gynecologist may be called to provide care for females who desire sex reassignment surgery, called FTM (female-to-male) transsexuals, or for women who have had their surgery who were previously phenotypic men, called MTF (male-to-female) transsexuals. All transsexuals should be referred to by the pronouns of their identified genders. The specific needs of each are different.

FTMs

Young heterosexual girls, lesbians, and girls who later become FTM males may all dress as tomboys to varying degrees;

however, girls who later become FTM males cross-dress more frequently and are more comfortable in boys clothes. In most survey reports, they describe themselves as the consummate tomboys, experiencing clear gender dysphoria and increasing discomfort with pubertal onset of thelarche and menarche [25, 59]. Clinicians should refer these young women, at their request, for supportive counseling to a center experienced with transsexualism and help her to begin to explore her status for possible hormones and possibly later sex reassignment surgery. Prior to surgery, an FTM must live ostensibly as a male for at least 1 year, self-injecting 200 mg testosterone every 2 weeks to suppress menses and induce masculine secondary sex characteristics. A laparoscopic hysterectomy/oophorectomy and possibly vaginectomy are part of the surgery in which the gynecologist can collaborate. Because these individuals may desire to have children, cryopreservation of unstimulated ovarian cortex during oophorectomy should be discussed as a means to preserve follicles for later insemination and gestation [68]. Serum cholesterol should be monitored in these individuals as usual for all men.

MTFs

Some young boys love to dress as women and actually may recognize themselves to have been born into the wrong body. After they have matured, they express a strong wish to be themselves, living their lives as women. Before initiating estrogen therapy to begin the transformation, cryopreservation of banked sperm should be offered to these phenotypic males [34]. Once they are stabilized on the dose of estrogen, which suppresses gonadotropins and produces serum estradiol levels of 200–400 pg/ml, spermatogenesis ceases; but it will resume in a few months if estrogen is discontinued [51] to allow for sperm banking if desired. The surgery, performed long after the MTF has been living as an overt female, usually involves remodeling the skin of the penile shaft into a vagina, preserving a portion of the glans penis as a clitoris, and fashioning an opening for the urethra beneath the clitoris.

Sometimes a vagina is extended by adding a split-thickness skin graft, or it can be made from a segment of colon. The final result usually forms a moist vagina and a functional orgasmic sexual response and has a good cosmetic effect. There are many transsexuals that do not seek out such extensive surgery and may not seek any surgery at all.

Squamous cell carcinomas have been documented in the neovagina of MTF transsexuals, usually occurring 10 or more years after vaginoplasty [41]. Papanicolaou smears should be performed per the usual risk profiles, and all suspicious lesions biopsied. Mammography is probably not indicated for MTF women until after 10 or more years of estrogen stimulation because the risk of breast cancer is cumulative over time. Reports of prostate cancer in MTF patients have been reported within 12 years of transition [86]. The yearly exam needs to also include an assessment of the prostate, as this is not removed in most surgeries but is often too small to identify. If any nodularity is identified, a serum prostate-specific antigen (PSA) assay and sonography should be obtained. The gynecologist may be consulted for the occasional stenosis of the vaginal graft and may need to surgically revise a contracted introitus to accommodate sexual activity.

References

1. Bailey JV, Farquhar C, Owen C, Mangtani P. Sexually transmitted infections in women who have sex with women. Sex Transm Infect. 2004;80(3):244–6.
2. Bailey JV, Kavanagh J, Owen C, McLean KA, Skinner CJ. Lesbians and cervical screening. Br J Gen Pract J R Coll Gen Pract. 2000;50(455):481–2.
3. Barnard AG. Effects of sexuality on lesbians' experiences of depression. J Psychosoc Nurs Ment Health Serv. 2005;43(10):36–43.
4. Berger BJ, Kolton S, et al. Bacterial vaginosis in lesbians: a sexually transmitted disease. Clin Infect Dis. 1995;21(6):1402–5.
5. Bradford J, Ryan C, et al. National Lesbian Health Care Survey: implications for mental health care. J Consult Clin Psychol. 1994;62(2):228–42.

6. Brogan D, Frank E, Elon L, O'Hanlan KA. Methodologic concerns in defining lesbian for health research. Epidimiology. 2001;12(1):109–13.
7. Bybee D. Michigan lesbian survey: a report to the Michigan Organization for Human Rights and the Michigan Department of Public Health. Detroit: Michigan Department of Health and Human Services; 1990.
8. Callahan EJ, Sitkin N, Ton H, Eidson-Ton WS, Weckstein J, Latimore D. Introducing sexual orientation and gender identity into the electronic health record: one academic health center's experience. Acad Med. 2015;90(2):154–60.
9. Case P, Austin SB, Hunter DJ, Manson JE, Malspeis S, Willett WC, et al. Sexual orientation, health risk factors, and physical functioning in the nurses' health study II. J Women's Health (Larchmt). 2004;13(9):1033–47.
10. Chu SY, Buehler JW, et al. Epidemiology of reported cases of AIDS in lesbians, United States 1980–89. Am J Public Health. 1990;80(11):1380–1.
11. Chute CG, Willett WC, et al. A prospective study of body mass, height, and smoking on the risk of colorectal cancer in women. Cancer Causes Control. 1991;2(2):117–24.
12. Cochran, Mays. Disclosure of sexual orientation to physicians by black and latino women. J West Med. 1988;149(5):616–9.
13. Cochran SD, Mays VM, Bowen D, Gage S, Bybee D, Roberts SJ, et al. Cancer-related risk indicators and preventive screening behaviors among lesbians and bisexual women. Am J Public Health. 2001;91(4):591–7.
14. Coker AL, Harlap S, Fortney JA. Oral contraceptives and reproductive cancers: Weighting the risks and benefits. Fam Plann Perspect. 1993;25(1):17.
15. Curmi C, Peters K, Salamonson Y. Barriers to cervical cancer screening experienced by lesbian women: a qualitative study. J Clin Nurs. 2016;25(23-24):3643–51.
16. Dancey C. Sexual orientation in women: an investigation of hormonal and personality variables. Biol Psychol. 1990;30(3):251–64.
17. Diamant A. Funding for more research is urgently needed. West J Med. 2000;172(6):384–5.
18. Diamant AL, Schuster MA, Lever J. Receipt of preventive health care services by lesbians. Am J Prev Med. 2000;19(3):141–8.
19. Diamant AL, Wold C. Sexual orientation and variation in physical and mental health status among women. J Women's Health (Larchmt). 2003;12(1):41–9.

20. Diamant AL, Wold C, Spritzer K, Gelberg L. Health behaviors, health status, and access to and use of health care: a population-based study of lesbian, bisexual, and heterosexual women. Arch Fam Med. 2000;9(10):1043–51.
21. Dibble SL. Government administrations must provide culturally appropriate care to all underserved groups. ONS News I Oncol Nurs Soc. 2003;18(10):3. author reply 3
22. Dibble SL, Roberts SA, Nussey B. Comparing breast cancer risk between lesbians and their heterosexual sisters. Women's Health Issues Off Publ Jacobs Inst Women's Health. 2004;14(2):60–8.
23. Dibble SL, Roberts SA, Robertson PA, Paul SM. Risk factors for ovarian cancer: lesbian and heterosexual women. Oncol Nurs Forum. 2002;29(1):El–7.
24. Ehrenfeld DC. The opportunity for medical systems to reduce health disparities among lesbian, gay, bisexual, transgender and intersex patients. J Med Syst. 2015;39(11):178.
25. Ehrhardt AA, Grisanti G, et al. Female-to-male transsexuals compared to lesbians: behavioral patterns of childhood and adolescent development. Arch Sex Behav. 1979;8(6):481–90.
26. Einhorn, Polgar. HIV risk behavior among lesbian and bisexual women. AIDS Educ Prev. 1994;6(6):514–23.
27. Elias AN, Valenta LJ. Are all males equal? Anatomic and functional basis for sexual orientation in males. Med Hypotheses. 1992;39(1):85–7.
28. Epstein S. Sexualizing governance and medicalizing identities: the emergence of "state-centered" LGBT health politics in the United States. [Electronic version]. Sexualities. 2003;6(2):131–71. Retrieved 5 Feb 2007
29. Fogarty S. Culturally competent care for the invisible minority. Mich Nurse. 2003;76(6):11–3.
30. Fry RD, Fleshman JW, et al. Cancer of the colon and rectum. Clin Symp. 1989;41(5):29–30.
31. Giordano G, Giusti M. Hormones and psychosexual differentiation. Minerva Endocrinol. 1995;20(3):165–93.
32. Giovannucci E, Rimm EB, et al. A prospective study of cigarette smoking and risk of colorectal adenoma and colorectal cancer in U.S. men. J Natl Cancer Inst. 1994;86(3):183–91.
33. Giovannucci E, Stampfer MJ, et al. Folate, methionine, and alcohol intake and risk of colorectal adenoma. J Natl Cancer Inst. 1993;85(11):875–84.
34. Hall C, Schaffer J. Gamete cryopreservation prior to sex reassignment. 1997. Unpublished manuscript from the Seahorse

Medical Clinic in San Jose, CA specializing in health for transsexuals.
35. Haynes S. Risk of breast cancer in lesbians. Annual Meeting of the National Gay and Lesbian Health Education Foundation, Los Angeles. 1992.
36. Herzog D, Newman K, et al. Body image satisfaction in homosexual and heterosexual women. Int J Eat Disord. 1992;11(4):391.
37. Holleb A, Fink D, et al. American Cancer Society textbook of clinical oncology. Atlanta: American Cancer Society; 1991.
38. Hughes C, Evans A. Health needs of women who have sex with women. BMJ (Clin Res Ed). 2003;327(7421):939–40.
39. Hughes TL. Alcohol use and alcohol-related problems among lesbians and gay men. Annu Rev Nurs Res. 2005;23:283–325.
40. Hughes TL, Jacobson KM. Sexual orientation and women's smoking. Curr Womens Health Rep. 2003;3(3):254–61.
41. Imrie J, Kennedy J, et al. Intraepithelial neoplasia arising in an artificial vagina. Case report. Br J Obstet Gynaecol. 1986; 93:886–8.
42. Institute of Medicine. The health of lesbian, gay, bisexual, and transgender people: building a foundation for better understanding. Washington, DC: National Academies Press; 2011. p. 362.
43. Johnson SR, Guenther SM, et al. Factors influencing lesbian gynecologic care: a preliminary study. Am J Obstet Gynecol. 1981;140(1):20–8.
44. Johnson SR, Smith EM, et al. Comparison of gynecologic health care problems between lesbians and bisexual women. A survey of 2,345 women. J Reprod Med. 1987;32(11):805–11.
45. Klitzman RL, Greenberg JD. Patterns of communication between gay and lesbian patients and their health care providers. J Homosex. 2002;42(4):65–75.
46. Koh AS. Use of preventive health behaviors by lesbian, bisexual, and heterosexual women: questionnaire survey. West J Med. 2000;172(6):379–84.
47. Koh AS, Ross LK. Mental health issues: a comparison of lesbian, bisexual and heterosexual women. J Homosex. 2006;51(1):33–57.
48. Lawrence, et al. Obstetrician and gynecologists beliefs about assisted reproductive technologies. Obstet Gynecol. 2010;116(1):127–35.
49. Leaverton PE, Sorlie PD, et al. Representativeness of the Framingham risk model for coronary heart disease mortality: a comparison with a national cohort study. J Chronic Dis. 1987;40(8):775–84.

50. London SJ, Colditz GA, et al. Prospective study of relative weight, height, and risk of breast cancer. JAMA. 1989;262(20):2853–8.
51. Lubbert H, Leo-Roberg I, et al. Effects of ethinyl estradiol on semen quality and various hormonal parameters in a eugonadal male. Fertil Steril. 1992;58(3):603–8.
52. Manson JE, Colditz GA, et al. A prospective study of obesity and risk of coronary heart disease in women. N Engl J Med. 1990;322(13):882–9.
53. Marmor M, Weiss LR, et al. Possible female-to-female transmission of human immunodeficiency virus [letter]. Ann Intern Med. 1986;105(6):969.
54. Marrazzo JM. Barriers to infectious disease care among lesbians. Emerg Infect Dis. 2004;10(11):1974–8.
55. Marrazzo JM, Stine K. Reproductive health history of lesbians: implications for care. Am J Obstet Gynecol. 2004;190(5):1298–304.
56. Matthews AK, Brandenburg DL, Johnson TP, Hughes TL. Correlates of underutilization of gynecological cancer screening among lesbian and heterosexual women. Prev Med. 2004;38(1):105–13.
57. Mays VM, Cochran SD. The black women's relationships project: a national survey of black lesbians. In: Shemoff M, Scott WA, editors. A sourcebook of gay/lesbian health care. Washington, DC: National Gay and Lesbian Health Foundation; 1988.
58. Mays VM, Cochran SD. Mental health correlates of perceived discrimination among lesbian, gay, and bisexual adults in the United States. Am J Public Health. 2001;91(11):1869–76.
59. McCauley EA, Ehrhardt AA. Role expectations and definitions: a comparison of female transsexuals and lesbians. J Homosex. 1977;3(2):137–47.
60. McNair R. Outing lesbian health in medical education. Women Health. 2003;37(4):89–103.
61. McNair R. Lesbian health inequalities: a cultural minority issue for health professionals. Med J Aust. 2003;178(12):643–5.
62. Meyer IH. Why lesbian, gay, bisexual, and transgender public health? Am J Public Health. 2001;91(6):856–9.
63. Meyer IH. Prejudice, social stress, and mental health in lesbian, gay, and bisexual populations: conceptual issues and research evidence. Psychol Bull. 2003;129(5):674–97.
64. Minority Health and Health Disparities Research and Education Act. United States public law 106–525, 2498. 2000.
65. Monzon OT, Capellan JM. Female-to-female transmission of HIV [letter]. Lancet. 1987;2(8549):40–1.

66. Narnnoum A. Obesity: a disease worth treating. Female Patient. 1993;18(33):33–44.
67. National Center for Cultural Competence. Cultural competence: definition and conceptual framework. Retrieved 23 Apr 2008 from definition.
68. Newton H, Aubard Y, Rutherford A, Sharma V, Gosden R. Ovary and ovulation: low temperature storage and grafting of human ovarian tissue. Hum Reprod. 1996;11(7):1487–91.
69. O'Hanlan KA. Risk of cancers and heart disease in the lesbian population. Annual Meeting of the Lesbian Physicians' Conference, Taos, NM. 1991.
70. O'Hanlan KA, Crum CP. Human papillomavirus-associated cervical intraepithelial neoplasia following lesbian sex. Obstet Gynecol. 1996;88(4 Pt 2):702–3.
71. Obedin-Maliver J, Goldsmith ES, Stewart L, et al. Lesbian, gay, bisexual, and transgender-related content in undergraduate medical education. JAMA. 2011;306(9):971–7.
72. Perry S, Jacobsberg L, et al. Orogenital transmission of human immunodeficiency virus (HIV) [letter]. Ann Intern Med. 1989;111(11):951–2.
73. Price JH, Easton AN, Telljohann SK, Wallace PB. Perceptions of cervical cancer and Pap smear screening behavior by women's sexual orientation. J Community Health. 1996;21:89–105.
74. Rizer AM, Mauery DR, Haynes SG, Couser B, Cindy G. LGBT Health. 2015;2(2):105–12. https://doi.org/10.1089/lgbt.2014.0122.
75. Roberts SA, Dibble SL, Nussey B, Casey K. Cardiovascular disease risk in lesbian women. Women's Health Issues Off Publ Jacobs Inst Women's Health. 2003;13(4):167–74.
76. Roberts SJ. Health care recommendations for lesbian women. J Obstet Gynecol Neonatal Nurs JOGNN I NAACOG. 2006;35(5):583–91.
77. Roberts SJ, Grindel CG, Patsdaughter CA, Demarco R, Tarmina MS. Lesbian use and abuse of alcohol: results of the Boston lesbian health project IL. Subst Abuse Off Publ Assoc Med Educ Res Subst Abuse. 2005;25(4):1–9.
78. Roberts SJ, Patsdaughter CA, Grindel CG, Tarmina MS. Health related behaviors and cancer screening of lesbians: results of the Boston lesbian health project IL. Women Health. 2004;39(4):41–55.
79. Roberts SJ, Sorensen L. Health related behaviors and cancer screening of lesbians: results from the Boston lesbian health project. Women Health. 1999;28(4):1–12.

80. Robertson MM. Lesbians as an invisible minority in the health services arena. Health Care Women Int. 1992;13(2):155–63.
81. Robertson P, Schachter J. Failure to identify venereal disease in a lesbian population. Sex Transm Dis. 1981;8(2):75–6.
82. Shaya FT, Gbarayor CM. The case for cultural competence in health professions education. Am J Pharm Educ. 2006;70(6):124.
83. Solarz AL. Lesbian health: current assessment and directions for the future. Washington, DC: National Academy Press; 1999.
84. Troncoso AR, Romani A, et al. Probable HIV transmission by female homosexual contact. Medicina (BAires). 1995;55(4):334–6.
85. Valanis BG, Bowen DJ, Bassford T, Whitlock E, Charney P, Carter RA. Sexual orientation and health: comparisons in the women's health initiative sample. Arch Fam Med. 2000;9(9):843–53.
86. van Haarst EP, Newling DW, Gooren LJ, Asscheman H, Prenger DM. Metastatic prostatic carcinoma in a male-to-female transsexual. Br J Ural. 1998;81:776.
87. Waterman L, Voss J. HPV, cervical cancer risks, and barriers to care for lesbian women. Nurse Pract. 2015;40(1):46–53. January 16
88. Willett WC, Stampfer MJ, et al. Moderate alcohol consumption and the risk of breast cancer. N Engl J Med. 1987;316(19):1174–80.
89. Yancey AK, Cochran SD, Corliss HL, Mays VM. Correlates of overweight and obesity among lesbian and bisexual women. Prev Med. 2003;36(6):676–83.
90. Young RM, Meyer IH. The trouble with "MSM" and "WSW": erasure of the sexual-minority person in public health discourse. Am J Public Health. 2005;95(7):1144–9.
91. Zhou JN, Hofinan MA, et al. A sex difference in the human brain and its relation to transsexuality. Nature. 1995;378(6552):68–70.

Chapter 22
Office Practice Risk Management

John S. Rinehart

Risk management can be viewed as preventative, and medical malpractice can be viewed as compensatory once an adverse event has occurred. Unfortunately, risk management has come to mean an attempt to avoid medical malpractice lawsuits. That is an unrealistic goal on its face and misses the real value of risk management. Risk management and medical malpractice center on undesired outcomes in the delivery of healthcare. Some undesired outcomes occur by the very nature of chance and illness, which make them unavoidable. Other undesired outcomes result from preventable causes. Risk management focuses on limiting the occurrence of preventable undesired outcomes. Medical malpractice, while ostensibly existing to compensate monetarily for negligent outcomes, acts as a means of attempting to derive compensation for both avoidable and unavoidable undesired outcomes. A more equitable system could be achieved if there was a

J. S. Rinehart (✉)
Division of Reproductive Endocrinology and Fertility, Department of Obstetrics and Gynecology, NorthShore University HealthSystem, Evanston, IL, USA

Pritzker School of Medicine, University of Chicago, Department of Obstetrics and Gynecology, Section of Reproductive Endocrinology and Infertility, Evanston, IL, USA
e-mail: jsrinehart@aol.com

J. V. Knaus et al. (eds.), *Ambulatory Gynecology*,
https://doi.org/10.1007/978-1-4939-7641-6_22

means of compensating injured parties where the injury was from unavoidable undesired outcomes and medical malpractice was reserved for those situations where true negligence exists. That seems highly unlike to occur anytime soon, if ever, so today's physician must deal with the system as it exists today.

A physician cannot devise a system the will eliminate all errors. Anytime errors occur, there will be a risk of liability. There does not exist a system that is suit-proof. A recent study by Jena et al. [1] reported that for physicians in a high-risk specialty, by age 45, 88% of the physicians will have a malpractice claim against them. For physicians practicing in a high-risk specialty to age 65, the chance of having a malpractice claim filed was 99%. So physicians practicing OB/GYN for a normal life period of time can plan on having at least one malpractice claim filed against them. However a physician can greatly reduce the risk of liability by organizing aspects of their practice, which will minimize these risks. By implementing a risk management program, a physician can reduce the number of lawsuits filed against them. There are a number of areas where lawsuits can occur. The legal and medical systems intersect in regulatory issues, criminal case, and civil lawsuits. Many physicians immediately think of medical malpractice whenever risk management is mentioned, but there are a number of other areas that can expose the physician to liability.

Physicians, however, owe a greater duty to their patients than simply trying to avoid malpractice suits, and risk management is much more than litigation prevention. Risk management applies to the fiduciary nature of medicine whereby a physician pledges to do the best possible to care for the patient. In return the patient gives the physician elevated standing, permitting them license into their lives, which denied other members of society. Risk management encompasses systems designed to maximize the care of the patient thus helping the healthcare team to meet its obligation to the patient. One approach to risk management is to consider two types of medical malpractice: negligently performed and

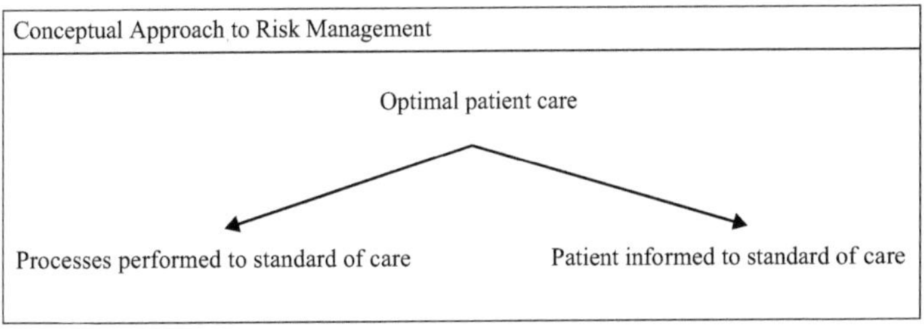

FIG. 22.1 Conceptual approach to risk management

negligently informed. While both apply to the physician, the performance is under the control of the physician, and the informed aspect requires both the healthcare provider and the patient interacting to reach an understanding by the patient of what healthcare is proposed. Risk management programs typically deal with the performance aspect of healthcare delivery. Informed consent processes typically address the issue of patient autonomy and understanding (Fig. 22.1).

What Is Risk Management?

Risk management refers to processes. The processes are ones of identification, assessment, evaluation, intervention, outcome monitoring, and adjustment. These processes are put in place to protect human safety with concerns for patients, employees, and the general community. The processes are also utilized to improve the quality of patient care by maximizing intended outcomes. Finally, many of the processes are used to reduce the exposure that the healthcare community has for professional liability. The processes rely upon data and data evaluation with application of statistical analysis whenever possible so that the practice of medicine can be more accurate in its predictions and more aware of the possibilities for preventive medicine to avoid unwanted outcomes rather than trying to correct the damage done by avoidable bad outcomes (Table 22.1).

Table 22.1 Risk management

Identification
Assessment
Evaluation
Intervention
Outcome monitoring
Adjustment

Risk management is imperative for a number of reasons. Medical error studies have demonstrated a need to reduce iatrogenic injury as demonstrated by the incidence of medically adverse events. A loud wake-up call was issued when the Institute of Medicine published *To Err is Human: Building a Safer Health System* [2]. The publication called for an evaluation of the causes of medical errors and then an application of computerized and other mechanical system in an attempt to reduce medical errors. However, the publication caused considerable concern when it estimated that between 44,000 and 98,000 people died each year in hospitals as a result of medical errors. The estimates about the number of deaths were in part derived from an article published in 1991, which studied records from 30,121 randomly selected from acute care hospitals in New York. The IOM study has been the subject of debate for the inferences it made (see McDonald [3]; Leape [4]). Nonetheless, the goal of reducing medical errors remains as one of the principle tenets of medicine in the form of the "do no harm." A second reason for implementing risk management approaches to medical practice is medical malpractice litigation. A recent report from the AMA demonstrated that surgeon and obstetrician/gynecologists were the most frequently sued specialties in medicine. The review reported that approximately 70% of the physicians in these specialties had been sued with over 200 career claims for every 100 physicians. The report also noted that more than 50% of OB/GYNs were sued before they turned 40. These data emphasize that obstetrician/gynecologist is at a real threat for being sued, and therefore any process which can minimize that threat becomes a valuable tool to limit malpractice litigation. One theory about poor-quality care hypothesizes that a limited number of physicians are responsible for a majority of the errors. Applying this theory to malpractice litigation should demonstrate that the majority of claims made are incurred by a limited number of physicians. However, the data from the AMA's survey contradict this theory since 69.2% of OB/GYNs had been sued at least once and 52.1% had been sued twice. Applying a risk management strategy that tried to single out the poor-quality physicians would target over half of the practicing OB/GYNs. Therefore a more system wide approach to limit malpractice litigation is needed [5].

Finally, patient satisfaction requires attention to risk management. In an age of electronic information sharing, poor outcomes can readily be revealed to a number of current and potential patients.

Why Do Errors Occur?

Understanding why errors occur forms a basis of approach to solutions that minimize errors. One theory concerning the cause of medical errors is that proposed by Gluck PA [6]. Gluck identified four factors that can cause medical errors: (1) human fallibility, (2) complexity, (3) system deficiencies, and (4) vulnerability of defensive barriers (Table 22.2).

The report by the Institute of Medicine emphasizes the impact that human errors happen, which are a result of human fallibility and cannot be reduced by human "trying harder." The solution for human errors is to devise systems that protect people from their own fallibility. Traditionally, the emphasis was on "person-centered" prevention. Van Beuzekom [7] three categories of human error: (1) knowledge-based,

TABLE 22.2 Gluck: causes of medical errors

Human fallibility
Complexity
System deficiencies
Vulnerability of defensive barriers

(2) rule-based, (3) skill-based. The approach for improving patient safety then, using this theory, concentrates on correcting these deficiencies in the form of extra supervision or retraining. A systems approach assumes that people are fallible and that this fallibility is not completely correctable by changing the person. The systems approach is designed to make it harder to do the wrong thing by designing hardwired systems that force certain functions to occur. Forced functions simply do not perm its certain functions to be performed unless they conform to the desired action. Many electronic medical systems have forced functions, which prevent further action until the correct choice has been made. Gluck gives as an example of another type of forced function, the introduction of the Pin Insertion Safety System, which physically prevents one type of gas line (e.g., oxygen) to be connected to another type of gas line (e.g., nitrous oxide). A recent example of preventing errors concerns the use of heparin in neonates. The example involved the overdose of twins because a pharmacy worker took the wrong bottle of heparin because the labels were similar. Changing the labeling and restricting where and how various concentrations of heparin were stored would reduce the risk of inadvertent overdosing of infants. Other examples of forced functions involve the use of checklists or internal programs for machines that have a complex sequence of steps that need to be done before the machine can be used. Some surgical instruments have a complex sequence that must be completed before the instrument can be used. Internal commands and demands prompt the surgical team as to the proper function and sequence before the machine can be activated. Finally, there are a number of reports where electronic medical records can be used to limit medication prescribing errors. One such publication by Saxena et al. J Yiii [8] reported that the use of a clinical decision support system alerts modified physician prescribing behavior in 41.75% of the times medication orders were placed. Electronic medical record systems designed for office use can be implemented to limit a variety of errors especially medication prescribing errors.

Healthcare is increasingly more complex. Complexity can lead to an increase in medical errors. Dain [9] suggests that in complex systems some errors are inevitable based upon the complexity itself, which results in many interactions some of which are unexpected. Dain asserts that healthcare is an industry in which there is interactive complexity, which refers to the fact that in healthcare there are many processes. Also, healthcare is tightly coupled meaning that the numerous processes are very dependent upon the other process. Given that healthcare has "interactive complexity" and "tight coupling," certain errors are inevitable, i.e., people make mistakes. Dain suggests four categories of errors: (1) error of execution, (2) error of planning, (3) active errors (effects are immediate), and (4) latent errors. Identifying the type of error can assist in determining methods to limit the occurrence of that error (Table 22.3).

Active errors are those that occur at the point of intersection between the patient and the healthcare system. Latent errors are those that occur in the systems, which provide healthcare services and do not cause immediate harm. Since this type of error does cause immediate harm, the system often tries to work around the problem until a number of these cause an error.

In healthcare, there has evolved a practice of establishing "defensive barriers" in an attempt to prevent harm.

A systems approach to this has been described by Reason [10], as the Swiss cheese theory of error. Conceptually, this proposes that a number of defensive barriers prevent harm by placing layers of protection between the activity and the outcome so that any one error has a limited chance of affecting the outcome to cause harm. If enough individual errors occur, then these layers of protection will be aligned like the

TABLE 22.3 Dain: categories of errors

Error of execution
Error of planning
Active error (effects are immediate)
Latent errors

holes in Swiss cheese, and an unlikely event will occur. Frequently, when a serious error occurs, a review of how it happened shows just this effect where a series of small errors eventually caused serious harm.

Getting Started

A systematic approach to risk management will maximize the success of the effort required for excel lent risk management. The goal is to both reduce errors and improve patient care. Reducing errors is not just clinical errors but any error that could compromise the practice. A physician can only practice medicine if they have a "practice" which includes not just patient care but also the business of medicine. The rapidly changing field of medicine exposes practices to new liabilities that can be just as harmful for good patient care as an error directly related to patient care. Initially, the areas of concern can be defined as (1) clinical, (2) laboratory, (3) compliance, (4) communication, and (5) financial (Table 22.4).

Once these areas have been identified, then establish a hierarchy of risks and priorities. Evaluate the practice by each of these categories and priorities to determine how much time and personnel will be required. Once the time and personnel are established, the estimated cost can be determined, and this information can be used to determine a cost-benefit analysis for the entire practice. Potential problems which may have initially created considerable concern may be found to be far less of a concern when their impact both financially and actually is determined.

Table 22.4 Categorizing areas of practice for evaluation of performance

Clinical
Laboratory
Compliance
Communication
Financial

The next step is to establish a "plan of action." This will require a review of existing protocols and practices, which is the retrospective analysis of the practice. This information will help determine prospectively how risk management processes will be developed. The process being reviewed will determine which personnel will perform the review and where possible; both someone familiar with the process and someone not familiar with the process will help achieve both an insiders and a new perspective on the issue under consideration. The prospective process creates revised or new protocol and processes. The new protocol and processes need to be implemented which involves education and monitoring for compliance. Monitoring the results perm its ongoing revision to meet change demands of the practice or adjust the policies to the needs of the practice.

Areas of Concern: Clinical Issues

Practice guidelines and protocols provide a prospective means of limiting errors either of commission or omission. The American College of Obstetricians and Gynecologists publishes extensive guidelines that can provide a starting point for establishing office practices that comply with the standard of care. Following guidelines is not sufficient to prevent liability, and thus guidelines need to be evaluated in relation to the individual practice. Guidelines provide starting point for analysis of liability. Plaintiff attorneys seek cases where there is evidence of negligence but then also have another factor – a malpractice plus – aspect that would make the case more sympathetic for the plaintiff if the case were to be tried by the jury. Guidelines can assist a defense by helping to establish a standard of care, which can be asserted by the defense and reinforced by an expert witness. However, failure to follow guidelines, especially if they were used to develop practice protocols, can be used by the plaintiff to add that malpractice plus factor. Any deviation from practice-accepted guidelines or practice-developed protocols needs thorough documentation as to why for this particular patient in a particular clinical setting the guidelines or protocols were not appropriate. The prospective use of guidelines and protocols can be a very valuable tool to Jim it adverse events and to limit risk from liability. Practice guidelines are constantly changing. Protocols need to change to comply with new guidelines since a disparity between what a practice accepts as valid guidelines and what a practice actually does can create errors and thus expose a practice to liability. Updating protocols and acquiring the most recent guidelines require considerable effort and expense. Large practices can designate a person to be their compliance person, but in a smaller practice this job usually falls to the physician or nursing staff. Nonetheless, the effort devoted to the constant updating and monitoring of practice guidelines and protocols can assure a practice that the care the patients are receiving meets the standard of care and limits the practice's risk of liability. There needs to be documentation of compliance with a practice's own guidelines and protocols so that if a case is brought against a practice, the practice has documentation that the protocols and guidelines were followed.

Patient education and compliance are frequently issues involved with adverse events and malpractice. Many practices use patient education material or refer a patient to a website for education about proposed treatments. Documentation that the patient received educational material and completed an online video is critical when malpractice claims are made especially when the claim is one for lack of informed consent. However, it is not sufficient to demonstrate by documentation that a patient received material or completed an online video. There needs to be some evidence that the patient actually understood what risks and benefits were involved with the procedure or treatment. The common form for informed consent is tell-ask-tell. Telling a patient about a procedure is not sufficient because many patients simply will not understand what is involved. So once told, the patient needs to be queried about what they understand about the treatment or procedure. Then there is an opportunity to correct or add to the information that the patient has been given. Documentation of this complete process provides excellent evidence for the defense. More importantly, this process provides the patient with the understanding that is necessary for the patient to make an autonomous informed decision, which is the core ethical mandate to the physician. Properly educated and motivated to comply with the requirements of the procedure or treatment, the patient becomes an active participant in their care, which should reduce error and improve desired outcomes.

Prospective risk management requires constant monitoring. Physicians have become very familiar with this approach since hospitals have implemented many risk management processes that monitor the outcome and may even give physicians individual scorecards as to how they are doing. The same concept can be successfully implemented in an office practice. Constant monitoring helps develop low-risk work habits, but any change will require effort and increased vigilance since changing one habit to a different habit takes time and constant effort.

Even with the best of guidelines, protocols, and compliance devices, errors and unwanted outcomes will occur. Prospective plans to deal with unwanted outcomes may help the patient minimize the damage of such errors and at the same time provide defense against litigation. Protocols need to have directions concerning how a deviation from the protocol will be handled. There also needs to be an acceptance and a process for reacting when a subpoena is served on the physician or a patient or their attorney request records. Most practices have at least one person who is excellent at dealing with unhappy patients or difficult situations. That person's early involvement with an escalating situation may avoid further conflict and can actually help the patient in arriving at the best possible solution to a difficult problem. Working together to solve a complicated problem or dealing with an adverse outcome is the goal. Adversarial approaches seldom allow for the optimal solution to complicated problems (Table 22.5).

TABLE 22.5 Elements for medical malpractice

1. The actor owes a duty of care
2. The actor breaches this duty
3. As a result of this breach, an injury results
4. The injury causes damages that the law considers compensable

For medical malpractice, the duty arises in the nature of the doctor-patient relationship, which is considered a fiduciary duty owed to the patient by the physician (healthcare provider). Determining if the healthcare provider meets the requirements of the duty is established by a standard of care. The standard of care is in relationship to what a physician would normally be expected to do or what a reasonable patient would expect be done. The establishment of that standard is usually determined by experts who provide instruction due to the complex nature of medicine. Many malpractice cases become a "war of the experts" in trying to establish just what the standard of care applies to the case in question. Damages are often difficult to define since the loss of function is difficult to quantitate for monetary compensation. The loss of wages can be determined from actuarial computations, but the value of the loss of an arm, or sight, or movement is almost impossible to standardize.

Medical malpractice can arise from two major areas of action: the actual procedural issues and the issue of informed consent. Malpractice litigation can be initiated, for example, if a lost lab report about a breast malignancy results in significant delay in treatment, which may have caused harm to the patient. But an injury during surgery may also trigger a malpractice claim if the patient thinks they were not informed about the possible risks or benefits from the surgery and that knowledge would have allowed them to make a different decision about the surgery, which then would have avoided the injury. The issue of a lost lab report falls under risk management in terms of designing systems to limit the occurrence of such losses. Following such a system even if there is an unintended outcome provides the defense with information that it can use to win the malpractice suit. Having systems in place and not following can be used by the plaintiff to bolster their case, so systems become critical if an unintended outcome results.

Informed consent has become a major source of litigation for medical malpractice claims. Informed consent is the result of a respect for a person. Informed consent acknowledges the fact that the healthcare provider has skills and knowledge not held by the patient, which places the patient at a disadvantage when considering their options for treatment. This establishes a fiduciary duty between the healthcare giver and the patient, which forms the basis for medical malpractice claims. The concept of informed consent includes more than just the malpractice facet in that there is an ethical component to informed consent. The ethical aspect refers to a set of moral principles established by a society, which define that society and established codes of conduct, which as professionals, healthcare givers attest to upholding. The moral principles identified for medicine, whether appropriate or not, include beneficence, nonmalificence, autonomy, and justice. The healthcare provider functions under the beneficence/nonmalificence, the patient under autonomy, and society under justice. The healthcare system in the USA focuses on patient autonomy, which is the overarching ethical principle for the delivery of healthcare. The legal manifestation of autonomy is defined through the legal concept of "privacy rights." The tension between the physician's ethical principles and the patient's ethical principles can create problems for both patients and healthcare providers when trying to make treatment plans for patients. A physician may have a clear idea of what is "best for the patient," while the patient may clearly not agree with this plan. The process of informed consent attempts to provide the patient with intelligible information so that they can make a decision about their healthcare, which agrees with the modem scientific basis for medicine. When the patient feels that they were not given enough information to make a good decision and a bad outcome results, they frequently seek compensation for that lack of information.

The core of informed consent is education. Most healthcare providers are not trained educators, which creates problems when asked to provide meaningful informed consent. Therefore, while there are lofty ethical ideals governing informed consent, the day-to-day task of informed consent is much more mundane and practical. The process of informed consent has many components, but three of them are (1) the discussion between healthcare provider and the patient, (2) the memorialization of that discussion in the form of a chart note, and (3) the signing of an informed consent form. The ethical obligation to the patient is complete with the discussion and education of the patient. The chart note is the physician's defense team's weapon when litigation arises. The formalized informed consent form is used by the plaintiff's legal team in an attempt to prove that the patient did not adequately understand what they had consented to since many forms are either overly complex or inadequate and easily attacked. From a risk management standpoint, the chart note becomes critical when a malpractice claim is made. Other forms of documentation that the patient was educated also become critical to the defense team such as written materials, videos, website usage, and collaborating healthcare team members chart notes such a nursing notes.

Informed consent is meaningless unless the patient actually understands the information that they are given. Listing risks and complications without providing a context for those risks and benefits does not satisfy either the ethical or legal requirements of providing adequate informed consent. Thus if the information given does not lead to understanding, there is no empowerment of the patient, and thus there is no informed consent. The definitive case for modem informed consent remains Canterbury [11] where the elements of the doctrine of informed consent were enumerated. In Canterbury, the plaintiff underwent a laminectomy by Dr. Spence. Subsequent to that, he injured himself when he slipped off of his bed and fell. The court initially dismissed the case because they could find no negligence by Dr. Spence.

However, the Appellate Court reversed on the grounds of a lack of informed consent. The court states: "True consent to what happens to one's self is the informed exercise of a choice, and that entails the opportunity to evaluate knowledgeably the options available and the risks attendant upon each. The average patient has little or no understanding of the medical arts, and ordinarily has only his physician to whom he can look for enlightenment with which to reach an intelligent decision. From these almost axiomatic considerations springs the need and in turn the requirement, of a reasonable divulgence by physician to patient to make such a decision possible" [12]. The court then defines the elements for informed consent as such: "In broad outline, we agree that a risk is thus material when a reasonable person, in what the physician knows or should know to be the patient's position, would be likely to attach significance to the risk or cluster of risks in deciding whether or not to forego the proposed therapy. ... The topics importantly demanding a communication of information are the inherent and potential hazards of the proposed treatment, the alternatives to that treatment, if any, and the results likely if the patient remains untreated" [13]. The court then established the need for a proximate cause when it states: "A causal connection exists when, but only when, disclosure of significant risks incidental to treatment would have resulted in a decision against it. The patient obviously has no complaint if he would have submitted to the therapy notwithstanding awareness that the risks was one of its perils" [14].

Informed consent laws are established on a state-by-state basis. That notwithstanding, Rozovsky defines five elements common to all consent processes [15]: (1) a description of the indications for treatment, (2) an explanation for the proposed test or treatment, (3) an explanation of the probable benefits and risks associated with the proposed test or treatment, (4) description of diagnostic or treatment alternatives and the attendant probable benefits and probable risks associated with these options, and (5) a description of the consequences of declining the proposed test or treatment or the alternatives.

Medical Malpractice

Medical malpractice is a negligent-based tort. A tort occurs when an unintended outcome occurs as a result of a breach of duty (not contractual) owed to someone. Tort is distinguished from a crime where the duty for a crime is to society in general. There are many goals for tort law, but three of them are compensation to the injured party, deterrence for bad behavior, and equitable justice. Tort law is responsible for defining what a tort is and what a legally compensable injury is so that an injured party can legally enforce their right to compensation. Injuries are not necessarily physical but can be emotional, economic, privacy invasion property, reputational, or even constitutional. Many areas of tort law exist, but the one most concerning to physicians is that of negligence from which springs medical malpractice. Negligence is defined in the Restatement (second) of Torts§ 282: "Conduct which falls below the standard established by law for the protection of others against unreasonable risk of harm."

Negligence in medical malpractice requires four things to have happened which are referred to as elements. All four must be proven by a "more probably than not" standard. The four elements are (1) the actor owes a duty of care; (2) the actor breaches this duty; (3) as a result of this breach, an injury results; and (4) the injury caused damages that the law considers compensable (Table 22.6).

Table 22.6 Rozovsky: elements common to all informed consent processes

1. A description of the indications for treatment
2. An explanation for the proposed test or treatment
3. An explanation of the probable benefits and risks associated with the proposed test or treatment
4. A description of diagnostic or treatment alternatives with the attendant probable benefits and risks associated with these options
5. A description of the consequences of declining the proposed test or treatment or the alternatives

Providing informed consent needs to consider a number of factors that may enhance or hinder the understanding by the patient. To begin with, can the patient communicate and are they capable of understanding the language that is being used for the informed consent? Not uncommonly, a patient may be somewhat conversational in a language but not truly fluent in that language. Thus a patient may be able to read a consent form given in English, may have nodded understanding when asked by a physician if they understood what was going to be done, and yet have no real understanding of what all those words meant. Practices that treat foreign-speaking patients need to provide informed consent processes that are in the language of the patient. That may mean obtaining a translator who is capable of translating the medical jargon into an understandable format for the patient. In addition, the patient's ability to understand is critical to the informed consent process. Medical personnel are comfortable with their language and level of conversation. But to a nonmedical person, it can sound like a bunch of acronyms and highly intelligent but unintelligible words. Consent forms need to be written for a sixth grader comprehension. Most people now would know what hypertension is, but many would not understand words like amenorrhea, endometrial hyperplasia, or cervical atypia. All of this needs to be placed in the context of the patient's cultural background. In some cultures, women remain subjugated to a male member of the social unit. Informed consent under these conditions can be both difficult and distressing to the healthcare team. Further complication arises when there are a number of members of the healthcare team providing the informed consent. There needs to be uniformity among all team members as to what is being communicated so that confusion can be minimized.

The consent process needs to be patient specific. Using boilerplate documents of discussions may not provide adequate informed consent. The evolution of prognostic models should help physician tailor the treatment for individual patients. As this becomes more standard of care, the information provided by these models can be present in levels of confidence that a patient can understand. For example, a physician may order a test and based upon that test may be able to say based upon literature data and personal experience of that physician (data which can be obtained form their own electronic medical record) that they are 50% confident that the disease they are diagnosing and the treatment they are recommending are appropriate. However, by adding a second or third test or an alternative or second treatment, they may be able to say that given the results of these tests, the physician is now 70% or 90% confident that their predictions are accurate. This approach would help a patient decide if taking the risk of more testing or treatment is worth assuming.

The internet and social media add other dimensions to the informed consent process. Patients gather information from a number of sources, some of which is accurate and useful and other information that is inaccurate and maybe even harmful. The duty of the healthcare team might become to be knowledgeable about what information the patient has amassed and address the accuracy of that information. Using the internet to help in the informed consent process can be extremely useful and can also often be documented. Furthermore, many programs can be structured to ask questions of the patient in an attempt to assess if the patient truly understood the concepts being presented by the informed consent program. All of this can be documented for the defense team if litigation arises. To provide meaningful informed consent, the informed consent process needs to be broken into understandable segments. People simply cannot retain or understand information if the session is too long or involves too much material. Providing written reminders are helpful, but relying upon the patient to read the handouts and then comprehend them does not assure the healthcare provider that the patient actually understood what was said or what would happen. Education is best accomplished using manageable segments where the information is given (teach) and then the person is asked questions to determine what was actually learned by the patient (ask) and, then, reiterating the information that was either not learned or learned incorrectly (teach).

The TAT method takes more time but allows the healthcare provider to assess just how adequate was the informed consent process. Central to teaching the material is that the material be presented in an understandable format. While the language should be at the eighth grade reading level and free from acronyms and technical jargon, the presentation of information should not be demeaning to the patient. Thus there is a precarious balance between making the information too complex or making it so simple that the healthcare provider is seen as "talking down" to the patient. An example of a well-constructed informed consent process is the Department of Veteran's Affairs electronic informed consent program. The program includes anatomical diagrams and information written at the sixth grade level. The patient can then electronically sign the consent form, which is stored in the patient's permanent record.

Patients having elective procedures are given this information before their surgery thus giving them time to study the information if they chose to do that. Utilizing some form of electronic informed consent can assure at least a basic understanding of what is proposed, provide a record that the patient actually was exposed to the information, and can be constructed in the teach-ask-teach mode. Providing feedback and evaluating the answers to questions allow the healthcare team to construct their information in a more effective manner. Asking the patient what their questions are about their proposed treatment would also provide information about what needs to be conveyed to the patient to complete their understanding of what is proposed.

Not only is the manner in which information is presented important, the person presenting the information can influence how the information is processed by the patient. The person presenting the information needs to be neutral to the patient and certainly not antagonistic to the patient. Having a healthcare worker who has had negative interactions with a patient will influence how the person receives the information and how they will use that perception if an unexpected outcome ensues.

Determining which information needs to be conveyed depends upon the standard of care in that community. The community may be local, but due to the trend toward globalization and medical tourism, for some information, the community may include the entire USA or even other countries. Each situation will have its standard of care requirements. Recent standards have required disclosure of costs and financial incentives for the healthcare team.

The National Cancer Institute has an interesting presentation of the informed consent process [16].

The presentation is aimed at the patient and it presents five myths about informed consent.

1. Informed consent is designed primarily to protect the legal interest of the research team.
2. The most important part of this process is signing the informed consent document.
3. My doctor knows best; he or she can tell me whether or not I should consent to participate.
4. Once I sign the consent form, I have to enroll and stay enrolled in the trial.
5. Medical personnel are busy, so I can't really expect them to keep me informed as the trial progresses or listen to my questions.

While these myths are related to research, they apply equally well to the everyday practice of OB/GYN.

Conclusion

The ethical standards for informed consent require that the patient is educated to a degree that they can make a knowledgeable decision about their healthcare. The legal standards require documentation that an acceptable informed consent process occurred. The key to successful risk management programs and informed consent is an understanding that both are processes. The processes require definition, organization, monitoring, adjustment, and, most importantly, documentation of what processes actually occurred.

Proactively established programs will improve patient care and limit the risks of successful physician-adverse malpractice litigation. No longer is it a question as to whether an OB/GYN will be sued. The issue is to provide a system that meets the standard of care and that provides documentation for the defense team when such litigation does happen.

References

1. Jena AB, Seabury S, Lakdawalla D, Chandra A. Malpractice risk according to physician specialty. NEJM. 2011;365:629–36.
2. Kohn LT, Corrigan JM, Donaldson M, editors. To err is human: building a safer health system. Washington, DC: Institute of Medicine; 1999.
3. McDonald CJ, Weiner M, Hui SL. Deaths due to medical errors are exaggerated in the Institute of Medicine report. JAMA. 2000;284:93–5.
4. Leape LL. Institute of medicine medical error figures are not exaggerated. JAMA. 2000;284:95–7.
5. Kane CK. Medical liability claim frequency: a 2007–2008 snapshot of physicians AMA 2010: policy research perspectives.
6. Gluck PA. Medical error theory. Obstet Gynecol Clin N Am. 2008;35:11–7.
7. Van Beuzekom M, Boer F, Akerboom S, Hudson P. Patient safety: latent risk factors. Br J Anaesth. 2010;105:52–9.
8. Saxena K, Lung BR, Becker JR. Improving patient safety by modifying provider ordering behavior using alerts (COSS) in CPOE system. AMIA Annu Symp Proc. 2011:1207–16.
9. Dain S. Normal accidents: human error and medical equipment design. Heart Surg Forum. 2002;5:254–7.
10. Reason J. Human error: models and management. BMJ. 2000;320:768–70.
11. Canterbury v. Spence, 464 F.2d 772 (1972).
12. Id. at 780.
13. Id. at 787.
14. Id. at 790.
15. Rozovsky FA. Consent to treatment: a practical guide. In: Rozovsky FA, editor. $th Ed/Wolters Kluwer Austin. 2007.
16. http://www.cancer.gov/ciinicaltrials/conducting/informed-consent-guide/page2.

Chapter 23
Domestic Violence

Gloria A. Bachmann, Nancy Phillips, and Janelle Foroutan

Definition

Domestic violence is a pattern of behavior intended to establish power and control over another person in a current or former relationship. This form of abuse has such a high prevalence, both nationally and internationally, that it can be considered an epidemic. Domestic violence affects persons of all ages, ranging from children to the elderly, and crosses all socioeconomic and cultural lines. It is estimated that one in four women will experience some type of domestic violence [1]. Types of abuse are categorized as noted in Table 23.1.

Intimate partner violence is a form of domestic violence specifically against adolescents or adults within the context of a past or current intimate relationship. Studies consistently show that 85–95% of cases of partner abuse are a male to female offense [2, 3]. IPV occurs as a repetitive cycle of [1]

G. A. Bachmann · N. Phillips (✉)
Rutgers Robert Wood Johnson Medical School, Department of OB/GYN and Reproductive Sciences, New Brunswick, NJ, USA
e-mail: phillina@rwjms.rutgers.edu

J. Foroutan
Rutgers Robert Wood Johnson Medical School, Saint Peter's University Hospital, Department of OB/GYN, New Brunswick, NJ, USA

J. V. Knaus et al. (eds.), *Ambulatory Gynecology*,
https://doi.org/10.1007/978-1-4939-7641-6_23

TABLE 23.1 Definitions

Domestic violence
The willful intimidation, assault, battery, or other abusive behavior perpetrated by one family member, household member, or intimate partner against another
Domestic violence includes intimate partner violence, child abuse, and elder abuse
Intimate partner violence
Violence within the context of a past or current intimate relationship
Child abuse
Violence of a child by its parents, guardians, or other adult
Elder abuse
A singe or repeated act or lack of appropriate action, occurring within any relationship where there is an expectation of trust, which causes harm or distress to an older person

the tension-building phase, [4] the violent phase, and [5] the honeymoon phase [6]. Over time, with repeated episodes of abuse, the violence tends to intensify, while the tension building and honeymoon phases tend to shorten. IPV may begin with psychological or verbal abuse, then progress to physical or sexual abuse [2].Other forms of abuse include economic, usually in the form of monetary restriction, and social control or isolation (Table 23.2).

Prevalence

The prevalence of domestic violence is difficult to estimate because it is underreported. Many victims do not report abuse to friends, family, or authority figures because of feelings of fear, hopelessness, economic retributions, and shame. Other victims accept abuse as a normal lifestyle variant, as exemplified in the message of Eminem's hit song, "Love the Way you Lie."

Table 23.2 Forms of abuse

Physical abuse	
Intentional use of physical force with the potential for causing injury, disability, or death	Biting, grabbing, choking, slapping, scratching, shoving, strangling, throwing, burning, punching, use of restraints
Sexual abuse	
Physical force to compel a person to engage in a sex act against their will, a sex act involving a person who is unable to decline willingness to engage in the sexual act because of illness, disability, or the influence of alcohol and/or drugs	Forced sexual contact, unprotected sex, painful sex acts, infidelity, including vaginal, oral, or anal intercourse as well as use of a foreign object
Psychological abuse	
Inflicting mental and emotional anguish as a means to control the victim. This type of abuse can be verbal and nonverbal and diminishes the victim's sense of self-worth	Putting down, name-calling, yelling, rages, jealousy, feelings of guilt, criticism, intimidation, coercion, threats, neglect, abandonment, brainwashing, broken promises, stalking
Economic abuse	
The use of money as a means to control the victim by ensuring either financial dependence on the abuser or shifting financial responsibility onto the victim while simultaneously denying the ability to work	Limited or no access to funds, giving an allowance, preventing aquisition of job or independent funds
Social abuse	
Preventing the victim from having contact with friends, family, children, and service providers. Also included restricting activities thereby	Isolation, public humiliation, restricting access to medical care

Approximately 4.8 million women are victims of physical assault by an intimate partner annually in the United States [7]. In the year 2000, approximately 3 women were murdered daily by a spouse or boyfriend in the United States, for a total of 1247 women [8]. This number remained fairly consistent with 1178 women dying in 2005 as the result of IPV [9]. The National Institute of Justice conducted the Violence against Women Survey from November 1995 to May 1996 in an effort to gather data on the epidemiology of abuse. They found that 51.9% of women surveyed said they were physically assaulted either by a caretaker as a child or as an adult by any abuser. Additionally, 17.6% of women reported they had been victims of an attempted or completed rape [1] (Available at www.ojp.usdoj.gov/nij/pubs-sum/181867.htm).

Intimate partner violence specifically has been reported by up to 31% of women, accounting for 22% of all violent crimes against women [10]. Women aged 20–24 are at the greatest risk for IPV.

Surveys also confirm a high incidence of physical assault in men (up to 66% according to the Violence against Women Survey) and a lifetime risk of sexual assault of 2.1%. Partners of either sex may be victimized in any context as outlined above. Child and elder abuse encompasses a high percentage of assaults against males.

Socioeconomic Impact

In addition to impacting a women's physical and mental well-being, domestic violence also has socioeconomic impacts. The cost of intimate partner violence exceeds $5.8 billion each year. The medical and mental healthcare costs alone are $4.1 billion annually. Victims often lose their jobs due to absenteeism related to violence and abuser control. This loss of productivity accounts for approximately $1.8 billion annually [11].

Victims of domestic violence who separate themselves from the abuser are often left without a place to stay and can eventually become part of the community's homeless population thereby increasing their risk of other types of victimization. More than 30% of women in need of housing are turned away from shelters due to lack of space. When faced with being homeless, these women often return to their homes where the domestic violence is taking place.

Risk Factors

Although females are more prone to be in domestic violence situations than males, certain populations of women have an increased likelihood of victimization. Factors that contribute are multilevel and include individual, relationship, community, and social factors (Table 23.3).

TABLE 23.3 Risk factors

Individual risk factors	
Low self-esteem	Being a victim of physical or psychological abuse (strong risk factor)
Low income	Having few friends and being isolated from other people
Low academic achievement	Unemployment
Young age, especially adolescents	Emotional dependence and insecurity
Pregnancy	Belief in strict gender roles, e.g., male dominance and aggression in relationships
Chronically ill or disabled	Desire for power and control in relationships
Aggressive or delinquent behavior as a youth	Perpetrating psychological aggression
Heavy alcohol and drug use	History of experiencing poor parenting as a child
Depression	History of experiencing physical discipline as a child
Anger and hostility	
Antisocial/borderline personality traits	
Prior history of being physically abusive	

(continued)

TABLE 23.3 (continued)

Relationship factors
Marital conflicts and instability – divorces or separations
Dominance and control of the relationship by one partner over the other
Economic stress
Unhealthy family relationships and interactions
Community factors
Poverty and associated factors, e.g., overcrowding
Low social capital – lack of institutions, relationships, and norms that shape a community's social interactions
Social factors
Traditional gender norms, e.g., women should stay at home, not enter workforce, and be submissive; men support the family and make the decisions
Culturally isolated, i.e., immigrants, illegal aliens
Geographically isolated, i.e., rural areas

Women in a dependent role, such as those with chronic medical or psychological illness, those who are solely economically reliant on their partner, and those living in poverty or social isolation, are at particular risk. Identifying the multilevel risk factors can be the key to identification and intervention.

Screening for Domestic Violence

In the medical field, domestic violence has been cited as a leading cause of preventable morbidity and mortality. Although risk factors and clinical presentations may raise the suspicion for domestic violence, often the victim will have no clearly identifiable signs or suggestions of abuse. For this reason, universal screening is recommended [12].

Reasons that clinicians often do not screed for DV include time constraints and not feeling equipped to handle DV patients. Additionally, physicians are concerned that the patient may perceive this questioning as proof that the clinician believes she is in an abusive situation.

TABLE 23.4 Domestic violence screening questions

Screening can be conducted by making the following statement and asking these three simple questions: **"Because violence is so common in many women's lives and because there is help available for women being abused, I now ask every patient about domestic violence:"** 1. Within the past year – or since you have been pregnant – have you been hit, slapped, kicked, or otherwise physically hurt by someone? 2. Are you in a relationship with a person who threatens or physically hurts you? 3. Has anyone force you to have sexual activities that made you feel uncomfortable?

Modified from Screening tools – domestic violence [12]

Routine DV screening by practitioners with clear evidence that this is standard practice of the office usually eliminates this concern. Screening questions have been suggested by various organizations (Table 23.4). Any information or inquiry by a healthcare professional concerning domestic violence provides the victim with a message that the healthcare provider is concerned and willing to help. Self-administered screening (Table 23.5) has been shown to be as effective as a face-to-face interview [13]. In fact, studies indicate that women prefer self-completed approaches over face-to-face questioning [14]. It is important to routinely rescreen all patients; initial denials of violence may be followed by admissions at subsequent visits.

Annual visits, family planning, contraception, and STI testing or treatment visits are opportunities for screening for DV. Obstetric patients should be screened at their initial prenatal visit, once every trimester and again at their postpartum visit. The issue of screening will become less awkward for clinicians as practices adopt electronic health records and these questions are a routine part of the intake questions.

The effects of abuse impact a woman's physical health and her emotional and behavioral well-being. Physicians should recognize the "battered woman syndrome" in which a woman

TABLE 23.5 "SAFE" questions

"SAFE" questions
Stress/safety – do you feel safe in your relationship?
Afraid/abused – have you ever been or are you in a relationship where you were/are threatened, hurt, or afraid?
Friends/family – if yes to the above, are your f/f aware that you've been hurt?
Could you tell them and would they help?
Emergency plan – if yes to the above, do you have a safe place to go and the resources you need in an emergency?

Modified from Ashur [15]

TABLE 23.6 "HITS" a domestic violence screening tool for use in the community

Please read each of the following, and fill in the circle that best indicates the frequency with which your partner acts in the ways depicted

How often does your partner:	Never	Rarely	Sometimes	Fairly often	Frequently
1. Physically hurt you?	( )	( )	( )	( )	( )
2. Insult or talk down to you?	( )	( )	( )	( )	( )
3. Threaten you with harm?	( )	( )	( )	( )	( )
4. Scream or curse at you?	( )	( )	( )	( )	( )

Each item is scored from 1 to 5. Thus, scores for this inventory range from 4 to 20. A score of greater than 10 is considered positive
Modified from Sherin et al. [16]

will present to a healthcare provider (or multiple healthcare providers) repeatedly, with varying vague complaints. She may undergo multiple medical evaluations and referrals without recognition of a clear etiology or resolution of her symptoms.

This syndrome is reflected in the high prevalence of abuse in patients who present with chronic pelvic pain, headaches, and recurrent GI complaints (Table 23.6).

Intervention/Physician's Role

Although healthcare professionals may feel ill-equipped to handle a situation in which domestic violence is revealed, in actuality they are institute-effective interventions. This requires that the provider has a supply of knowledge of appropriate safety information and availability of referral algorithms.

Victims often have compelling social, economic, or psychological reasons for remaining in an abusive relationship. Healthcare providers should express their concerns for the patient staying in the abusive situation but should also remain supportive of women who decide to stay.

The healthcare provider should first assess the patients' immediate safety and that of any dependent children within the household. If danger is imminent, the patient should be offered immediate referral to social services and/or other available community services.

For patients who report they are not in immediate danger, strategies such as having a packed bag, stored in a secret location or with a trusted friend or neighbor, should be offered (Table 23.7). The patient should be provided educational

TABLE 23.7 Clinical presentation

Symptoms commonly associated with victimization	**Somatic complaints commonly associated with victimization**
Depression	Insomnia
Anxiety	Headaches/migraines
Post-traumatic stress disorder	GI symptoms
Eating disorders	Dyspareunia
Sleep disturbances	Chest pain
Substance abuse	Back pain
Somatization disorders	Hyperventilation
Sexual dysfunction, promiscuity	
Self-neglect – failure to thrive, malnutrition	
Suicide attempts	
Poor adherence to medical recommendations	

Table 23.8 Safety bag

Prepacked bag hidden in a safe place contents should include:
Cash or credit cards
A change of clothes[a]
Extra set of keys
Documentation[b]
Birth certificates
Health insurance cards
Proof of residency (phone bill, credit card bill, copy of lease)
Social security card, green card
Driver license or other photo ID

[a]Self and children
[b]Certified copies may be made if originals cannot be removed from household

Table 23.9 If you need help

The National Domestic Violence Hotline: 1-800-799-7233
(SAFE) The National Sexual Assault Hotline: 1-800-656-4673
The National Teen Dating Abuse Hotline: 1-866-331-9474
Local police department
Local hospital/emergency department
Local social worker

materials and phone numbers, including toll-free hotlines, to have on hand if immediate help is needed (Table 23.8).

Physicians should not confront nor advise the patient to confront the abuser. This should be approached only when the patient has a safety plan available. Similarly, the abuser should not be referred for interventional therapy, as this has been shown not only to potentially increase the violence but also to be of limited success. Marital counseling is also contraindicated for similar reasons [6, 17] (Table 23.9).

A practice that is equipped to handle DV should have a standard operating procedure in place so that the issue is routinely addressed with each patient, DV guidelines are well described for the clinician, and office staff and management is initiated in a timely manner, in order to insure the best outcomes for the patient and, when applicable, her children.

Documentation

Medical records are legal documents. In the case of domestic violence, medical records can be used as evidence for obtaining protective relief (such as a restraining order), can corroborate police evidence, and can support a victim's claim of abuse to help qualify for welfare, public housing, victim relief, etc. [18].

Photographs, drawings, and inclusion of a "body map" will help to increase medical record documentation to higher legal standards needed for evidence of domestic violence. If using nonelectronic health records, writing should be legible and patient complaints recorded verbatim, identified as such in quotation marks. The patient's demeanor should be recorded, for example, withdrawn, tearful, etc. Avoid terms which imply doubt about the patient's statements, such as "claims and alleges," or imply hostility, such as "denies and refuses" (Table 23.10).

Table 23.10 The physician's responsibility in addressing intimate partner violence and domestic violence

Implement universal screening
Acknowledge trauma
Assess immediate safety of patient and children
Help establish a safety plan
Review options
Offer educational materials and a list of community and local resources (including toll-free hotline)
Provide referrals
Document interactions
Provide ongoing support at subsequent visits

Modified from Intimate partner violence and domestic violence. Special Issues in Women's Health [6]

Mandatory Reporting

Physicians should be familiar with mandatory reporting requirements in their state. There is no state mandate to report domestic violence. In general, child abuse, elder abuse, or abuse of an incapacitated patient (mentally or physically disabled) must be reported. Additionally, any injury resulting from attack with a gun, knife, or a deadly weapon requires reporting. Sexual assault requires reporting without identifying the victim. Both medical professionals and victims of domestic violence can research laws concerning domestic violence and sexual assault in their state at www.womenslaw.org [3] (Table 23.11).

TABLE 23.11 Physician do's and don'ts

Screening	Screen everyone Screen on multiple visits	Screen by perceived risk factors
Documentation	Use patient's exact words	Paraphrase
	Write "declines, reports"	Use vague descriptions of injuries
	Include photos, drawings	Write patient "denies, refuses"
		Make patient appear hostile
Intervention: abuse confirmed	Express concern	Judge decisions to stay/leave
	Provide support	Encourage patient to "just leave"
	Initiate safety plan	Confront or have patient confront abuser
	Refer to social worker	Refer to marital counselor
	Document findings	Refer abuser to interventional treatment

(continued)

Table 23.11 (continued)

Intervention: abuse suspected but denied	Express concern Provide support Provide resources Schedule follow-up appointment Document findings Offer social work referral	Report to authorities
Report to authorities	Child abuse, elder abuse Injury with knife, gun As required by state law	If adult patient declines intervention

References

1. Tjaden P, Thoennes N. National Institute of Justice and the Centers of Disease Control and Prevention, "extent, nature and consequences of intimate partner violence: findings from the national violence against women survey. 2000.
2. Toohey JS. Domestic violence and rape. Med Clin N Am. 2008;92(5):993.
3. National coalition against domestic violence. Domestic violence facts. 2007. Available at www.ncadv.org.
4. The National Center for victims of Crime. Washington, DC; 2010. Available at www.ncvc.org.
5. Action on Elder Abuse. South London, UK; 2006. Available at www.elderabuse.org.uk.
6. Intimate partner violence and domestic violence. Special Issues in Womens Health. Washington, DC: ACOG; 2005.
7. Understanding Intimate Partner Violence – fact sheet. 2009. Available at www.cdc.gov/violenceprevention.
8. Tjaden P, Thoennes N. Full report of the prevalence, incidence, and consequences of violence against women; findings from the national violence against women survey. Criminologist. 1999;24(3):1,4, 13–14.

9. Dept of Justice, Bureau of justice statistics. Homicide trends in the United States. 2007. Available at www.ojp.usdoj.gov/bjs/homicide/tables/intimatestab.htm.
10. Scott CK, Schoene, Joseph S, et al. Health concerns across a women's lifespan: the Commonwealth Fund 1998 survey of Women's health. Available at http://www.cmwf.org/usr_doc/HealthConcerns_surveyreport.pdf.
11. Intimate Partner Violence: Consequences. CDC; 2003. Available at www.cdc.govNiolencePrevention/intimatepartner violence/consequences.html.
12. Screening tools – domestic violence. ACOG; 2009. Available at violence@acog.org.
13. Ping HC, Ravi S, Washington J, et al. Randomized comparison of 3 methods to screen for domestic violence in family practice. Ann Fam Med. 2007;5(5):430.
14. MacMillian HL, Wathen CN, et al. Approaches to screening for intimate partner violence in health care settings: a randomized trial. JAMA. 2006;296(5):530.
15. Ashur ML. Asking about domestic violence: SAFE questions. JAMA. 1993;268(18):2367.
16. Sherin KM, Sinacore JM, Li QX, et al. HITS: a short domestic violence screening tool for use in a family practice setting. Fam Med. 1998;30(7):508–12.
17. Cognitive behavioral therapy for men who physically abuse their female partner. Cochrane Libr. 2009:4.
18. Isaac NE, Enos VP. Documenting domestic violence: how health care providers can help victims, National Institute of Justice, research in brief. 188564. 2001. Available at www.ncjrs.gov.

Chapter 24
Psychiatric Disorders in Women's Health

Shambhavi Chandraiah

Introduction

The global burden of psychiatric disorders is growing. Common disorders, like major depression, can be as debilitating as many chronic medical illnesses such as coronary artery disease or diabetes [1] on family, work, and social functioning. Depression displays high rates of lifetime prevalence, early age of onset, high chronicity, and role impairment [2]. Nevertheless, the stigma of psychiatric disorders continues to keep patients from seeking care or opting to delay care. Primary care physicians and obstetrician/gynecologists are often the only health-care professionals whom women see, and thus they frequently encounter and have to manage psychiatric illnesses in their practices. The most common psychiatric disorders seen in primary care are depressive and anxiety disorders. However, these disorders are sometimes masked presenting as somatic symptoms such as headache, constipation, diarrhea, chest pain, shortness of breath, numbness, dizziness, and weight changes leading to lack of or delayed recognition.

S. Chandraiah (✉)
Quillen College of Medicine, Department of Psychiatry and Behavioral Sciences, East Tennessee State University, Johnson City, TN, USA
e-mail: chandraiah@etsu.edu

J. V. Knaus et al. (eds.), *Ambulatory Gynecology*,
https://doi.org/10.1007/978-1-4939-7641-6_24

Mood Disorders

Mood disorders are the highest disability causing psychiatric illnesses worldwide in terms of quality of life, work days lost, and death [3]. About 10% of the US population aged 18 and older in a given year have a mood disorder. The common mood disorders seen in women are, respectively, major depression, dysthymia, and bipolar disorder [4]. The full criteria for diagnosing the different mood disorders can be found in the *Diagnostic and Statistical Manual* (DSM 5) [6] (Fig. 24.1).

Major Depressive Disorder

The National Comorbidity Survey Replication (NCS-R) found that major depression has a 17% lifetime prevalence in adults [4]. Major depressive disorder (MDD) can be remembered by the pneumonic SIG E CAPSS [6], which stands for persistent S (sad mood), and/or I (decreased interest) for two or more weeks, accompanied by three to four of the following: G (guilt), E (decreased energy), C (decreased concentration), A (appetite change), P (psychomotor retardation or agitation), S (suicidal ideation), and S (sleep changes). Often, feelings of inadequacy with hopelessness for the future may be present. These symptoms must cause significant disruption of one or more aspects of one's normal daily functioning and must not be due to a medical condition (e.g., hypothyroidism), substance use (e.g., alcohol), or medications (e.g., sedatives) to meet diagnostic criteria for MDD. The PHQ-9 (which is in the public domain) can be used to screen for depression, with a score of greater than 10 suggestive of significant depression [7]. Additional specifiers can include with anxious distress (worried and tense), mixed (concurrent manic symptoms), atypical (with hyperphagia and hypersomnia), melancholic, psychotic, postpartum (within 4 weeks of delivery), and seasonal (usually fall/winter depression) features which may dictate more specific treatments [5].

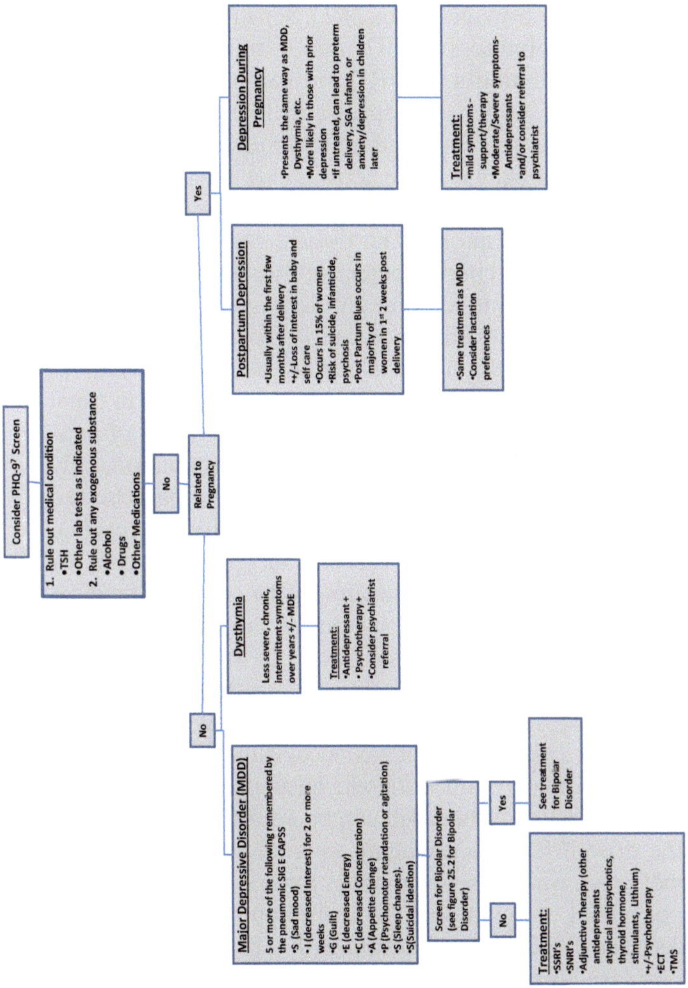

FIG. 24.1 Depressive disorders

For mild depression, medication or psychotherapy can be considered but for severe major depression, medication is indicated. The current first-line antidepressants are selective serotonin reuptake inhibitors (SSRI) because of their safety, ease of use, and cost (see Tables 24.1). Serotonin norepinephrine reuptake inhibitors (SNRI) and norepinephrine dopamine reuptake inhibitor (NDRI) are second-line treatment (see Table 24.2). Older antidepressants like tricyclic antidepressants and monoamine oxidase inhibitors are rarely used because they may cause more serious side effects and overdose sequelae. Medications may take 4–6 weeks to show improvement in symptoms. The dosage can be increased if there is only a partial improvement in 4 weeks (at least 25%); otherwise, switching to another antidepressant from another class or augmenting with a medication from another class is recommended. The NIMH Sequenced Treatment Alternatives to Relieve Depression (STAR*D)) trial showed that in usual outpatient practices even after four successive trials of antidepressants or psychotherapy alone or in combination, only about two thirds of patients with major depression achieved remission [8]. Remission should be aimed for as residual symptoms impair quality of life and increase the risk for relapse. Patients should be encouraged to continue medication, despite improvement in symptoms, in order to prevent relapse of their depression. Side effects of SSRIs and SNRIs include headache, nausea, insomnia, nervousness, and sexual dysfunction. Most side effects of antidepressants will subside over the first 2 weeks except sexual dysfunction (decreased libido or orgasmic dysfunction) which can occur in up to 40% of patients. Sexual dysfunction can be addressed by decreasing the dose if feasible, changing to an antidepressant from another class, waiting a few months for spontaneous resolution, or a trial of low-dose concurrent bupropion– the latter for decreased libido. Consultation with a psychiatrist should be considered if symptoms do not improve despite treatment with two different classes of antidepressants or if suicidal ideation, psychosis, or bipolar disorder is present. Maintenance treatment for several years or longer should be considered

TABLE 24.1 Selective serotonin reuptake inhibitor antidepressants

Generic name	FDA pregnancy category	Dose (mg)
Citalopram	C	20–40
Escitalopram	C	10–20
Fluoxetine[a]	C	20–60
Fluvoxamine[b]	C	100–300
Paroxetine[b]	D	20–60
Sertraline[a]	C	50–200

Categories used by US FDA to classify drug safety for use during pregnancy:

A – Controlled human studies show no risk

B – No risk in animals but no data in humans

C – Risk in animals but no human studies

D – Evidence of human risk but benefits may outweigh risks

X – Evidence of human risk and risks exceed benefits (contraindicated in pregnancy)

Side effects:

All can cause nausea, vomiting, diarrhea, and sexual side effects (drive, arousal, orgasm)

[a]Activation

[b]Sedation

for those with three or more episodes of major depression or for those with severe depression with past serious suicide attempt or psychosis. Atypical antipsychotics, namely, low-dose aripiprazole, brexpiprazole, or quetiapine extended release, added to the primary antidepressant, or fluoxetine and olanzapine combination are currently FDA-approved for treatment of severe major depression. The FDA in 2007 issued a warning about an increased risk of suicidal thinking and behavior in young adults during initiation of antidepressant treatment [9]. For psychosis associated with depression, any antipsychotic at the usual higher doses used to treat psychosis can be used.

Cognitive behavioral therapy (CBT)) can be as effective as medication for mild to moderate depression, but availability of trained mental health professionals as well as patients'

TABLE 24.2 Other antidepressants (SNRI, NDRI, other)

Generic name	Pregnancy risk category	Dose (mg)
Bupropion	C	300–450
Duloxetine[a]	C	60–120
Mirtazapine[b]	C	15–45
Nefazodone[b]	C	400–600
Trazodone[b]	C	400–600
Venlafaxine[a]	C	75–375
Desvenlafaxine[a]	C	50–100
Vilazodone	C	20–40
Vortioxetine	C	10–20
Levomilnacipran[a]	C	40–120

Side effects:
Most can cause nausea, diarrhea, and dry mouth except mirtazapine
[a]Hypertension, tachycardia, activation, sweating, dizziness, and sexual side effects
[b]Sedation

lesser acceptance of this alternative treatment may limit its use. CBT, generally conducted over 12–20 weeks, involves changing the patient's negative view of herself, the world, and the future and also includes activation strategies [10]. Other types of psychotherapies can also be helpful. Early morning light therapy for 20–30 min with special light boxes emitting greater than 2500 LUX (usually 10,000 LUX) can be helpful for seasonal (fall/winter) exacerbation of depression, which is most commonly seen in the Northern United States [11]. Other FDA-approved treatment modalities for treatment-resistant major depression include electroconvulsive therapy (ECT), transcranial magnetic stimulation, and vagal nerve stimulation [12].

Persistent Depressive Disorder (Dysthymia)

Pure dysthymic syndrome is a less severe but long-standing, intermittent form of depression and is often reactive to stressors in the patient's life. These women may report that they have always felt this way seeing this dysphoric state as their normal level of functioning and thus may not seek treatment until a major life stressor or a major depressive episode occurs. The symptoms can be similar to major depression but of lesser quantity or quality. Persistent depressive disorder (PDD) can be a pure dysthymic syndrome or may have concomitant intermittent or persistent major depressive episodes that last more than 2 years. The lifetime prevalence of pure dysthymia in adults is 2.5% [5]. Treatment of PDD usually involves a combination of psychotherapy along with antidepressants to attempt to achieve remission. Maintenance treatment is the norm due to the chronicity of the illness.

Bipolar Disorder

Bipolar disorder (BD) is characterized by alternating periods of major depressive episodes and either manic or hypomanic (less severe manic) episodes with interspersed euthymic (normal) moods of varying lengths. Mania can consist of a combination of the following symptoms noted by the pneumonic STRAP E GooD [13] which stands for decreased need for sleep, talkative, racing thoughts, increased activity, pleasurable activities, elevated mood, grandiosity, and distractibility. A manic episode can onset within a week with impulsive and sometimes risky sexual and financial behaviors that can have a major negative impact on the patient's social or work functioning, at times necessitating hospitalization. As with MDD, BD has specifiers like anxious distress, mixed, atypical, psychotic, peripartum, and seasonal. Rapid cycling (more than four separate manic hypomanic and/or depressive episodes within a single year) is more common in women particularly when underlying (often subclinical) hypothyroidism is present. The lifetime prevalence of adult BD is 4% [4]. The 13-item MDQ (mood disorder questionnaire) can be used to screen for BD where a score of 7 or more suggests possible BD [14] (Fig. 24.1).

The treatment options for bipolar disorder are divided into acute treatment and maintenance treatment. Acute manic episodes may be treated with traditional mood stabilizers (like lithium, valproate, or carbamazepine) or atypical antipsychotics, alone or in combination (see Tables 24.3 and 24.4). Adjunctive treatment with benzodiazepines or hypnotics may be necessary for specific symptoms (see Tables 24.5 and 24.6).

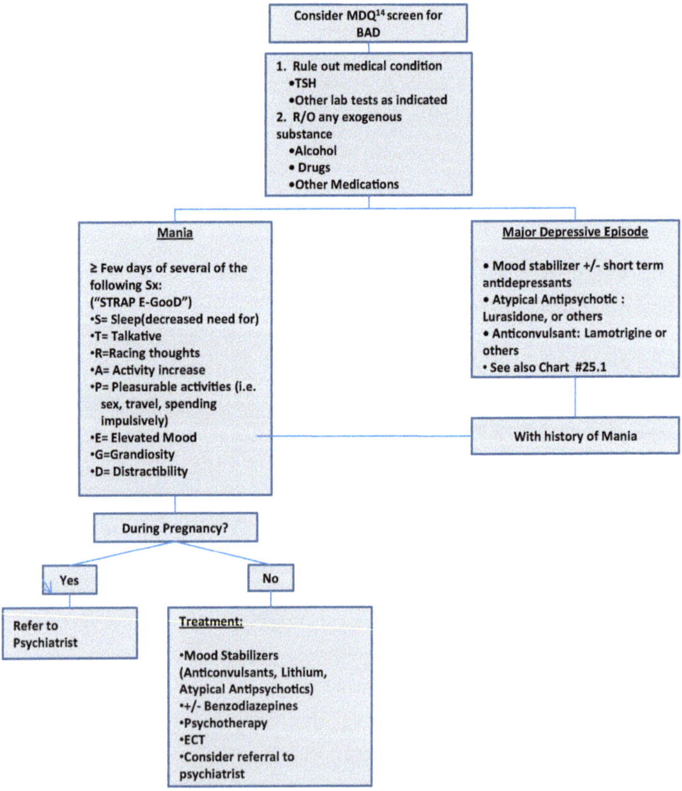

FIG. 24.2 Bipolar disorder

Table 24.3 Antipsychotics

Generic name	FDA pregnancy category	Dose (mg)
Risperidone[a]	C	2–4
Olanzapine[a,b]	C	10–20
Quetiapine[a,b]	C	400–800
Ziprasidone[a]	C	80–160
Aripiprazole[a,b]	C	10–30
Paliperidone[a]	C	6–12
Asenapine[a]	C	10–20
Iloperidone[a]	C	12–24
Lurasidone[a]	B	40–80
Brexpiprazole[a,b]	–	2–3
Cariprazine[a]	C	1.5–6
Chlorpromazine	C	400–800
Haloperidol	C	2–10
Clozapine[c]	B	300–900

Side effects:
[a]Atypical antipsychotics-> FDA warning of diabetes, hyperglycemia, also variable EPS, weight gain, sedation
[b]FDA-approved augmentation for MDD at lower doses but olanzapine only with fluoxetine combination
[c]Agranulocytosis with weekly to monthly CBC monitoring needed

The NIMH Systematic Treatment Enhancement Program for Bipolar Disorder (STEP-BD) trial did not show greater recovery with antidepressant addition to a mood stabilizer for treatment of bipolar depression [15]. Thus, antidepressants should be discontinued (or used for a limited time only for depressive symptoms) to prevent cycling into mania or induction of rapid cycling. Bupropion and SSRIs are less likely to cause manic switch. Lithium carbonate is most useful for mania and decreases suicidal thinking [16]. Valproate or carbamazepine is more helpful for manic or mixed states or for

TABLE 24.4 Anticonvulsant mood stabilizers

Generic name	Side effects	Pregnancy risk category	Dose
Lithium	Mild diarrhea Nausea Tremor Weight gain Hypothyroidism Renal toxicity	D	900–1800 mg Level 0.8–1.2
Valproate	Weight gain Nausea Tremor Hepatotoxicity Pancreatitis	D	750–3000 mg Level 50–150
Carbamazepine	Aplastic anemia Agranulocytosis Rash	D	800–1600 Level 4–12
Lamotrigine	Rash Stevens-Johnson syndrome	C	100–200 mg
Topiramate	Nephrolithiasis Weight loss Cognitive dulling	D	50–200 mg

TABLE 24.5 Benzodiazepine anxiolytics

Generic name	FDA pregnancy category	Dose (mg)
Diazepam	D	2–40
Alprazolam	D	3–6
Clonazepam	D	2–4
Lorazepam	D	2–6
Clorazepate	D	30–60

rapid cycling. Lamotrigine is best for maintenance prevention of bipolar depression. There are significant adverse effects of traditional mood stabilizers which may include weight gain, tremor, and rash (see Table 24.4 for side effects).

Table 24.6 Hypnotics

Generic name	FDA pregnancy category	Dose (mg)
Zolpidem	C	5–10
Eszopiclone	C	1–3
Zaleplon	C	5–10
Ramelteon	C	8
Suvorexant	C	10–20

Atypical antipsychotics are better for manic or mixed states, but lurasidone with or without lithium or valproate, olanzapine with fluoxetine combination, and quetiapine monotherapy have indications for bipolar depression (with the consequent FDA warning of a potential increase in suicidal ideation/behavior in young adults and adolescents). Atypical antipsychotics have the potential to cause a metabolic syndrome with increases in cholesterol, triglycerides, serum glucose, blood pressure, and weight gain necessitating regular monitoring of these parameters. Among current atypical antipsychotics, ziprasidone, aripiprazole, asenapine, iloperidone, and lurasidone are less likely to cause such side effects. Atypical antipsychotics have an FDA warning about the potential for hyperglycemia and diabetes. All atypical antipsychotics have a very small risk of causing tardive dyskinesia, a potentially permanent movement disorder; this risk is greater in older women and non-Caucasian women [17]. Older antipsychotics such as haloperidol, perphenazine, chlorpromazine, etc. have greater overall side effects (including extrapyramidal symptoms, sedation, tardive dyskinesia) and are rarely used now. Clozapine may be used off label as a tertiary agent for patients with schizoaffective disorder (those with BAD and schizophrenia) who do not respond to other atypical antipsychotics and/or mood stabilizers. However, clozapine is very rarely used as a third-line agent due to an increased risk for agranulocytosis and a requirement of CBC monitoring every 1–4 weeks. Patients may benefit from concomitant supportive psychotherapy, while ECT may be considered in treatment-resistant cases [18].

Long-term maintenance treatment involves using traditional mood stabilizers and/or atypical antipsychotics as the primary mode of treatment. Maintenance of a regular sleep cycle and adherence to medication as well as family support is critical to minimize relapses. Maintenance treatment is the goal when remission is achieved as BD is a serious chronic, relapsing psychiatric disorder. The chronicity and complexity of managing BD would suggest that most physicians should refer these patients to a psychiatrist for management.

Anxiety Disorders

The NCS-R found that about 30% of adults develop an anxiety disorder in their lifetime [4]. Almost all anxiety disorders are more common in females especially generalized anxiety disorder (GAD), panic disorder, social anxiety disorder, and post-traumatic stress disorder (PTSD). The full criteria for diagnosing the various anxiety disorders can be found in the DSM-5 [5]. More than half of patients have co-occurring anxiety and depressive disorders with anxiety presenting in adolescence and depression in adulthood. Anxiety disorders can also be associated with substance abuse [4] (Fig. 24.3).

Generalized Anxiety Disorder

GAD is a long-standing illness (more than 6 months) characterized by unwarranted worrying most days about common things in a patient's life and can disrupt the patient's sleep, concentration, or be associated with symptoms of fatigue, restlessness, irritability, or muscle tension [4] (Fig. 24.3). The lifetime prevalence of GAD is about 6% in adults (5). The GAD-7 can be used to screen for GAD with a score of ≥10 suggestive of GAD [19].

GAD can be treated with individual psychotherapy and/or medication. SSRI antidepressants continue to be the first-line of treatment. Since more than 50% of patients with anxiety

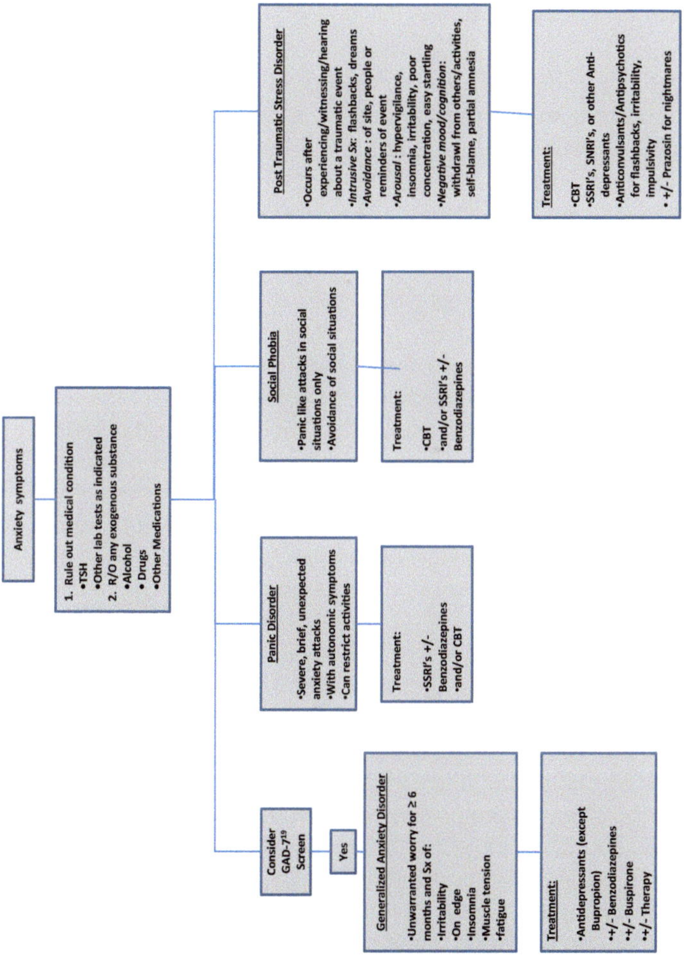

FIG. 24.3 Anxiety disorders

disorders have comorbid depression, all antidepressant medications have the added advantage of also treating any concurrent depression that may be present. The only exception is the antidepressant bupropion which lacks any anxiolytic serotonergic action. Benzodiazepines can be used alone or in conjunction with antidepressants for any residual symptom relief (see Table 24.5). Buspirone can be particularly relevant for patients with the potential for addiction as it is a non-benzodiazepine anxiolytic [20]. As noted before, antidepressants have an FDA warning about the possible onset of or increase in suicidal ideation in adolescents and young adults.

Post-traumatic Stress Disorder

PTSD may occur after a traumatic event (involving serious bodily injury or risk of such injury) is experienced, witnessed, or learned about. These events may include natural disasters, physical or sexual assault, motor vehicle accidents, or combat situations [5]. For women, the most common causes are childhood sexual abuse, physical abuse, or rape. The core symptoms are *intrusive* symptoms associated with the event (through flashbacks, recurring dreams, memories), *avoidance* of stimuli associated with the trauma (sites, individuals, activities that are a reminder of the trauma), increased *arousal* (insomnia, irritability, poor concentration, easy startling, hypervigilance, reckless behavior), and *negative mood and cognition* due to the trauma (partial amnesia, self-blame, negative emotional state, withdrawal from others or activities) [5]. The lifetime prevalence is about 7% [4]. The nature of the boundary violations of sexual and physical abuse of women usually results in persistence of the PTSD symptoms for an extended period of time and interferes significantly with their work, family, and/or social functioning.

Treatment modalities for PTSD consist of therapy as well as medications. CBT is often used in treating PTSD and can involve learning relaxation techniques, graduated exposure to the trauma images, and cognitive restructuring [21]. SSRIs at usual doses are considered the first-line treatment for PTSD [22]; sertraline and paroxetine are FDA-approved for PTSD. Since the majority of patients with PTSD also develop depression, antidepressants can also help this comorbid condition. Mood stabilizers such as valproate and lamotrigine may be effective in decreasing the symptoms of irritability, violent behavior, impulsivity, and flashbacks. Antipsychotics may be useful for flashbacks or anger problems, but the risk of tardive dyskinesia and the metabolic syndrome can be a problematic side effect [22]. Prazosin may be helpful for decreasing nightmares in PTSD [23]. Hypnotics may be helpful for transient insomnia (Table 24.6). Benzodiazepines are not generally recommended because of concerns of potential disinhibition, difficulty integrating the traumatic experiences during psychotherapy, and addiction risks [24].

Panic Disorder

Panic disorder is characterized by recurrent, unexpected panic attacks followed by at least a month of worrying about further attacks or avoidance of situations that might cause such attacks. Panic attacks typically consist of sudden fear with four or more symptoms of tachycardia, sweating, shortness of breath, chest pain, dizziness, nausea, paresthesia, or fear of going crazy or dying that peak in minutes [5]. The avoidance (agoraphobia) may include public places like buses, malls, bridges, crowds, or standing in line. The autonomic symptoms can escalate quickly and can sometimes be misinterpreted as an impending heart attack resulting in emergency room visits. The lifetime prevalence is about 5% [4]. The first-line treatment is SSRIs with some patients needing early concurrent benzodiazepines, given as a standing or as a prn regimen. Notably, the SSRI must be started at a much lower dose and increased much slower to avoid initial increased panic symptoms. CBT is also very effective; it can give a sense of control over the symptoms and can be used first line if the patient is willing [25].

Social Anxiety Disorder

Also called social phobia, this disorder is characterized by 6 months or more of a fear of social situations (e.g., parties, giving speeches, eating in public) where the person may be scrutinized by others or fears negative evaluation, leading to avoidance of such situations or anxious endurance. The lifetime prevalence is 12% [4]. Treatment is best addressed with psychotherapy (e.g., CBT) and/or medications like SSRIs augmented with short-term or intermittent benzodiazepines if needed. Social phobia starts in adolescence, and without treatment, these patients may not reach their full potential professionally or socially.

Psychiatric Disorders Linked to the Reproductive Cycle

Women who have reproductive cycle associated psychiatric problems, e.g., premenstrual dysphoric disorder (PMDD), postpartum depression (PPD), and perimenopausal depression, show a greater likelihood of psychiatric problems at other times in their life, e.g., MDD [65]. Thus, it is important to ask a woman about past episodes of PMDD or MDE if she presents with current depression during pregnancy. As well, if a woman has had a past MDE, a heightened awareness of possible future perinatal depression is necessary (Fig. 24.4).

Premenstrual Dysphoric Disorder

Premenstrual syndrome (PMS) is a common syndrome of primarily physical symptoms that can occur in a third of women during many menstrual cycles. PMS can include very transient psychological symptoms such as irritability, tension, or dysphoria, as well as physical symptoms such as breast tenderness, weight gain, bloating, and joint/muscle pain. However, only about 5% of women experience premenstrual

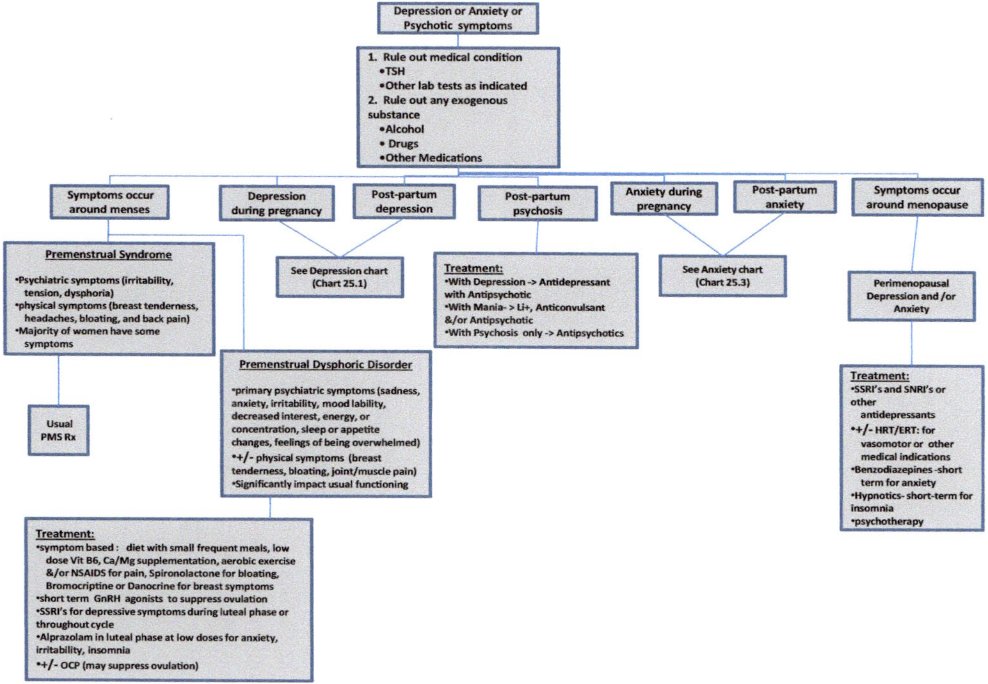

FIG. 24.4 Reproductively linked psychiatric disorders

dysphoric disorder (PMDD). PMDD is characterized by at least five primarily psychiatric symptoms of (a) sadness, anxiety, irritability, or mood lability and (b) decreased interest, energy, concentration, feelings of being overwhelmed, sleep or appetite changes, or physical symptoms as noted above; these symptoms must significantly impact a woman's usual functioning. A 1 week symptom free time after menses is essential to differentiate cyclical PMDD from premenstrual exacerbation of pre-existing anxiety and mood disorders [5]. PMDD symptoms can onset any time after cycle day 14 and crescendos to menses with rapid relief of symptoms thereafter. A prospective daily log of symptoms over at least two symptomatic cycles is needed to confirm the diagnosis. About two thirds of those who report cyclical PMDD are confirmed on prospective log keeping. PMDD can also be familial. PMDD symptom presence or intensity can vary over the reproductive lifetime of a woman with onset or offset of PMDD symptoms often linked to times of hormonal flux such as with oral contraceptive use or cessation, or after a pregnancy.

A number of past theories regarding PMDD include progesterone deficiency or estrogen excess, vitamin B6 deficiency, prolactin excess, hypoglycemia, endogenous opiate withdrawal, alteration in the renin-angiotensin system, calcium and magnesium deficiency, and serotonin deficiency [26]. Current thinking about PMDD suggests an increased sensitivity to usual changes in gonadal hormones over the menstrual cycle with symptoms ensuing in the luteal phase as a result of changes originating in the follicular phase [27].

Treatment of PMS is symptom based and can include a diet with small frequent meals, low-dose vitamin B6, calcium or magnesium supplementation, aerobic exercise and/or NSAIDs to alleviate pain, spironolactone for bloating, and bromocriptine or danocrine for breast symptoms. For severe symptoms of PMS or PMDD, short-term gonadotropin-releasing hormone agonists may be useful to suppress hypothalamic gonadal cyclicity that triggers symptoms. Of course, the risks of inducing a medical menopause are considerable with respect to their negative impact on lipid profile, bone density, etc. Danocrine or oral contraceptives (OCP) may help prevent ovulation leading to a decrease in PMDD symptoms [26]. Drospirenone/ethinylestradiol has an FDA indication for PMDD. Notably, for some patients, the use of sequential OCP may initiate or exacerbate PMS/PMDD symptoms. For significant psychiatric symptoms, studies have shown efficacy of cyclical luteal phase or full cycle treatment with SSRIs as the optimal mode of treatment [28]. Fluoxetine, paroxetine controlled release, and sertraline have FDA indications for PMDD. Buspirone was shown to have a beneficial effect in one study [29]. Low-dose alprazolam use in the luteal phase has also been shown to have efficacy in controlled trials for PMDD symptoms of anxiety, irritability, and insomnia [30].

Psychiatric Disorders in Pregnancy and Postpartum

There are a number of important roles for physicians during this time. Patients may present before pregnancy to consult about management of their psychiatric illness, impact of illness or medications on the fetus and during breastfeeding, or to assist in discontinuing medications on a trial basis. Others may present after exposure to psychotropics has already occurred. Additionally, new onset of psychiatric disorders may occur during pregnancy or in the postpartum. Some women may also seek prophylactic treatment for recurrent postpartum depression, mania, or psychosis.

The risk assessment during pregnancy involves considering the base frequencies of developmental anomalies, the timeline of embryonic/fetal development, potential risks of exposure to psychiatric and nonpsychiatric medications, and obstetrical complications, as well as the potential risks of untreated maternal psychiatric illness. It is important to note that some type of medication is used in the majority of pregnancies, and more than a third of women receive psychotropics [31].

The general adage is not to use any medication, including psychotropics, during the first trimester due to the risk of major congenital malformations. However, due to the continued development of the fetal nervous system throughout pregnancy and even after birth, the impact of medication use during the last trimester and in the perinatal period should be assessed. Additionally, prior effective medications are preferred unless there are specific contraindications to their use during pregnancy or postpartum. The least effective dose should be used and monotherapy is preferred. Since 1979, the FDA has classified medications based on drug safety using the following categories (which will remain till July 2018): A, controlled studies show no risk in humans; B, no evidence of risk in animals but no studies in humans; C, evidence of risk in animals but no studies in humans; D, positive evidence of human fetal risk but benefits may be worth the risks; X, positive evidence of human fetal risks outweigh any benefits. Most psychotropics are category C, suggesting that their use be considered if the potential benefit warrants it [32]. All medications approved by the FDA after July 2015 will have descriptive information about the impact of drugs on pregnancy (including labor and delivery), lactation (including nursing mothers), and a new subsection on female and male infertility intended to allow physicians and patients to make more meaningful decisions about medication use [33]. It is thus recommended that clinicians review the latest available data when considering the use of psychotropics in pregnancy or during breastfeeding. For some patients who choose to discontinue medication, psychotherapy may be a good potential alternative treatment.

Depression in Pregnancy

Depression may present as a major depressive episode or as minor depression during pregnancy although studies are not consistent that there is any increased occurrence of depression during pregnancy [34]. Symptoms of major depression can be similar to what has previously been described. The somatic changes of pregnancy may include fatigue, sleep, and appetite changes such that inquiring about sadness, guilt, anxiety symptoms, or suicidal thoughts become more important in establishing the diagnosis of major depression. Unfavorable outcomes of untreated major depression during pregnancy may include inadequate prenatal care, low birth weight, preterm delivery, fetal hyperactivity, and neonatal depressive symptoms [35]. Over 7% of women have used antidepressants in the first trimester of pregnancy a tripling over the last 20 years, notably SSRIs [31]. There is a greater likelihood of relapse if medications are discontinued during pregnancy in women who are on maintenance antidepressant treatment for recurrent major depression [36]. Usual antidepressants at typical doses may generally be used to treat depression.

Effects of antidepressant during pregnancy may include the following: a one and a half times greater likelihood of spontaneous abortions, unlikely major congenital malformations except slight possible increase in cardiovascular malformations with paroxetine, minimal preterm risk (<1 week), unlikely small for gestational age births, and unlikely persistent pulmonary hypertension with later pregnancy SSRI or SNRI use. The neonatal behavioral syndrome may occur due to SSRI/SNRI use in the third trimester with neonates experiencing jitteriness, increased reflexes, and vomiting that resolve within 2 weeks, while more severe symptoms may need special care nursery admission [37]. For severe depression, when antidepressants have been unsuccessful or when urgent response is needed (e.g., active suicidal ideation or serious psychotic symptoms), ECT can be considered, as it results in rapid and major symptom relief. Antidepressants usually have to be continued after a course of six to eight ECT treatments to maintain benefit. The risks of ECT include some potential residual retrograde memory impairment. For mild to moderate depression and for women who choose to discontinue antidepressants, CBT or interpersonal therapy can be a useful treatment.

Bipolar Disorder in Pregnancy

Bipolar disorder in expectant mothers presents itself in much the same way as in a woman who is not pregnant. There may be prominent mood episodes of depression, mania, or hypomania. Women of childbearing age with bipolar disorder should be educated regarding the possible effects of pregnancy on the course of their illness, treatment options during pregnancy, postpartum and lactation, and effective contraceptive practices, to allow them to make informed decisions. Untreated mania, in general, poses clear risks due to associated impulsivity, poor judgment, and possible non-compliance with treatment and may require hospitalization. The risk of recurrence of bipolar disorder is extremely high during pregnancy and is doubled when maintenance medications are discontinued, especially precipitously [38, 39].

Patients with bipolar disorder are often treated with multiple medications including anticonvulsant mood stabilizers, antidepressants, anxiolytics, hypnotics, and antipsychotics. All psychotropic medications diffuse readily across the placenta after the first 2 weeks of pregnancy. Most of the psychotropic medications used to treat bipolar disorder have been categorized as C or D.

Lithium (Cat D) was the earliest mood stabilizer available to treat bipolar disorder. Ebstein's anomaly with first trimester lithium use has been recognized to be much less than formerly thought, at only 0.1% (despite being 20 times greater than the usual risk of 0.005%) [40]. There is also a 2.5 times greater risk of overall congenital malformations and a five times greater risk of cardiac abnormalities with first trimester exposure to lithium. A 16-week fetal echocardiogram is suggested to look for cardiac anomalies. Exposure to lithium in the last trimester has also been shown to be rarely associated with neonatal cardiac arrhythmia, nephrogenic diabetes insipidus, transient hypothyroidism, premature delivery, and birth complications such as low muscle tone, lethargy, respiratory difficulty ("floppy baby syndrome"), and polyhydramnios [41]. Lithium levels should be monitored frequently due to changes in blood volume, and dosing should be decreased to prepregnancy dose at delivery.

Anticonvulsants may pose a more serious teratogenic risk with higher doses and polytherapy with multiple anticonvulsants further increasing the risk of congenital malformations. Valproate (Cat D) is associated with a 4% risk of neural tube defects, such as spina bifida when exposure occurs in the first 4 weeks of development. Neural tube defects also increase with doses greater than 1000 mg of valproate or when combinations of anticonvulsants are used. Other congenital anomalies (6%) include developmental delay, cleft lip and/or palate, craniofacial abnormalities, and cardiac defects. Valproate use later in pregnancy may lead to toxicity in the newborn with impact on muscle tone, liver toxicity, and coagulation problems. As well, neurodevelopmental impact on cognition including decreased IQ and behavioral problems are significant although many of the studies are with mothers with epilepsy [42]. Maternal carbamazepine (Cat D) use during pregnancy carries an increased risk of major congenital malformations (3%) including cardiovascular and urinary tract abnormalities as well as craniofacial defects, neural tube defects (1%), neonatal toxicity, and neurodevelopmental problems. Although oxcarbazepine is category C, the manufacturer notes that it may be a teratogen due to its similarity to carbamazepine. If used, these anticonvulsants should be used at the lowest effective dosage with frequent monitoring of drug levels. In addition, prenatal screening for congenital malformations is recommended including careful fetal monitoring with ultrasonography. Folic acid supplementation in early pregnancy may help mitigate some of the effects on the nervous system. Lamotrigine (Cat C) does not appear to increase overall risk of major congenital malformations associated with first trimester exposure, although conflicting reports exist regarding increased risk of oral clefts. There are also no clear increased risk of perinatal or neurodevelopmental adverse outcomes with monotherapy use of lamotrigine [42]. Topiramate, another anticonvulsant used off label for BD or to treat the side effects of weight gain from other psychotropics, is category D due to an increased risk of cleft lip or palate [43]. Gabapentin and tiagabine may sometimes be used off label for BD. All anticonvulsant mood stabilizers have a warning about an increased risk of suicidal ideation [44].

Benzodiazepines (Cat D), which are used on an as needed basis with bipolar disorder, have been associated with a small 0.001% risk of cleft lip or palate [45]. Buspirone (Cat B) can be used for anxiety but requires a daily maintenance dose for efficacy and is not as effective for most patients as the immediately effective benzodiazepines. For patients with severe depression, acute suicidal ideation or homicidal ideation, severe mania, or psychosis, ECT may be the treatment of choice for rapid improvement of symptoms.

Antipsychotics have also been used for acute and maintenance management of BD. The older typical antipsychotics, like haloperidol and perphenazine, have not been shown to have any major congenital malformations. Newer atypical antipsychotics like risperidone, olanzapine, and quetiapine appear not to cause a material increase in congenital malformations [46]. However, they may cause weight gain and gestational diabetes with large for gestation babies resulting in premature or caesarian deliveries [47] especially when polypharmacy (e.g., atypical antipsychotic with SSRI) occurs [48]. Limited data suggest that early developmental delays may resolve over time [47]. All antipsychotics are category C except for clozapine and lurasidone (which are Cat B). Clozapine may be used off label as a tertiary agent for patients with schizoaffective disorder. Recent prospective and large-scale retrospective studies have noted that there may be a slight increase in congenital malformations with antipsychotic polypharmacy resulting in more prematurity, poor neonatal adaptation, and more NICU admissions [46, 48]. The FDA has a warning about the use of antipsychotics in the third trimester posing a risk for the development of abnormal muscle movements (extrapyramidal symptoms) and withdrawal symptoms in neonates, which can present as increased or decreased muscle tone, tremor, sleepiness, difficulty with feeding or breathing, and agitation. These symptoms may subside within hours or days without treatment, while some neonates may require longer hospital stays [49]. Because of the complexity of treating BD, referral for psychiatric consultation or concurrent management should be considered, particularly if symptoms of bipolar disorder are inadequately controlled or if the patient has a history of severe bipolar disorder or has suicidal, homicidal, or psychotic symptoms.

Anxiety Disorders in Pregnancy

The same anxiety disorders that occur at other times can occur during pregnancy in vulnerable women. Anxiety during pregnancy will typically continue and may worsen in the postpartum but may also predict increased likelihood of postpartum depression [50]. Untreated anxiety during pregnancy can also lead to increase in fetal heart patterns [51]. Psychotherapy (CBT, interpersonal therapy) would be the first treatment choice if there is availability of psychotherapy providers, the patient is receptive to this, and if psychotherapy can adequately treat the anxiety disorder. The use of SSRIs at usual doses can be considered – see also earlier section on use of these during pregnancy. Benzodiazepines are not recommended for regular use during pregnancy (Cat D) due to the rare occurrence of oral clefts with first trimester exposure [45] as well as potential neonatal withdrawal symptoms upon delivery. Late pregnancy benzodiazepine use may also lead to neonatal floppy syndrome with hypotonia, apnea, poor feeding, and temperature regulation problems.

Psychotic Disorders in Pregnancy

Non-mood-related psychoses such as schizophrenia or delusional disorder may be treated with antipsychotics at the same dosages as described in the sections under depression and bipolar disorder with psychosis. Mothers with psychosis may have a higher risk of poor self-care and compliance with medications and may require closer monitoring due to the risk of postpartum psychosis.

Postpartum Disorders

New mothers undergo multiple changes associated with childbirth, including sleep deprivation, breastfeeding, adjustment in existing relationships, social isolation, and the formation of the mother-infant relationship. Untreated or undertreated postpartum psychiatric disorders could potentially lead to an increased risk of insecure attachment or developmental delays, cognitive (e.g., decreased IQ [52]) and behavioral problems in the infant, and, in rare severe cases, a risk of infanticide and/or suicide.

Postpartum Depression

Onset of symptoms in postpartum depression (PPD) typically occurs within the first 4 weeks following delivery, but the risk period can be up to 2 years post-delivery. The prevalence of PPD is approximately 10–15% although this may vary cross-culturally [53]. "Baby blues" with symptoms such as weeping, sadness, irritability, anxiety, and occasionally confusion, occur in the majority of new mothers and is a transient mood disturbance that peaks by the fourth day after delivery and resolves by the tenth day. Unlike "baby blues", postpartum depression typically persists beyond the first several months after delivery and is more severe. Common symptoms are those seen in major depression and include depressed mood, loss of interest, and disturbance of sleep, appetite, and cognition. Postpartum depression may be associated with maternal disengagement, marital conflict, low self-esteem, impaired social or occupational functioning, and a poor quality of life.

Antidepressants at usual doses are appropriate for treatment of PPD. Consideration for prophylactic use of antidepressants in the postpartum period (if no antidepressants were used during pregnancy) should be considered for women who have had a prior PPD due to the doubled risk of developing depression in the postpartum. Discussion of risks of treatment in breastfeeding women with postpartum depression includes a potential risk to the child of not treating maternal depression (delayed psychomotor, cognitive, or emotional development) as well as a risk through the limited exposure the infant typically receives to antidepressant medication [54]. Efficacy of 12-week interpersonal psychotherapy for women with PPD has been shown [55]. Other types of individual or group therapy can also be helpful.

Postpartum Bipolar Disorder

The risk of having a postpartum mood episode for a patient with BD increases to 35% if the patient has had a prior mood episode at any time in her life. If she has had a prior postpartum episode, whether depression, mania, or hypomania, then the risk increases to 50% or more [38, 56]; therefore, prophylactic treatment (if no psychotropics were used during pregnancy) should be seriously considered [38]. Prophylactic treatment with lithium has shown greater protection against postpartum BD recurrence in women who chose this than those who did not [57]. For depression, transient antidepressant use can be considered as long as a mood stabilizer is also added. For mania, anticonvulsant mood stabilizers or atypical antipsychotics can be used (see the BD section).

Postpartum Psychosis

Postpartum psychosis (PPP) represents a psychiatric emergency requiring immediate intervention due to an increased risk of suicide and infanticide. PPP can occur as a component of major depression, bipolar depression or mania, or as the onset or recurrence of a primary psychotic disorder. The relapse risk after an initial PPP is about 35% [58].

The presentation in a patient with PPP can involve more unusual psychotic symptoms such as mood-incongruent delusions about the baby, command hallucinations, aggression to others, and rapid onset with a fluctuating picture including cognitive disorganization that may resemble delirium [59]. Organic causes of psychosis should be considered. Neurologic workup and possible evaluation with a CT or MRI should be considered. Mood stabilizers as well as antipsychotics may be considered for treatment of bipolar psychosis. For postpartum depression with psychosis, antidepressants with concomitant antipsychotic use or ECT can be considered. Other primary postpartum psychosis (such as with schizophrenia) respond best to antipsychotic therapy. The mother's breastfeeding preference should be considered when considering pharmacologic interventions. The patient's family should also be educated regarding the patient's illness to help recognize signs of relapse and to provide a support system. Supportive therapy can also help to build parenting skills to promote better infant-maternal bonding.

Postpartum Anxiety Disorders

Some anxiety disorders may worsen or onset for the first time in the postpartum, notably GAD and obsessive compulsive disorder (OCD). OCD consists of obsessions (recurring thoughts) or compulsions (recurring actions) that are recognized as irrational but consume time, cause distress, and interfere with usual functioning [51].The obsession postpartum may be a fear of harming the baby, but this is recognized as unreasonable, unwanted ideas such that the patient will go to great lengths to ensure that no harm comes to the baby. Such obsessions are different from the very serious postpartum psychosis where infanticidal ideation is an emergency as the mother believes the infant is dangerous and may act on such thinking (see PPP section). The use of SSRI or SNRIs in usual doses would be the first preference. There is a high comorbidity with depression which these medications would also treat (see also prior section on anxiety disorders for details of use). Concurrent, standing, or as needed use of benzodiazepines can be considered. Some retrospective reports have suggested that weaning may exacerbate panic attacks [51]. Ruling out new onset of anemia or thyroid dysfunction is relevant since these can onset in the postpartum. Psychotherapy is always an important option as postpartum mothers often need more support, and new motherhood may evoke earlier conflicted issues with one's own rearing.

Lactation and Psychotropic Medications

The American Academy of Pediatrics (AAP) committee on drugs views medications present in breast milk at less than 10% of the maternal dose as acceptable choices for use in breastfeeding [60]. The use of psychotropics during lactation carries less risk than during pregnancy, as usually only a very small amount of medication (<2%) gets into the breast milk. This amount varies with the particular medication's qualities. Infant medication exposure may be decreased by breastfeeding before the next maternal dose of the medication is taken and by avoiding breastfeeding at peak medication concentration in the breast milk, which differs for the various medications. Antidepressants can usually be used by the mother during breastfeeding as infant exposure is very low, with sertraline and paroxetine being considered first choice. However, case reports of sedation or agitation, etc. may be seen occasionally in individual infant/mother dyads [60]. Lithium should not be used if a woman wishes to breastfeed because the level in breast milk can be as high as one-half that of the mother's serum level. As well, lamotrigine can be present at high levels in breast milk and should not be used. The AAP views carbamazepine and valproate as medications that are compatible with breastfeeding. Generally, very low doses of antipsychotic medication are present in breast milk, except for clozapine [61]. Benzodiazepines may lead to sedation in the neonate so caution is warranted. Monitoring for any changes in infant behavior may best dictate whether a particular medication is affecting an infant or not.

Perimenopausal Depression and Anxiety

The perimenopausal period refers to the time when a woman's menstrual cycle becomes irregular, typically occurring between the ages of 45 and 50. The perimenopause involves vasomotor symptoms such as hot flashes and night sweats. Other related symptoms include sleep disturbance, mood fluctuations, cognitive changes, sexual dysfunction, and an associated increased risk for osteoporosis and cardiovascular disease [62]. Studies have suggested that there is a higher likelihood of developing depression in the perimenopause if there is a past history of major depression particularly if hot flashes are also present. In addition, the timing of depression, which has been shown to occur during relatively elevated FSH levels, suggests that endocrine mechanisms may be associated with the pathophysiology of perimenopausal depression [63].

The treatment for perimenopausal depression can vary from patient to patient. Since comorbid anxiety can also occur at this time, the first line of treatment is antidepressants, namely, SSRIs, SNRIs, or other antidepressants at usual doses and duration. Estrogen replacement may augment the response to antidepressants for patients with perimenopausal depression, although addition of progesterone diminished this effect. However, the use of gonadal hormones in the perimenopause should be dictated by their need primarily for vasomotor or other medical indications due to exogenous gonadal hormones potentially increasing heart attacks and strokes as well as breast and uterine cancer [64]. Anxiety can also occur at this time in a woman's life (middle age) due to a number of psychosocial stressors including caring for aging parents, self or family ill-health, children leaving or returning home, divorce, return to the job market, retirement, financial problems, and a negative view of aging. Thus, short-term benzodiazepines can be utilized as well as individual supportive psychotherapy or marital or family therapy as relevant.

Summary

Some psychiatric disorders are more common in women, in particular depressive and anxiety disorders. The risk for mood disorder recurrence is particularly linked to the female reproductive cycle. Having a reproductively linked mood disorder increases the likelihood of a mood episode at other times in a woman's life and the converse is true as well [65]. Treatment with psychotropics and/or psychotherapy to achieve remission decreases the risk of recurrence with some women needing maintenance treatment. Obstetrician/gynecologists and primary care physicians are uniquely positioned to assess and treat most common psychiatric disorders in women.

Acknowledgment Thank you to Drs. Umesh Bhandari and Holly Kinget for their early contributions to this chapter.

References

1. Cassano P, Fava M. Depression and public health: an overview. J Psychosom Res. 2002;53(4):849–57.
2. Sansone RA, Sansone LA. Psychiatric disorders: a global look at facts and figures. Psychiatry (Edgmont). 2010;7(12):16–9.
3. Murray CJ, Atkinson C, Bhalla K, Birbeck G, Burstein R, Chou D, Murray. The state of US health, 1990–2010: burden of diseases, injuries, and risk factors. JAMA. 2013;310(6):591–608.
4. Kessler RC, Berglund P, Demler O, Jin R, Merikangas KR, Walters EE. Lifetime prevalence and age-of-onset distributions of DSM-IV disorders in the National Comorbidity Survey Replication. Arch Gen Psychiatry. 2005;62(6):593–602.
5. American Psychiatric Association. Diagnostic and statistical manual of mental disorders. 5th ed. Arlington: American Psychiatric Publishing; 2013.
6. Carlat DJ. The psychiatric review of symptoms: a screening tool for family physicians. Am Fam Physician. 1998;58(7):1617–24.
7. Spitzer RL, Kroenke K, Williams JB. Validation and utility of a self-report version of PRIME-MD: the PHQ primary care study. Primary care evaluation of mental disorders. Patient Health Questionnaire. JAMA. 1999;282(18):1737–44.
8. Rush AJ. STAR*D: what have we learned? Am J Psychiatry. 2007;164(2):201–4.
9. US Food & Drug Administration. FDA proposes new warnings about suicidal thinking, behavior in young adults who take antidepressant medications [press release]. Retrieved from http://www.fda.gov/NewsEvents/Newsroom/PressAnnouncements/2007/ucm108905.htm. 2007.

10. Rupke SJ, Blecke D, Renfrow M. Cognitive therapy for depression. Am Fam Physician. 2006;73(1):83–6.
11. Lam RW, Levitt AJ, Levitan RD, Enns MW, Morehouse R, Michalak EE, Tam EM. The Can-SAD study: a randomized controlled trial of the effectiveness of light therapy and fluoxetine in patients with winter seasonal affective disorder. Am J Psychiatry. 2006;163(5):805–12.
12. George MS, Nahas Z, Borckardt JJ, Anderson B, Foust MJ, Burns C, Short EB. Brain stimulation for the treatment of psychiatric disorders. Curr Opin Psychiatry. 2007;20(3):250–4. discussion 247–259
13. Chandraiah S. STRAP E GooD. 2011.
14. Hirschfeld RM, Williams JB, Spitzer RL, Calabrese JR, Flynn L, Keck PE Jr, Zajecka J. Development and validation of a screening instrument for bipolar spectrum disorder: the Mood Disorder Questionnaire. Am J Psychiatry. 2000;157(11):1873–5.
15. Bowden CL, Perlis RH, Thase ME, Ketter TA, Ostacher MM, Calabrese JR, Sachs GS. Aims and results of the NIMH systematic treatment enhancement program for bipolar disorder (STEP-BD). CNS Neurosci Ther. 2012;18(3):243–9.
16. Machado-Vieira R, Manji HK, Zarate CA Jr. The role of lithium in the treatment of bipolar disorder: convergent evidence for neurotrophic effects as a unifying hypothesis. Bipolar Disord. 2009;11(Suppl 2):92–109.
17. Morgenstern H, Glazer WM. Identifying risk factors for tardive dyskinesia among long-term outpatients maintained with neuroleptic medications. Results of the Yale Tardive Dyskinesia Study. Arch Gen Psychiatry. 1993;50(9):723–33.
18. Geddes JR, Miklowitz DJ. Treatment of bipolar disorder. Lancet. 2013;381(9878):1672–82.
19. Spitzer RL, Kroenke K, Williams JB, Löwe B. A brief measure for assessing generalized anxiety disorder: the GAD-7. Arch Intern Med. 2006;166(10):1092–7.
20. Durham RC. Treatment of generalized anxiety disorder. Psychiatry. 2004;3(4):30–4.
21. Nemeroff CB, Bremner JD, Foa EB, Mayberg HS, North CS, Stein MB. Posttraumatic stress disorder: a state-of-the-science review. J Psychiatr Res. 2006;40(1):1–21.
22. Berger W, Mendlowicz MV, Marques-Portella C, Kinrys G, Fontenelle LF, Marmar CR, Figueira I. Pharmacologic alternatives to antidepressants in posttraumatic stress disorder: a systematic review. Prog Neuro-Psychopharmacol Biol Psychiatry. 2009;33(2):169–80.

23. Kung S, Espinel Z, Lapid MI. Treatment of nightmares with prazosin: a systematic review. Mayo Clin Proc. n.d.;87(9):890–900.
24. Guina J, Rossetter SR, De Rhodes B, Nahhas RW, Welton RS. Benzodiazepines for PTSD: a systematic review and meta-analysis. J Psychiatr Pract. 2015;21(4):281–303.
25. Otto MW, Deveney C. Cognitive-behavioral therapy and the treatment of panic disorder: efficacy and strategies. J Clin Psychiatry. 2005;66(Suppl 4):28–32.
26. Chandraiah S. Premenstrual syndrome. In: Blackwell RE, editor. Women's medicine. New York: Blackwell Science Publishing; 2002. p. 503–17.
27. Schmidt PJ, Nieman LK, Grover GN, Muller KL, Merriam GR, Rubinow DR. Lack of effect of induced menses on symptoms in women with premenstrual syndrome. N Engl J Med. 1991;324(17):1174–9.
28. Yonkers KA, Kornstein SG, Gueorguieva R, Merry B, Van Steenburgh K, Altemus M. Symptom-onset dosing of sertraline for the treatment of premenstrual dysphoric disorder: a randomized clinical trial. JAMA Psychiat. 2015;72(10):1037–44.
29. Rickels K, Freeman E, Sondheimer S. Buspirone in treatment of premenstrual syndrome. Lancet. 1989;1(8641):777.
30. Freeman EW. Luteal phase administration of agents for the treatment of premenstrual dysphoric disorder. CNS Drugs. 2004;18(7):453–68.
31. Mitchell AA, Gilboa SM, Werler MM, Kelley KE, Louik C, Hernández-Díaz S. Medication use during pregnancy, with particular focus on prescription drugs: 1976–2008. Am J Obstet Gynecol. n.d.;205(1):51.e51–51.e58.
32. Koren G, Sakaguchi S, Klieger C, Kazmin A, Osadchy A, Yazdani-Brojeni P, Matok I. Toward improved pregnancy labelling. J Popul Ther Clin Pharmacol. 2010;17(3):e349–57.
33. US Food & Drug Administration. FDA issues final rule on changes to pregnancy and lactation labeling information for prescription drug and biological products [press release]. Retrieved from http://www.fda.gov/NewsEvents/Newsroom/PressAnnouncements/ucm425317.htm. 2014
34. Ryan D, Milis L, Misri N. Depression during pregnancy. Can Fam Physician. 2005;51(8):1087–93.
35. Gentile S. Untreated depression during pregnancy: short- and long-term effects in offspring. A systematic review. Neuroscience. 2017;242:154–166.
36. Cohen LS, Altshuler LL, Harlow BL, Nonacs R, Newport DJ, Viguera AC, Stowe ZN. Relapse of major depression during

pregnancy in women who maintain or discontinue antidepressant treatment. JAMA. 2006;295(5):499–507.
37. Yonkers KA, Blackwell KA, Glover J, Forray A. Antidepressant use in pregnant and postpartum women. Annu Rev Clin Psychol. 2014;10(1):369–92.
38. Wesseloo R, Kamperman AM, Munk-Olsen T, Pop VJ, Kushner SA, Bergink V. Risk of postpartum relapse in bipolar disorder and postpartum psychosis: a systematic review and meta-analysis. Am J Psychiatry. 2016;173(2):117–27.
39. Viguera AC, Whitfield T, Baldessarini RJ, Newport DJ, Stowe Z, Reminick A, Cohen LS. Risk of recurrence in women with bipolar disorder during pregnancy: prospective study of mood stabilizer discontinuation. Am J Psychiatry. 2007;164(12):1817–24. quiz 1923
40. Cohen LS, Friedman JM, Jefferson JW, Johnson EM, Weiner ML. A reevaluation of risk of in utero exposure to lithium. JAMA. 1994;271(2):146–50.
41. Epstein RA, Moore KM, Bobo WV. Treatment of bipolar disorders during pregnancy: maternal and fetal safety and challenges. Drug Healthc Patient Saf. 2015;7:7–29.
42. Yonkers KA, Wisner KL, Stowe Z, Leibenluft E, Cohen L, Miller L, Altshuler L. Management of bipolar disorder during pregnancy and the postpartum period. Am J Psychiatry. 2004;161(4):608–20.
43. Mines D, Tennis P, Curkendall SM, Li DK, Peterson C, Andrews EB, Chan KA. Topiramate use in pregnancy and the birth prevalence of oral clefts. Pharmacoepidemiol Drug Saf. 2014;23(10):1017–25.
44. US Food & Drug Administration. Suicidal behavior and ideation and antiepileptic drugs. Retrieved from http://www.fda.gov/Drugs/DrugSafety/PostmarketDrugSafetyInformationforPatientsandProviders/ucm100190.htm. 2009.
45. Dolovich LR, Addis A, Vaillancourt JM, Power JD, Koren G, Einarson TR. Benzodiazepine use in pregnancy and major malformations or oral cleft: meta-analysis of cohort and case-control studies. BMJ. 1998;317(7162):839–43.
46. Huybrechts KF, Hernandez-Diaz S, Patorno E, Desai RJ, Mogun H, Dejene SZ, Bateman BT. Antipsychotic use in pregnancy and the risk for congenital malformations. JAMA Psychiat. 2016;73(9):938–46.

47. Galbally M, Snellen M, Power J. Antipsychotic drugs in pregnancy: a review of their maternal and fetal effects. Ther Adv Drug Saf. 2014;5(2):100–9.
48. Sadowski A, Todorow M, Yazdani Brojeni P, Koren G, Nulman I. Pregnancy outcomes following maternal exposure to second-generation antipsychotics given with other psychotropic drugs: a cohort study. BMJ Open. 2013;3(7) pii: e003062. https://doi.org/10.1136/bmjopen-2013-003062.
49. US Food & Drug Administration. FDA drug safety communication: antipsychotic drug labels updated on use during pregnancy and risk of abnormal muscle movements and withdrawal symptoms in newborns [press release]. Retrieved from http://www.fda.gov/Drugs/DrugSafety/ucm243903.htm. 2011.
50. Heron J, O'Connor TG, Evans J, Golding J, Glover V. The course of anxiety and depression through pregnancy and the postpartum in a community sample. J Affect Disord. 2004;80(1):65–73.
51. Ross LE, McLean LM. Anxiety disorders during pregnancy and the postpartum period: a systematic review. J Clin Psychiatry. 2006;67(8):1285–98.
52. Sui G, Pan B, Liu G, Liu G, Wang L. The long-term effects of maternal postnatal depression on a child's intelligence quotient: a meta-analysis of prospective cohort studies based on 974 cases. J Clin Psychiatry. 2016;77:e1474–82.
53. Halbreich U, Karkun S. Cross-cultural and social diversity of prevalence of postpartum depression and depressive symptoms. J Affect Disord. 2006;91(2):97–111.
54. Berle JØ, Spigset O. Antidepressant use during breastfeeding. Curr Womens Health Rev. 2011;7(1):28–34.
55. O'Hara MW, Stuart S, Gorman LL, Wenzel A. Efficacy of interpersonal psychotherapy for postpartum depression. Arch Gen Psychiatry. 2000;57(11):1039–45.
56. Jones I, Chandra PS, Dazzan P, Howard LM. Bipolar disorder, affective psychosis, and schizophrenia in pregnancy and the postpartum period. Lancet. 2014;384(9956):1789–99.
57. Viguera AC, Nonacs R, Cohen LS, Tondo L, Murray A, Baldessarini RJ. Risk of recurrence of bipolar disorder in pregnant and nonpregnant women after discontinuing lithium maintenance. Am J Psychiatry. 2000;157(2):179–84.
58. Bergink V, Rasgon N, Wisner KL. Postpartum psychosis: madness, mania, and melancholia in motherhood. Am J Psychiatry. 2016;173(12):1179–88.

59. Sit D, Rothschild AJ, Wisner KL. A review of postpartum psychosis. J Womens Health (Larchmt). 2006;15(4):352–68.
60. American Academy of Pediatrics Committee on Drugs. Transfer of drugs and other chemicals into human milk. Pediatrics. 2001;108(3):776–89.
61. Fortinguerra F, Clavenna A, Bonati M. Psychotropic drug use during breastfeeding: a review of the evidence. Pediatrics. 2009;124(4):e547–56.
62. Seritan AL, Iosif AM, Park JH, DeatherageHand D, Sweet RL, Gold EB. Self-reported anxiety, depressive, and vasomotor symptoms: a study of perimenopausal women presenting to a specialized midlife assessment center. Menopause. 2010;17(2):410–5.
63. Parry BL. Perimenopausal depression. Am J Psychiatry. 2008;165(1):23–7.
64. Parry BL. Optimal management of perimenopausal depression. Int J Womens Health. 2010;2:143–51.
65. Chandraiah S, Richter H, Holley R. Relationship of reproductive cycle-associated and non-reproductive cycle-associated psychological problems in women. Int J Fertil Womens Med. 2005;51(1):33–7.

Index

J. V. Knaus et al. (eds.), *Ambulatory Gynecology*,
https://doi.org/10.1007/978-1-4939-7641-6

MIX
Papier aus verantwortungsvollen Quellen
Paper from responsible sources
FSC® C105338

If you have any concerns about our products, you can contact us on
ProductSafety@springernature.com

In case Publisher is established outside the EU, the EU authorized representative is:
Springer Nature Customer Service Center GmbH
Europaplatz 3, 69115 Heidelberg, Germany

Printed by Libri Plureos GmbH
in Hamburg, Germany